Bovine Neonatology

Guest Editor

GEOF W. SMITH, DVM, MS, PhD

VETERINARY CLINICS OF NORTH AMERICA: FOOD ANIMAL PRACTICE

www.vetfood.theclinics.com

Consulting Editor
ROBERT A. SMITH, DVM, MS

March 2009 • Volume 25 • Number 1

SAUNDERS an imprint of ELSEVIER, Inc.

W.B. SAUNDERS COMPANY
A Division of Elsevier Inc.

1600 John F. Kennedy Boulevard • Suite 1800 • Philadelphia, PA 19103-2899

http://www.vetfood.theclinics.com

VETERINARY CLINICS OF NORTH AMERICA: FOOD ANIMAL PRACTICE Volume 25, Number 1
March 2009 ISSN 0749-0720, ISBN-13: 978-1-4377-0559-1, ISBN-10: 1-4377-0559-6

Editor: John Vassallo; j.vassallo@elsevier.com
Developmental Editor: Theresa Collier

Veterinary Clinics of North America: Food Animal Practice (ISSN 0749-0720) is published in March, July, and November by Elsevier Inc., 360 Park Avenue South, New York, NY 10010-1710. Business and Editorial Offices: 1600 John F. Kennedy Blvd., Suite 1800, Philadelphia, PA 19103-2899. Customer Service Office: 11830 Westline Industrial Drive, St. Louis, MO 63146. Periodicals postage paid at New York, NY and additional mailing offices. Subscription prices are $163.00 per year (domestic individuals), $260.00 per year (domestic institutions), $81.00 per year (domestic students/residents), $189.00 per year (Canadian individuals), $339.00 per year (Canadian institutions), $239.00 per year (international individuals), $339.00 per year (international institutions), and $123.00 per year (international and Canadian students/residents). To receive student/resident rate, orders must be accompanied by name of affiliated institution, date of term, and the *signature* of program/residency coordinator on institution letterhead. Orders will be billed at individual rate until proof of status is received. Foreign air speed delivery is included in all *Clinics* subscription prices. All prices are subject to change without notice. **POSTMASTER:** Send address changes to *Veterinary Clinics of North America: Food Animal Practice*, 11830 Westline Industrial Drive, St. Louis, MO 63146. Customer Service (orders, claims, online, change of address): Elsevier Periodicals Customer Service, 11830 Westline Industrial Drive, St. Louis, MO 63146. Tel: 1-800-654-2452 (U.S. and Canada). Fax: 314-523-5170. E-mail: journalscustomerservice-usa@elsevier.com (for print support); journalsonlinesupport-usa@elsevier.com (for online support).

Reprints. For copies of 100 or more, of articles in this publication, please contact the Commercial Reprints Department, Elsevier Inc., 360 Park Avenue South, New York, NY 10010-1710. Tel.: 212-633-3812; Fax: 212-462-1935; E-mail: reprints@elsevier.com.

Veterinary Clinics of North America: Food Animal Practice is covered in *Current Contents/Agriculture, Biology and Environmental Sciences, MEDLINE/PubMed (Index Medicus),* and *Excerpta Medica.*

Printed and bound in the United Kingdom
Transferred to Digital Print 2011

Contributors

GUEST EDITOR

GEOF W. SMITH, DVM, MS, PhD
Diplomate, American College of Veterinary Internal Medicine; Associate Professor
of Ruminant Medicine, Department of Population Health and Pathobiology, College
of Veterinary Medicine, North Carolina State University, Raleigh, North Carolina

AUTHORS

JOACHIM BERCHTOLD, Dr Med Vet
Diplomate, European College of Bovine Health Management; Veterinary Practice,
Drs. Prechtl and Berhtold, Obing, Germany

ULRICH BLEUL, DMV
Diplomate, European College of Bovine Health Management; Clinic of Reproductive
Medicine, Department of Farm Animals, Vetsuisse-Faculty, University of Zurich, Zurich,
Switzerland

PETER D. CONSTABLE, BVSc (Hons), MS, PhD, MRCVS
Diplomate, American College of Veterinary Internal Medicine; Professor and Head,
Department of Veterinary Clinical Sciences, School of Veterinary Medicine, Purdue
University, West Lafayette, Indiana

VICTOR S. CORTESE, DVM, PhD
Diplomate, American Board of Veterinary Practitioners (Dairy); Director, Cattle
Immunology, Pfizer Animal Health, Simpsonville, Kentucky

G. ARTHUR DONOVAN, DVM, MSc
Diplomate, American Board of Veterinary Practitioners; Professor, Department of Large
Animal Clinical Sciences, College of Veterinary Medicine, University of Florida, Gainesville,
Florida

GILLES FECTEAU, DMV
Diplomate, American College of Veterinary Internal Medicine; Professor, Faculté de
Médecine Vétérinaire, Université de Montréal, St. Hyacinthe, Québec, Canada

D.M. FOSTER, DVM, MS
Diplomate, American College of Veterinary Internal Medicine; Clinical Instructor,
Department of Population Health and Pathobiology, North Carolina State College
of Veterinary Medicine, Raleigh, North Carolina

LISLE W. GEORGE, DVM, PhD
Diplomate, American College of Veterinary Internal Medicine; Professor, St. Matthew's
University, Grand Cayman, British West Indies

JOHN K. HOUSE, BVMS, PhD
Diplomate, American College of Veterinary Internal Medicine; Associate Professor, Livestock Veterinary Teaching and Research Unit, Faculty of Veterinary Science, University of Sydney, Camden, Australia

MATTHEW M. IZZO, BVSc
Resident, Livestock Veterinary Teaching and Research Unit, Faculty of Veterinary Science, University of Sydney, Camden, Australia

TESSA S. MARSHALL, BVSc, MS
Diplomate, American Board of Veterinary Practitioners (Dairy Practice); Assistant Teaching Professor, University of Missouri–Columbia, Columbia, Missouri

FIONA P. MAUNSELL, BVSc, PhD
Diplomate, American College of Veterinary Internal Medicine (Large Animal); Research Assistant Professor, Department of Infectious Diseases and Pathology, College of Veterinary Medicine, University of Florida, Gainesville, Florida

SHEILA M. McGUIRK, DVM, PhD
Diplomate, American College of Veterinary Internal Medicine (Large Animal); Professor, Department of Medical Sciences, University of Wisconsin-Madison School of Veterinary Medicine, Madison, Wisconsin

VIRGINIA L. MOHLER, BS, BVSc
Resident, Livestock Veterinary Teaching and Research Unit, Faculty of Veterinary Science, University of Sydney, Camden, Australia

DUSTY W. NAGY, DVM, PhD
Diplomate, American College of Veterinary Internal Medicine; Department of Veterinary Medicine and Surgery, University of Missouri College of Veterinary Medicine, Columbia, Missouri

KEITH P. POULSEN, DVM
Diplomate, American College of Veterinary Internal Medicine (Large Animal); Clinical Instructor and PhD Candidate, Department of Medical Sciences; Department of Pathobiological Sciences, University of Wisconsin-Madison School of Veterinary Medicine, Madison, Wisconsin

BRADFORD P. SMITH, DVM
Diplomate, American College of Veterinary Internal Medicine; Professor Emeritus, School of Veterinary Medicine, University of California, Davis, Davis, California

GEOF W. SMITH, DVM, MS, PhD
Diplomate, American College of Veterinary Internal Medicine; Associate Professor of Ruminant Medicine, Department of Population Health and Pathobiology, College of Veterinary Medicine, North Carolina State University, Raleigh, North Carolina

Contents

Neonatal morbidity and mortality are major economic concerns in both beef and dairy cattle in the United States. In both beef and dairy most calf death occurs in the early neonatal period, particularly in calves born following dystocia. This article focuses on the resuscitation of calves after delivery and highlights some therapeutic points for the care of critical calves.

Infectious diarrhea in calves is most commonly associated with enterotoxigenic *Escherichia coli*, *Cryptosporidium parvum*, rotavirus, coronavirus, or some combination of these pathogens. Each of these agents leads to diarrhea through either secretion or malabsorption/maldigestion, though the specific mechanisms and pathways may differ. Specific pharmacologic control and treatment are dependent on gaining a greater understanding of the pathophysiology of these organisms.

Salmonellae are endemic on most large intensive farms and salmonellosis is a common cause of neonatal morbidity and mortality. Disease and mortality usually reflect a variety of management events and environmental stressors that contribute to compromised host immunity and increased pathogen exposure. The diversity of salmonella serovars present on farms, and the potential for different serovars to possess different virulence factors, require the implementation of broad prophylactic strategies that are efficacious for all salmonellae. This article discusses strategies to promote host immunity and minimize pathogen exposure at the farm level. The benefits of control include a reduction in disease incidence and mortality, reduced drug and labor costs, and improved growth rates.

respiratory disease. This article describes respiratory conditions in new-born calves that veterinarians are most likely to encounter, along with diagnostic and treatment options that can be applied to both herd investigations and individual animals.

Mycoplasma bovis Infections in Young Calves 139

Fiona P. Maunsell and G. Arthur Donovan

Mycoplasma bovis has emerged as an important pathogen of young intensively reared calves in North America. A variety of clinical diseases are associated with M bovis infections of calves, including respiratory disease, otitis media, arthritis, and some less common presentations. Clinical disease associated with M bovis often is chronic, debilitating, and poorly responsive to antimicrobial therapy. Current control measures are centered on reducing exposure to M bovis through contaminated milk or other sources, and nonspecific control measures to maximize respiratory defenses of the calf. This article focuses on the clinical and epidemiologic aspects of M bovis infections in young calves.

Respiratory Distress Syndrome in Calves 179

Ulrich Bleul

Respiratory disease syndrome (RDS) is a condition of neonatal calves in which insufficient oxygen uptake and increased retention of carbon dioxide result in respiratory acidosis. This condition is more common in premature calves and seems to be associated with a deficiency of surfactant. Although there is no uniform definition of RDS, clinical signs appear as tachypnea and expiration accentuated by an abdominal lift and expiratory grunt, and they occur in association with characteristic blood gas changes. This article discusses the pathophysiology of RDS in calves, along with the clinical findings, diagnosis, and treatment options.

Septicemia and Meningitis in the Newborn Calf 195

Gilles Fecteau, Bradford P. Smith, and Lisle W. George

Neonatal infections and sepsis occur most frequently in calves with failure of passive transfer. If the invading bacteria are not rapidly controlled, they can set up focal infections, such as in growth plates, joints, or meninges, or generalized sepsis may occur. If not successfully treated, sepsis can lead to a systemic inflammatory response, multiple organ dysfunction syndromes, septic shock, and death. Treatments are based on selecting an appropriate antimicrobial drug and dosage, supportive therapy, fluid therapy, nonsteroidal anti-inflammatory drugs, and plasma transfusion. Preventing the failure of passive transfer through good colostrum management is essential.

THE CLINICS ARE NOW AVAILABLE ONLINE!

Access your subscription at:
www.theclinics.com

Preface

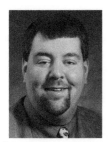

Geof W. Smith, DVM, MS, PhD
Guest Editor

Calf health should be a priority on beef and dairy farms. Despite this importance, surveys from the United States and other countries continue to show a preweaned heifer calf mortality rate close to 10% in the dairy industry. Only a small percentage of farms are able to supply adequate numbers of replacement animals from their own herd. Although mortality is slightly less in beef calves, 4% to 5% still die prior to weaning. Other than dystocia, the major causes of mortality in the bovine neonate continue to be the same as they have for decades—diarrhea, respiratory disease, and septicemia.

A renewed emphasis on the calf is occurring globally as diseases (such as bovine spongiform encephalopathy) have restricted animal movement between countries. The demand for beef and dairy heifers is strong, and there are many situations where replacement animals can no longer be imported economically from other countries. There has been a global increase in the importance of calf welfare. Since most of the diseases of the bovine neonate are related primarily to management, improving biosecurity, calf housing, nutrition, and immunity, combined with the early diagnosis and treatment of diseases, will increase the health and welfare of the calf. Producers and veterinarians must re-examine calf management programs at the individual farm level and make changes to improve health and decrease mortality.

This issue of *Veterinary Clinics of North America: Food Animal Practice* was written by ruminant clinicians for the practicing veterinarian. The articles focus on the pathophysiology, clinical signs, diagnosis, treatment, and prevention of the major diseases affecting calf health around the world, using the important principles of evidence-based medicine. All authors are internationally recognized specialists in ruminant internal medicine and have published extensively in the field of bovine neonatology. Many advances in bovine neonatology have been made in the past 10 years, and we have attempted to incorporate "state of the art" information in each article.

Conspicuous by its absence, an article dedicated to colostrum management recently was covered in detail in the March 2008 *Veterinary Clinics of North America: Food Animal Practice* issue titled "Dairy Heifer Management." In many ways, this issue can be viewed as a companion to the "Dairy Heifer Management" issue, with an increased focus on diseases affecting the bovine neonate.

Vet Clin Food Anim 25 (2009) xi–xii
doi:10.1016/j.cvfa.2008.10.005   **vetfood.theclinics.com**
0749-0720/08/$ – see front matter © 2009 Elsevier Inc. All rights reserved.

I extend my sincere thanks to all the authors for participating in this project and for sharing their knowledge and clinical experience. I hope that this issue proves to be a useful reference for practitioners in the field.

Geof W. Smith, DVM, MS, PhD
Department of Population Health and Pathobiology
College of Veterinary Medicine
North Carolina State University
4700 Hillsborough Street
Raleigh, NC 27606, USA

E-mail address:
geoffrey_smith@ncsu.edu (G.W. Smith)

Resuscitation and Critical Care of Neonatal Calves

Dusty W. Nagy, DVM, PhD

KEYWORDS

• Calf • Dystocia • Resuscitation • Critical care • Bovine

Neonatal morbidity and mortality are major economic concerns in both beef and dairy cattle. In dairy cattle it has been estimated that 75% of perinatal mortality occurs within 1 hour of birth.[1] In beef cattle, 69% of calf deaths between birth and weaning occur within 96 hours of birth.[2] This makes immediate evaluation and treatment, if indicated, a critical control point for ensuring calf health. Dystocia is a well-documented risk factor for morbidity and mortality in calves.[3] Beef calves born following dystocia are up to six times more likely to become ill than calves that have been through a normal birthing process.[4,5]

Unlike calves born following dystocia, mortality in calves with a normal birth is generally secondary to prematurity, dysmaturity, congenital defects, and infectious processes. This article focuses on the resuscitation of calves following dystocia and highlights some therapeutic points for the care of critical calves.

RESUSCITATION OF CALVES FOLLOWING DYSTOCIA

With most calf loss occurring in the first few days postpartum, adequate resuscitation of the newborn is critical to decreasing calf losses in both beef and dairy herds. Despite the importance, there are very little critically evaluated data available to aid in protocol development. Establishing a patent airway, initiating breathing, and establishing adequate circulation are the cornerstones to resuscitation in any species. In cattle, postdystocia resuscitation of the calf focuses on establishing breathing and correction of acid-base abnormalities. In general, cardiac resuscitation is not attempted because animals born without a heart rate are unlikely to be viable. Additional attention may be required to address specific ailments that occur during calving, maintaining appropriate body temperature, and ensuring adequate colostral intake.

Cardiopulmonary adaptations to the extrauterine environment are some of the most dramatic changes that must occur for calf survival. Rupture of the umbilical cord initiates hypoxia. Decreased oxygen tension and increased carbon dioxide

Department of Veterinary Medicine and Surgery, University of Missouri College of Veterinary Medicine, 900 East Campus Drive, Columbia, MO 65201, USA
E-mail address: nagyd@missouri.edu

Vet Clin Food Anim 25 (2009) 1–11
doi:10.1016/j.cvfa.2008.10.008
0749-0720/08/$ – see front matter © 2009 Elsevier Inc. All rights reserved.

concentrations stimulate gasping reflexes with subsequent inflation of the lungs. Increased oxygen tension in the blood and increased peripheral vascular resistance initiate closure of the ductus arteriosus, foramen ovale, and ductus venosus preparing the neonatal cardiovascular system for extrauterine life.[6,7] If dystocia is prolonged and a substantial hypercapnia or acidosis develops before expulsion of the fetus, central nervous system depression may be severe enough to impair the reflexes that initiate respiration.[7]

Removal of fluid from the pulmonary system is critical for normal ventilation and oxygenation of blood. Some fluid is eliminated from the body during the calving process. However, most is rapidly reabsorbed across the alveolar walls into the interstitium on the initiation of respiration.[8,9] Complete absorption of pulmonary interstitial fluid generally occurs within several hours postpartum.[8,9] Thoracic pressures between 35 and 40 cm H_2O optimize fluid removal.[8] Alterations from this optimum level in either direction may impair fluid removal or subsequent lung function.[8]

Clear Airway

Immediately after delivery (first 30 seconds), the calf should be placed in sternal recumbency to maximize ventilation and minimize ventilation-perfusion inequalities (**Fig. 1**). To ensure a patent airway, calves should have their upper respiratory tract (nose and mouth) cleared of any fluid or physical obstruction (by hand or by suctioning). Calves should never be suspended by the rear legs for an extended period of time (**Fig. 2**) or swung around by their back legs. These methods have been advocated by some practitioners over the years to allow for removal of fluids from the respiratory tract by gravity flow;[1,10] however, the safety of suspending the calf for both the animal and handler has been questioned. One study evaluated body position in 101 calves born by elective caesarian surgery demonstrated improved respiratory parameters in calves that were placed in sternal recumbency or suspended for less than 90 seconds immediately after birth when compared with calves placed in lateral recumbency.[11] In a very controlled manner, this study demonstrated that body position can have a positive impact on ventilation in calves. An additional study demonstrated improved respiratory parameters associated with pharyngeal and nasal suction

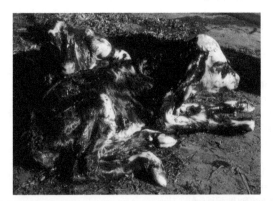

Fig. 1. Immediately following delivery, calves should be placed in sternal recumbency to maximize ventilation. Compared with other postural positions, this more efficiently enables the calf initially to expand its lungs and minimizes ventilation-perfusion mismatches. (*Courtesy of* Peter Constable, BVSc(Hons), MS, PhD, MRCVS, West Lafayette, IN.)

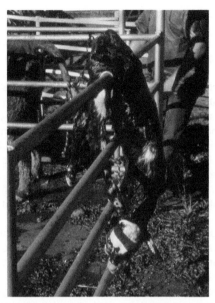

Fig. 2. Calves should never be suspended by the rear legs for an extended period of time or swung around by their back legs to drain fluid from the lungs. This increases the intrathoracic pressure making it more difficult for the calf to expand its lungs. It also causes the gastrointestinal organs to press against the diaphragm, making it harder for the calf to breath. (*Courtesy of* Peter Constable, BVSc(Hons), MS, PhD, MRCVS, West Lafayette, IN.)

immediately following birth.[12] From these studies it can be concluded that removal of pulmonary interstitial fluid is beneficial for appropriate postpartum respiratory adaptation in the calf. The improvement in respiratory parameters in calves postcesarean suggests that placing calves in sternal recumbency immediately after birth should be a minimum recommendation.

Stimulation of Respiration

Calves should make active respiratory movements within 30 seconds of being delivered. Primary apnea is defined as the absence of spontaneous breathing for 1 to 5 minutes. It is important to stimulate respiration in newborn calves, and when hypoventilation or apnea is present, assistance is generally indicated.

Mechanical

There are many methods that have been advocated for establishing respiration and airway patency in calves. Rubbing calves with bedding or towels is an attempt to stimulate the phrenic nerve.[7] Placing a finger, piece of straw, or other implement in the nose initiates a gasping reflex and helps aerate the lungs.[13] The use of acupuncture points on the muzzle has been advocated.[14] Pouring cold water over the calf's head or ear has been recommended for hypothermic respiratory stimulation.[15,16] Many of these methods are practiced on a regular basis. Very little information is available, however, as to their efficacy in calves.

One recent study evaluated the use of cold water to resuscitate calves.[12] Approximately 5 L of cold water (approximately 40°F or 5°C) was poured over the calf's head immediately after birth. Respiratory and metabolic parameters were then measured over 24 hours. This study demonstrated an improvement in respiratory rate, tidal volume, and total pulmonary resistance in treated calves. These changes were not significantly different when compared with control calves. Regardless, vigorous stimulation of the calf by rubbing around the head or body, and by placing a finger in the calf's nostrils or pharynx should be done immediately after placing the animal in sternal recumbency.

Positive pressure ventilation has also been advocated in calves. This is primarily used to initiate respiration as opposed specifically to treat hypoxia. Mouth-to-nose or mouth-to-mouth resuscitation is commonly initiated when presented with a calf that is not breathing; however, it is difficult to establish a normal respiratory pattern by this method. Establishing a tight enough seal to prevent air leakage is difficult. In addition, air often travels down the esophagus filling the abomasum, further impeding the calf's ability to breathe. Placing digital pressure over the esophagus may help divert the air to the trachea during this process. Mouth-to-mouth and mouth-to-nose procedures are also less ideal because of the potential of contracting zoonotic diseases.

Many other methods have been described that overcome calf-resuscitator cross-contamination. Unfortunately, most of the methods do not overcome the relative lack of resistance of air flow into the abomasum. The use of masks and nasal tubes requires digital pressure to impede air flow into the abomasum. A similar problem is present for compressed air devices.[1] A homemade oropharyngeal resuscitator composed of a teat cup liner, a one-way valve, and a tube to enter the larynx has also been described.[17] A flange present on the tube is designed to form an oral and nasal seal to allow for pressure build up. This method also requires occlusion of the esophagus to prevent air movement into the abomasum. At least one veterinary facility found it impossible to use with one person because inadequate seal formation at the mouth and nose requires an additional hand to operate the equipment.[1] The use of a laryngeal mask airway that has a cuff to obstruct the oroesophageal sphincter has also been described for use in humans;[18,19,20] however, difficulty in tube placement has been documented in calves.[1]

A cuffed endotracheal tube can be used to provide positive pressure ventilation while avoiding many of the problems encountered with previously described procedures.[21] The cuff prevents the passage of air into the esophagus and the ability to blow on the tube or use a resuscitation bag prevents cross-contamination of fetal and resuscitator fluids. A 5.5- to 9.5-mm tube is appropriate for use in calves and can be easily passed with the use of a long-bladed laryngoscope. Most average size (40–50 kg) calves take a 7- to 8-mm tube; however, a 5.5-mm tube might be needed for small calves (ie, Jerseys) or twins. Opening airways and displacing pulmonary fluid is critical to establishing oxygen tensions required to initiate circulatory changes that are compatible with extrauterine life. High pressure is required only for the first few breaths. It is important to remember with any positive pressure ventilatory procedure that overventilation or prolonged high-pressure ventilation can be damaging to the alveolar epithelium. When an oxygen supply is available, flow rates of 150 to 200 L/min with a 50-psi line pressure have been recommended. This yields a maximum pressure of 39 mm Hg through the endotracheal tube.[7] When the calf becomes strong enough to fight it, the endotracheal tube should be removed.

Pharmacologic

Doxapram hydrochloride stimulates peripheral chemoreceptors and medullary respiratory centers of the brain. The drug has a wide margin of safety and has been used successfully to stimulate respiration. Multiple studies have demonstrated improved respiratory parameters and survivability in calves and lambs with intravenous or sublingual administration of doxapram.[22,23,24,25,26] No studies have included un-treated controls, so it is difficult to determine if the animals would have survived without this intervention. In addition, several studies have demonstrated improvements only in mildly depressed newborns.[25,26] Severely affected calves and lambs do not seem to respond to the agent. Doxapram may also have some benefit in stimulating respiration in calves that have respiratory depression caused by drugs, particularly from xylazine given to the dam during calving. The use of doxapram in calves born to sedated cows is supported by a study in cattle demonstrating rapid reversal of the respiratory depression seen in juvenile animals sedated with xylazine.[27] It is unlikely to have a positive effect in calves with profound central nervous system depression secondary to hypercapnia. These animals are likely to require ventilatory support. Secondary ap-nea is defined as the absence of spontaneous breaths 5 minutes or more after delivery. This is a grave prognosis and doxapram is ineffective in these calves.

Cardiac stimulation In general, cardiac resuscitation is not undertaken in animals born without a heart beat. Successful resuscitation is unlikely in these settings. In foals, the likelihood for revival is approximately 50% if cardiac resuscitation is begun before development of a nonperfusing rhythm. Survival of less than 10% is expected when resuscitation efforts begin after asystole.[28] In calves that are profoundly bradycardic, epinephrine (0.2 mL/kg of 1:10,000 solution IM or 0.1 mL/kg of 1:10,000 solution IV or intracardiac) can be administered. This produces a rapid tachycardia; however, the calf likely still needs to be intubated and its ventilation assisted.

Trauma Fractures caused by excessive obstetrical force may occur and require attention. Fractures of the limbs, ribs, and spine are all possible, as are luxations of the hip and spine. Fractures of the distal limb can be economically stabilized with the use of fiberglass casting tape. Fractures located proximally on the limb often require internal fixation and as such are generally reserved for valuable calves. Crushing injuries carry a poor prognosis because of the propensity for vascular compromise with subsequent necrosis and sloughing of the affected regions of the limb. The extent of these types of injuries is not always obvious at birth and may take 10 to 14 days before they are clearly present as the effects of diminished vascular supply become apparent.

Swelling of the tongue or head Calves that become wedged in the pelvic canal for prolonged periods of time may suffer from poor venous return with subsequent regional swelling and edema. This is most often present in the tongue or head. Delivery of the calf helps re-establish venous return, and swelling resolves within a few days. Massage may help decrease the fluid retention. Furosemide (2.2 mg/kg IV) or mannitol (1 g/kg) may also be used to aid in the resolution of edema, although these diuretics are unproved for this use. If the calf is unable to generate a coordinated suckle response, nutritional support is required.

Care of the umbilicus Occasionally, trauma during dystocia may lead to excessive hem-orrhage from the umbilicus. Ligation to control the hemorrhage should be instituted immediately. Routine ligation of the umbilicus should be discouraged because it may prevent normal drainage. Applying caustic substances to the umbilicus is com-monplace, although little to no peer reviewed literature supports the practice. Mild an-tiseptics can be used, but strong agents should be avoided because these are often associated with irritation and inflammation of the umbilicus and surrounding struc-tures. Maintaining a clean, dry umbilicus and ensuring adequate high-quality colos-trum ingestion are the best ways to ensure appropriate umbilical health in calves.

Thermal In moving from an intrauterine to extrauterine environment, neonatal calves experience dramatic shifts in environmental temperature. In the normal calf, shivering and nonshivering thermogenic processes ensure adequate adaptation to extrauterine life.[29] Rapid decreases in body temperature and a failure of thermostatic regulatory mechanisms completely to restore normal rectal temperatures are characteristic of calves born following severe dystocia.[30] Some changes are also seen in calves born following mild complications. Moderate to severe metabolic disturbances can also mirror the changes seen in body temperature. This highlights the need to ensure that adequate body temperatures are maintained in neonates. A recent study evaluated how the use of infrared heaters on normal postpartum calves affected their adaptation to extrauterine life.[12] Calves exposed to an infrared heater for 24 hours postpartum had significantly improved rectal temperature, arterial hemoglobin oxygen saturation, tidal volume, dynamic lung compliance, and respiratory rate as compared with control calves. The authors postulated that the lower energy expenditures required for thermogenesis in these calves allowed for the increased energy demands required for the increased respiratory work needed to produce the improvement in respiratory parameters.

Colostrum The importance of colostrum ingestion on the immune health of calves has been well documented. The ingestion and absorption of maternally derived colostral components plays a large role in the immunologic capability of the neonate. Bovine colostrum contains many substances that support immune function in the neonatal calf. Immunoglobulins are the most commonly studied molecules, but maternal-derived immune cells, complement factors, lactoferrin, insulin-like growth factor-1, transforming growth factor, interleukin-2, and other soluble factors are present. In addition to immune support, colostrum is an excellent source of nutrients vital to the survival of the newborn including sugars and fat-soluble vitamins. Colostrum management and administrative practices have been recently reviewed.[31]

CRITICAL CARE OF SICK CALVES
Evaluation of the Sick Neonate

It is critical that a complete physical examination be performed on sick calves. Some diseases of the neonate are relatively easy to correct in an economic fashion, whereas others are not. Adequate patient evaluation is critical to determining an appropriate course of therapy. Hypothermia, hypoglycemia, dehydration, and acidosis are common causes of poorly responsive calves that are easy to correct as long as the underlying cause is addressed. Unlike these, the treatment of sepsis is often prolonged and unrewarding. Routine diagnostic examinations, such as auscultation of the thorax, can and should be performed. Pneumonia is a common finding in septicemic calves. Heart and respiratory rates, however, are poor predictors of sepsis in the bovine neonate.[32] Rectal temperature should also be determined, but the absence of fever does not preclude the possibility of septicemia.[33] Neonates seem less prone to developing a fever than adult cattle, particularly in environments with cool ambient temperatures.[34] The most consistent signs of septicemia are scleral injection; swollen joints; an enlarged, inflamed umbilicus; hypopyon; and evidence of meningitis (including opisthotonus, teeth grinding, and seizures).[35,36,37] Normal physical examination parameters in calves vary somewhat based on age and environmental parameters.

Establishing vascular access allows for the administration of intravenous fluids and drugs to neonates in septic or hypovolemic shock. Intravenous fluid therapy is contraindicated in animals during a cardiac arrest because of the decrease in cardiac output caused by the nonperfusing rhythm. Increased fluid administration at this time serves to increase venous pressure and impair coronary perfusion. The jugular vein is the vessel of choice in calves that require large volumes of fluids or the administration of caustic drugs. A 16-gauge 3.5-in catheter should provide adequate access in any size calf. In animals with profound hypovolemia, dropping the head below the level of the heart may help facilitate jugular filling for catheter placement. Administration of hypertonic (7.2%) saline (4 mL/kg IV slowly) temporarily increases intravascular volume and aids in IV catheter placement. Electrolyte derangements and acid-base abnormalities should be corrected. A thorough review of fluid therapy in calves is presented elsewhere in this issue.

In addition to electrolyte and acid-base correction, adequate nutritional and thermal support should be addressed. Unlike adults, young calves have minimal energy reserves to combat prolonged anorexia. The use of dextrose in intravenous fluids cannot be viewed as a replacement to adequate enteral nutrition in the sick calf. High-quality milk replacer or cow's milk should be provided at approximately 10% to 15% of body weight per day. The lower range of this estimate (10%) does not support growth and may not be adequate if increased energy demands are present because of pathologic processes or hypothermia. The higher end of the range may promote diarrhea in some calves. This author prefers to provide multiple small meals per day (0.5–1 L feedings depending on calf size) to avoid engorgement and minimize the potential for osmotic diarrhea. For calves that do not suckle, an oroesophageal feeder can be used. If prolonged feeding is anticipated, a nasoesophageal tube can be placed instead of passing an oroesophageal feeder multiple times. Care must be taken to ensure that calves are in sternal recumbency or standing to limit the potential for regurgitation and overflow into the lungs. Overfeeding should also be avoided because milk may sit for prolonged periods of time and putrefy in the rumen, resulting in a D-lactic (metabolic) acidosis.

Newborn calves often thermoregulate poorly, particularly if neurologic disease is present. Rectal temperature should be routinely monitored, especially when heating devices are being applied. Circulating water heating pads can be used, but these often warm slowly and animals that are struggling may puncture the pad. Electric heating pads should be monitored closely if they are used because they can get hot enough to induce local burns, particularly in animals that cannot move from the pad when they get too hot. Care should also be taken when using heat lamps because burning is possible. Calves often continue to warm after heating devices are removed, so consider discontinuing the use of heating devices or decreasing the intensity of the applied heat when calves attain a rectal temperature of 98°F to 99°F (36.5°C–37°C).

Cardiopulmonary Failure

In calves, cardiopulmonary failure is generally caused by systemic disease as opposed to disease inherent to the organ system. The on-farm nature of cattle practice makes aggressive treatment of arrest unlikely unless the veterinarian is present at the time it occurs. The economic feasibility and likelihood of successfully treating the underlying cause also needs to be considered. There has not been a critical evaluation of cardiopulmonary resuscitation (CPR) techniques in calves, and as a result most information presented here is extrapolated from techniques described for humans and foals.

The basics of establishing an airway are covered earlier in this issue. In humans, establishing an airway is considered of secondary importance to cardiac compressions when initiating CPR because blood flow (not hypoxia) is typically the primary determinant of oxygen delivery during early arrest.[38,39,40] In cattle, this is unlikely to be true because primary cardiac disease is rarely the cause of arrest. If a patient is hypoxic at the time of arrest, establishing an adequate airway and oxygenation becomes much more important for positive outcomes. No information exists on adequate parameters for respiratory rate, tidal volume, oxygenation, or cardiac compression rate in calves. In humans, a compression rate of 100 per minute with respirations provided at 8 to 10 per minute is recommended, with no attempt to coordinate respirations to cardiac compressions.[39] This is likely a reasonable goal for calves.

Many drugs have been used historically in CPR. It is important to recognize that the data surrounding many of the medications administered during CPR are contradictory. Prospective and retrospective studies and meta-analyses have found significant disagreement regarding the immediate and long-term outcomes associated with the administration of most commonly used drugs.[39,40] Furthermore, some drugs are incorporated into protocols based on physiologic principles as opposed to hard data. Drugs can be administered by IV or endotracheally if venous access has not been established. Endotracheal administration requires an increased dosage of drugs. In general 2 to 2.5 times the IV dose is administered endotracheally, although no data exist to substantiate this practice.[41]

Epinephrine hydrochloride is commonly used (1 mg IV every 3–5 minutes) during cardiopulmonary arrest in people.[41,42] The vasoconstrictive alpha adrenergic effects are able to increase coronary blood and cerebral blood flow during CPR. Administration of epinephrine is commonplace and various low- and high-dose regimens exist in the human literature. Despite this, there are very little data available that demonstrate improved rates of hospital discharge in patients that have been administered epinephrine at the time of resuscitation.

The use of vasopressin (40 U IV, repeat once if necessary), which is a nonadrenergic peripheral vasoconstrictor, in patients with asystole has been associated with positive outcomes when used alone or after one dose of epinephrine.[41] Atropine (1 mg IV repeated every 3–5 minutes for a maximum of three doses) is an anticholinergic that may have positive effects on heart rate, blood pressure, and systemic vascular resistance in patients in cardiac arrest. As a vagolytic agent, it may have benefit in patients that have prolonged asystole associated with increased vagal tone.[41] Lidocaine, amioderone, and magnesium have all been used in human cardiac arrest. Lidocaine has long been used for the treatment of ventricular arrhythmias. There are some human studies that demonstrate improved short-term survival with its use in patients with cardiac arrest. Amioderone seems to be associated with better short-term survival rates, however, than lidocaine. Magnesium has shown particular promise when administered to humans with torsades des pointes.

The on-farm nature of most cattle practice makes the use of advanced CPR uncommon. It is important to remember that even with the rapid, well-equipped responses in human medicine, the single biggest predictor of positive outcome is the time to the initiation of cardiac compressions. When considering CPR in calves, initiating an appropriate compression rate and establishing an airway are the two most critical procedures. The administration of drugs should be considered secondary to cardiac compressions and breathing. It is important to recognize that eliminating breaks in compressions is vital to maintaining blood pressure and perfusion.[39,40] This requires that all equipment and medications be in a single place and ready for use. It is also critical to remember that re-establishing a perfusing heart rhythm and voluntary breathing does not necessarily solve the whole problem. Animals often have electrolyte and acid-base abnormalities that require correction. In addition, if the underlying cause of arrest is not addressed it is likely that the animal will rearrest.

SUMMARY

Immediately after delivery, calves should be placed in sternal recumbency to maximize ventilation. The nose and mouth can then be cleared of any fluids or obstruction by hand or using suction. The calf should then be vigorously stimulated by rubbing around the head or body, and by placing a finger in the calf's nostrils or pharynx. A lack of response to these stimuli or an inability of the calf to remain stable in sternal recumbency after 10 minutes generally indicates a poor prognosis. Seizure activity, characterized by abnormal eye movement, paddling of limbs, and bawling, also constitutes a poor prognosis.

REFERENCES

1. Mee JF. Resuscitation of newborn calves: materials and methods. Cattle Practice 1994;2:197–210.
2. Patterson D, Bellows R, Burfening P, et al. Occurrence of neonatal and postnatal mortality in range beef cattle. I: calf loss incidence from birth to weaning, backward and breech presentation and effects of calf loss on subsequent pregnancy rates in dams. Theriogenology 1987;28:557–71.
3. Laster DB, Gregory KE. Factors influencing peri- and early postnatal mortality. J Anim Sci 1973;37:1092–7.
4. Toombs RE, Wikse SE, Kasari TR, et al. The incidence, causes, and financial impact of perinatal mortality in North American beef herds. Vet Clin North Am Food Anim Pract 1994;10:137–46.
5. Wittum TE, Perino LJ. Passive immune status at postpartum hour 24 and long-term health and performance of calves. Am J Vet Res 1995;56:1149–54.
6. Detweiler DK, Riedesel DH. Regional and fetal circulations. In: Swenson MJ, Reece WO, editors. Dukes' physiology of domestic animals. 11th edition. Ithaca (NY): Cornell University Press; 1993. p. 227.
7. Brunson DB. Ventilatory support of the newborn calf. Compendium on Continuing Education for the Practicing Veterinarian 1981;3:S47–52.
8. Egan EA, Olver RE, Strang LB. Changes in non-electrolyte permeability of alveoli and the absorption of lung liquid at the start of breathing in the lamb. J Physiol 1975;224:161–79.
9. Humphreys PW, Normand ICS, Reynolds EOR, et al. Pulmonary lymph flow and the uptake of liquid from the lungs of lambs at the start of breathing. J Physiol 1967;193:1–29.
10. Johnston NE, Stewart JA. The effect of glucocorticoids and prematurity on absorption of colostral immunoglobulins in the calf. Aust Vet J 1986;63:191–2.
11. Uystepruyst CH, Coghe J, Dorts TH, et al. Sternal recumbency or suspension by the hind legs immediately after delivery improves respiratory and metabolic adaptation to extra uterine life in newborn calves delivered by caesarean section. Vet Res 2002;33:709–24.
12. Uystepruyst CH, Coghe J, Dorts TH, et al. Effect of three resuscitation procedures on respiratory and metabolic adaptation to extra uterine life in newborn calves. Vet J 2002;163:30–44.
13. Tsuobone H. Nasal pressure receptors. Japanese Journal of Veterinary Science 1990;52:225–32.
14. Rogers PAM. Revival in collapse, shock, respiratory failure and narcotic overdose. Vet Rec 1977;101:215.

15. Dunn JM, Miller JA. Hypothermia combined with positive pressure ventilation in resuscitation of the asphyxiated neonate: clinical observations in 28 infants. Am J Obstet Gynecol 1969;104:58–67.
16. DeKruif A, Benedictus G. Perinatal mortality and the birth of weak calves. Tijdschr Diergeneeskd 1993;118:684–8.
17. Weaver BMQ, Angell-James J. A simple device for respiratory resuscitation of newborn calves and lambs. Vet Rec 1986;119:86–8.
18. Brain AI. The laryngeal mask: a new concept in airway management. Br J Aneasth 1983;55:801–6.
19. Davies PRF, Tighe SQM, Greenslade GL, et al. Laryngeal mask airway and tracheal tube insertion by unskilled personnel. Lancet 1990;336:977–9.
20. Anonymous. Laryngeal mask airway. Lancet 1991;338:1046–7.
21. Grove-White D. Resuscitation of the newborn calf. In Pract 2000;22:17–23.
22. Ayers MW, Besser TE. Evaluation of colostral IgG1 absorption in newborn calves after treatment with alkalinizing agents. Am J Vet Res 1992;53:83–6.
23. Bisgard GE, Ruiz AV, Grover RF, et al. Ventilatory control in the Hereford calf. J Appl Phys 1973;35:220–6.
24. Szenci O. The use of Dopram-V, Lobelin, and Respirot in newborn calves: a preliminary note. In: Proceeding of the 14th World Congress Dis Cattle 1986. p. 1283.
25. Brown LA. Improving survival rate of dyspneic neonatal lambs. Vet Med 1987;82: 421–2.
26. Szenci O, Fazekas Z, Tores I, et al. Treatment of asphyctic newborn calves with Dopram-V. Magyar Allatorvosok Lapja 1980;35:420–2.
27. Holenweger Dendi JA, Parada HL, et al. Analeptic effect of doxapram after Rompun treatment in cattle. Vet Med Rev 1981;1:70–4.
28. Palmer JE. Neonatal foal resuscitation. Vet Clin North Am Equine Pract 2007;23: 159–82.
29. Carstens GE. Cold thermoregulation in the newborn calf. Vet Clin North Am Food Anim Pract 1994;10:69–106.
30. Vermorel M, Vernet J, Dardillat C, et al. Energy metabolism and thermoregulation in the newborn calf: effect of calving conditions. Canadian Journal of Animal Science 1989;69:113–22.
31. Godden S. Colostrum management for dairy calves. Vet Clin Food Anim 2008;24: 19–39.
32. Vaala WE, House JK. Neonatal infection. In: Smith BP, editor. Large animal internal medicine. 3rd edition. St. Louis (MO): Mosby Inc; 2002. p. 303–18.
33. Roussel AJ. Principles and mechanisms of fluid therapy in calves. Compendium on Continuing Education for the Practicing Veterinarian 1983;5:332–6.
34. Terra RL. Ruminant history, physical examination and records. In: Smith BP, editor. Large animal internal medicine. 3rd edition. St. Louis (MO): Mosby Inc; 2002. p. 3–5.
35. Aldridge BM, Garry FJ, Adams R. Neonatal septicemia in calves: 25 cases (1985–1990). J Am Vet Med Assoc 1993;203:1324–9.
36. Radostits OM, Gay CC, Blood DC, et al. Diseases of the meninges. In: Veterinary medicine. 9th edition. London: W B Saunders Co Ltd; 2000. p. 538–9.
37. Fecteau G, VanMetre DC, Paré J, et al. Bacteriological culture of blood from critically ill neonatal calves. Can Vet J 1997;38:95–100.
38. Anonymous. American heart association guidelines for cardiopulmonary resuscitation and emergency cardiac care, part 7.1 Adjuncts for airway control and ventilation. Circulation 2005;112(Suppl IV):51–7.

39. Anonymous. American heart association guidelines for cardiopulmonary resuscitation and emergency cardiac care, part 7.2 management of cardiac arrest. Circulation 2005;112(Suppl IV):58–66.

40. Anonymous. American heart association guidelines for cardiopulmonary resuscitation and emergency cardiac care, part 7.4 monitoring and medications. Circulation 2005;(Suppl IV):78–83.

41. Andreka P, Frenneaux M. Haemodynamics of cardiac arrest and resuscitation. Curr Opin Crit Care 2006;12:198–203.

42. Aufderheide TP. The problem with and benefit of ventilations: should our approach be the same in cardiac and respiratory arrest? Curr Opin Crit Care 2006;12:207–12.

Pathophysiology of Diarrhea in Calves

D.M. Foster, DVM, MS*, Geof W. Smith, DVM, MS, PhD

KEYWORDS

- Rotavirus • Cryptosporidium • Enterotoxigenic *Escherichia coli*
- Coronavirus • Torovirus

Infectious diarrhea remains one the biggest health challenges in both the beef and dairy industries. More than 20% of beef cattle owners feel that calf diarrhea has a significant impact on their economic productivity,[1] and diarrhea accounts for more than half of all calf mortality on dairy farms.[2] Currently, enterotoxigenic *Escherichia coli* (ETEC), *Cryptosporidium parvum*, rotavirus, and coronavirus appear to be the most significant infectious causes of calf diarrhea. Research into the pathophysiology of these organisms may ultimately lead to more specific treatment and control recommendations.

ENTEROTOXIGENIC *ESCHERICHIA COLI*

Epidemiologic studies of both beef and dairy calves have implicated ETEC as the major cause of neonatal diarrhea occurring in the first 4 days of life; however it rarely leads to diarrhea in older calves or adult cattle.[3-6] Immediately after birth, oral exposure to fecal coliforms leads to colonization of the gut with the normal commensal flora, and these organisms continue to move caudally through the gastrointestinal tract with ingesta.[7,8] If environmental contamination is high, ETEC organisms are ingested at this same time and are able to produce disease caused by the presence of two virulence factors, K99 fimbria and heat stable toxin. Because nonpathogenic *E coli* are extremely common, fecal cultures as a diagnostic test are of little value unless the presence of these two virulence factors can be demonstrated.

Attachment of Escherichia coli *to Intestinal Epithelium*

Attachment to the intestinal epithelium allows the bacteria to maintain residence in the small intestine and multiply instead of being passed though with the ingesta. Studies have shown that up to 80% of the organisms are attached in calves with ETEC diarrhea, instead of only 10% to 20% in normal calves.[3,9,10] This attachment is mediated by the presence of fimbrial antigens. The antigen most commonly associated with

Department of Population Health and Pathobiology, College of Veterinary Medicine, North Carolina State University, 4700 Hillsborough Street, Raleigh, NC 27606, USA
* Corresponding author.
E-mail address: derek_foster@ncsu.edu (D. Foster).

Vet Clin Food Anim 25 (2009) 13–36
doi:10.1016/j.cvfa.2008.10.013
0749-0720/08/$ – see front matter. Published by Elsevier Inc.

vetfood.theclinics.com

ETEC diarrhea in calves is K99, which is more appropriately referred to as F5.[6,11] The F41 and 987P antigens can also be found in calf ETEC isolates, often in conjunction with F5.[12,13] Because the K99 antigen is only expressed at an environmental pH level of less than 6.5, the distal small intestine is the initial site of colonization. This is because the pH level of the intestinal fluid increases as it moves caudally, and it only reaches this threshold at the ileum.[14–18] The ability of K99 ETEC to bind to the small intestinal epithelium is age dependent and gradually decreases from 12 hours of age to 2 weeks of age. However, there is not a precipitous drop in the binding ability that would explain the age resistance to ETEC.[19] The attachment of ETEC allows the bacteria to colonize the ileum, proliferate, and spread proximally through the small intestine.[3,17,18,20] Once established in the gut, ETEC produces heat stable toxin leading to secretory diarrhea.

Heat Stable Toxin–Mediated Secretory Diarrhea

Classically, mechanistic discussions of enterotoxin-mediated secretory diarrhea have focused on the cholera toxin of *Vibrio cholerae* and the heat labile toxin (LT) of *E coli*. These are both significant causes of diarrhea in humans, and have a similar mechanism of action involving increases in intracellular cyclic adenosine monophospate (cAMP), which activates the cystic fibrosis transmembrane conductance regulator (CFTR) and ultimately causes secretion of chloride. This movement of chloride ions osmotically draws water into the lumen of the intestine, leading to diarrhea.[21,22] These models of human diarrhea have less bearing on toxin-mediated secretory diarrhea in the calf because the heat stabile toxin (STa) of ETEC is the primary mediator.[11,23,24] STa is an 18- or 19-amino-acid peptide that is secreted by many strains of ETEC; however, the production can vary up to 1,000 fold between strains when cultured under identical conditions.[25,26] After being secreted by *E coli*, STa binds to guanylyl cyclase-C (GCC), a brush border membrane enzyme that is present throughout the villi and crypts.[27,28] The concentration of GCC appears to be highest in the lower villous,[28] but this may vary by species,[27] and its precise location on the villous has not yet been determined in the calf. In contrast to rodents and humans, in which concentrations of GCC decrease in the distal small intestine,[28] GCC is present throughout the gastrointestinal tract of calves and is concentrated in the ileum.[29,30] In both mice and humans, the density of this receptor declines after birth,[26,31] and it remains present in pigs until up to 7 weeks of age.[32] No specific research has been done detailing the expression of GCC at various ages of calves, however inoculation with STa induces diarrhea in animals up to 15 days of age.[25] This indicates that GCC is present until at least 2 weeks of age and down-regulation of the receptor is not the reason for age-dependent resistance to ETEC diarrhea.

Binding of STa to GCC leads to the production of intracellular cyclic guanylyl monophospate (cGMP), which acts as a second messenger to activate cGMP-dependent protein kinase II (cGKII). This kinase phosphorylates CFTR, inducing movement of the protein to the cell surface and activation, which in turn leads to chloride secretion.[33] This up-regulation of chloride secretion osmotically pulls water into the intestinal lumen, which outweighs the absorptive ability of the villous (**Fig. 1**).[21] Blocking the CFTR dramatically decreases intestinal fluid secretion, indicating the importance of this protein in the pathogenesis of ETEC diarrhea. However, secretion is not completely prevented,[34] indicating that STa may have additional effects in the small intestine.

Further research has shown that STa can induce bicarbonate secretion through a tyrosine kinase that is independent of the GCC/cGMP/CFTR pathway, and this secreted bicarbonate can act as an osmotic agent to pull water into the lumen of the

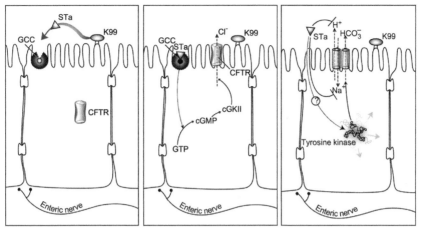

Fig. 1. Frame 1: K99 ETEC binds to an intestinal epithelial cell, and heat stable toxin (STa) is secreted, which binds to the receptor GCC. The enteric nervous system becomes activated by the secretion of STa, but the mechanism of this activation is unclear. At this point, CFTR is not active. Frame 2: STa binds to GCC, which converts guanylyl triphosphate (GTP) to cGMP. cGMP activates cGKII to phosphorylate the CFTR, and the CFTR moves to the luminal surface and is activated, leading to chloride (Cl) secretion. Frame 3: Secreted STa activates tyrosine kinase through an unknown pathway, which leads to bicarbonate (HCO_3) secretion. STa also directly inhibits the sodium–hydrogen exchanger, decreasing the movement of sodium (Na) and hydrogen (H) across the membrane.

intestine.[35,36] The receptor and other messengers in this pathway have not been elucidated. An opposing model of STa-induced diarrhea has also been proposed that is not based on fluid secretion caused by movement of chloride or bicarbonate, but which instead is caused by decreased fluid absorption. In addition to activating the CFTR, STa inhibits the apical Na-H exchanger, leading to failure of sodium absorption. This failure of sodium absorption decreases fluid movement from the intestinal lumen to the interstitial space. The importance of this mechanism of ETEC diarrhea in calves is unknown because this has been most conclusively shown in the duodenum and proximal jejunum of rodent models.[37,38]

Similar to expression of K99, production of STa is pH dependent. When the environmental pH is less than 7.0, toxin production is severely limited.[18,39] Therefore, toxin production is maximized in the distal small intestine because the pH level is greatest in this segment. Although it has not been directly investigated, it can be theorized that STa-mediated secretion of bicarbonate and inhibition of the Na-H exchanger would have the net effect of alkalinizing the proximal small intestine. This would create an environment more hospitable to ETEC promoting its spread to the proximal small intestine.

The autonomic and enteric nervous systems are known to be involved in the secretory response to cholera toxin through the actions of prostaglandin E_2 (PGE$_2$), 5-hydroxytriptamine (5-HT), and vasoactive intestinal polypeptide (VIP).[40–42] STa-mediated secretion may also involve local reflex arcs in the enteric nervous system (ENS); however, it does not involve the autonomic nervous system.[43] Most of the support for this idea comes from studies that inhibit the ENS and subsequently reduce the secretory effect of STa.[44–46] The neurotransmitters critical in these responses are nitric oxide (NO) and VIP,[40,46] whereas PGE$_2$ and 5-HT are not involved.[41] Furthermore, a well-defined example of the influence of the ENS in ETEC is its role in exacerbating

STa-mediated secretory diarrhea in states of malnutrition,[47–49] however the importance of these mechanisms in the calf is unknown because this was found in a rodent model of human disease.

Ultimately, the pathophysiology of ETEC is dependent on several factors. First is the exposure to and ingestion of the organism. Once ingested, ETEC must survive the acidic pH of the abomasum. This is facilitated in neonatal calves because the pH level of their abomasum ranges from approximately 6 to 7, which enables survival of ETEC. The pH of the abomasum decreases to less than 2 by 5 days of age, which is low enough to kill ETEC strains.[18,50] Once ETEC reaches the ileum, both the K99 antigen and STa are expressed as a result of the increased pH level, yet this may occur sooner because the pH level can be higher in the proximal GI tract of neonatal calves. K99 allows attachment of the organism, leading to colonization of the ileum. Production of STa induces secretion and may increase the luminal pH level, which would make the normally acidic proximal small intestine more hospitable for the organism. ETEC bacteria then move proximally toward the duodenum, and secretion dramatically increases, leading to diarrhea and dehydration.[18,51]

Treatment of Escherichia coli Diarrhea

The focus of treatment for ETEC diarrhea should be to remove the organism from the gastrointestinal tract and combat dehydration until normal absorption is restored. Based on an extensive review on the topic by Constable in 2004, the only antibiotic with documented efficacy and legal use in food animals in the United States is amoxicillin trihydrate, which is recommended at a dose of 10 mg/kg, orally every 12 hours. Ideally, this would only be used in calves with signs of systemic illness caused by diarrhea.[52]

Oral electrolyte solutions remain the mainstay of on-farm fluid replacement therapy for most calves with ETEC diarrhea. Based on the pathophysiology of the organism, two characteristics of oral replacement fluids are critical. The first is to maximize sodium absorption through means other than the Na-H exchanger, because this may be inhibited by STa. Most oral electrolyte solutions take advantage of the sodium-glucose cotransporters to improve sodium absorption, which bypasses the inhibited Na-H exchanger. Although this will not reduce the secretory response (and diarrhea), it will improve the hydration status of the calf.[21]

Second, increasing the pH of the abomasum and proximal small intestine favors the survival of ETEC, as discussed above. Hence, oral replacement fluids with bicarbonate as the alkalinizing agent may favor the proliferation of ETEC, expression of the K99 antigen, and secretion of STa.[18] If secretion of bicarbonate caused by STa is a significant component of the disease in calves, as it appears to be in some models, the additional bicarbonate load from an oral electrolyte solution could even exacerbate the secretory response. Because of the potential harm of bicarbonate, oral electrolyte solutions containing acetate are recommended for treatment of ETEC diarrhea. Additional approaches for increasing the abomasal pH are discussed in the article by Marshall found elsewhere in this issue.

CRYPTOSPORDIUM PARVUM

C parvum is one of the most commonly isolated gastrointestinal pathogens from dairy calves and immunosuppressed humans[53] and is a significant cause of waterborne diarrhea outbreaks.[54] Infection occurs when oocysts are ingested from the environment. Once in the host, the organism goes through a complicated life cycle that involves multiple stages. The cycle starts with exposure to gastric acid and bile salts, leading to excystation of the oocyst to the first life stage, the sporozoite. The sporozoites invade the intestinal epithelial cells of the ileum, where the infection is typically concentrated, but they can infect the gastrointestinal tract anywhere from the abomasum to the colon. The sprorozoites create an invagination of the luminal membrane, allowing them to maintain an extracytoplasmic but intracellular location known as a parasitophorous vacuole. From this location, the sporozoites transform into trophozoites. At this stage, asexual reproduction occurs and Type I meronts are formed. Merozoites are then released into the lumen. These organisms can form additional Type I meronts or Type II meronts, which form micro- and macrogamonts. Micro- and macrogamonts reproduce sexually to create thin- and thick-walled oocysts. The thin-walled oocysts lead to autoinfection, whereas the thick-walled oocysts pass out with feces to contaminate the environment. These oocysts are infective immediately, and remain viable in the environment for extended periods of time.[55–57]

C parvum oocyst shedding occurs as early as 3 days of age, peaks at 2 weeks of age, and can continue to occur in adult cattle. However, diarrhea caused by C parvum rarely occurs after 3 months of age.[57–63] After infection, clinical signs peak at 3 to 5 days and last 4 to 17 days.[60,64] Some studies have shown that up to 100% of dairy calves become infected with C parvum,[58,65] and become the major source of environmental contamination because calves shed up to 10^7 oocysts per gram of feces.[60] Shedding in beef calves is much less frequent and occurs in less than 5% of calves.[59,66] Calves appear to be resistant to subsequent infection after the initial episode of C parvum diarrhea.[63] Severity of diarrhea and incidence of clinical signs in calves shedding oocysts can be variable within and between farms, leading some to question the true importance of C parvum as a primary pathogen;[67] however, it has been repeatedly isolated independent of other known pathogens in clinical cases.[57]

Malabsorptive Diarrhea Caused by Cryptospordium parvum

Infection with C parvum has been shown to induce severe villous atrophy (**Fig. 2**) in calves and other food animal species.[64,68,69] This atrophy is caused by the loss of villous enterocytes and the subsequent retraction of the villous to maintain a continuous epithelial barrier. Crypt hyperplasia also occurs in an effort to replace the lost epithelial cells, however in severe infections, disruption of the epithelial barrier can occur despite these efforts.[64,70,71] Furthermore, both cell culture and animal models have shown an increase in epithelial permeability after C parvum infection when the loss of epithelial surface area is taken into account.[70,72] In spite of this well recognized consequence of C parvum infection, the precise mechanism of cell loss remains elusive. It is still not understood whether the cell loss is an effect of the pathogen or is part of the host response in an effort to resolve the infection.

There are two potential mechanisms for the increased loss of epithelial cells in C parvum infections. The first is a direct cytotoxic effect of the organism on the intestinal epithelium, but this is not well supported by the current literature. In a few cell culture models of C parvum infection, the cytosolic enzyme, lactate dehydrogenase, has been shown to leak into the cell media.[73–75] However, this may simply be caused by the deformation of the apical membrane by the organism as it attaches to and is enveloped by the membrane.[70]

The second and more likely mechanism for cell loss is apoptosis because apoptotic cells are consistently found in both in vitro and in vivo models of infection.[76–82] Yet there is evidence in cell culture models that the loss of epithelial cells is minimized by the inhibition of apoptosis during the infection,[78,83] and many infected cells are not apoptotic.[79] Specifically, research has shown that the activation and inhibition of apoptosis is

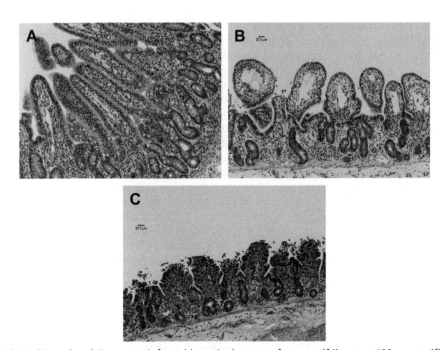

Fig. 2. Normal and *C parvum*–infected intestinal mucosa from a calf ileum at 100× magnification. (*A*) Normal calf ileal mucosa. (*B*) and (*C*). Calf ileal mucosa experimentally infected with *C parvum*. Note the blunting of the villi and the hyperplasia of the crypts. There are more severe histologic changes in (*C*), because the villi are more atrophied and the mucosa no longer completely covers the lamina propria (hematoxylin and eosin).

related to the life stage of *C parvum*, and that apoptosis is inhibited during the trophozoite stage when the organism is most dependent on the host, but then increases later during the infection. Furthermore, the incidence of apoptosis will vary over time between infected cells and uninfected neighboring cells. This may be beneficial to the host to limit spread of the organism, limit the severity of cell loss, and/or speed clearance of the organism.[83] Pharmacologically induced apoptosis in infected cell cultures is also prevented, indicating that apoptosis mechanisms are actively inhibited,[78,83] which has been shown to be mediated by NF-κB.[78] Additional research is needed to elucidate the ultimate beneficiary of this apoptotic regulation: the organism, to maintain its intracellular habitat, or the host, to limit cell loss and spread of infection.

Irrespective of how or why epithelial cell loss and villous atrophy occurs, this leads to a malabsorptive diarrhea. The net absorption of fluid is caused by the movement of sodium coupled with either chloride or other nutrients in the villous tip versus the secretion of anions in the crypts. Therefore, absorption is impaired because of the loss of the mature villous epithelial cells and their associated transporters as well as a decrease in total surface area.[64,70,84,85] Absorption of sodium and water can still occur to some degree in the crypts when coupled with glucose or neutral amino acids (eg, glutamine), which can be used to improve absorption of oral rehydration solutions,[86,87] but overall absorption of carbohydrates, lipids, and amino acids is reduced.[88–91] This malabsoption leads to diarrhea that can range from very mild to life threatening, depending on the dose of organism and coinfection with other pathogens. However *C parvum* has not been shown to decrease overall growth in calves once the infection has resolved.[55]

Prostaglandin-Mediated Diarrhea Due to Cryptospordium parvum

Epithelial cell loss, villous atrophy, and malabsorption cannot account for all the fluid loss seen in *C parvum* infections, and studies have documented a prostaglandin-mediated anion secretion (Cl^- or HCO_3^-) and inhibition of neutral NaCl absorption (**Fig. 3**). The prostaglandins PGE_2 and prostaglandin I_2 (PGI_2) are found at higher concentrations in infected tissue, and blocking the secretion of these prostaglandins reverses the anion secretion and inhibition of NaCl absorption.[70,84] However, in vivo, inhibition of prostaglandins exacerbated the villous atrophy, indicating that this approach is unlikely to be useful therapeutically.[92] The source of prostaglandins in the infected tissue is unknown, but is believed to be leukocytes that infiltrate the lamina propria in the infection. Macrophages appear to be the most likely source because they invade the lamina propria after infection and can induce prostaglandin secretion from mesenchymal cells,[64,70,92,93] whereas inhibition of neutrophil migration into infected tissue had no effect on prostaglandin synthesis.[94] Furthermore, NO, which has been shown to be important in defense against *C parvum* infections,[95] stimulates prostaglandin-mediated secretion when NO production is augmented by arginine supplementation.[96]

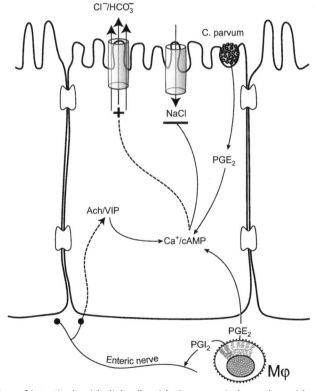

Fig. 3. Infection of intestinal epithelial cells with *C parvum* induces the epithelial cell to secrete PGE_2 and leads to activation of macrophages (M4) in the lamina propria. This leads to secretion of PGE_2 and PGI_2 from the mesenchymal cells. PGI_2 activates the enteric nervous system to secrete acetylcholine (Ach) and VIP. The secretion of Ach, VIP, and PGE_2 leads to an increase in intracellular calcium and cAMP, which activates anion secretion (Cl and HCO_3) and inhibits neutral sodium and chloride absorption (NaCl).

The mechanism of action of the two prostaglandins differs because PGE_2 acts on the enterocyte directly, whereas PGI_2 exerts its effect through the ENS. PGI_2 causes 75% of the secretion in *C parvum* infection by stimulating the nicotinic ganglia and the VIP-ergic and cholinergic motor neurons that innervate the intestinal mucosa. Prostaglandin secretion ultimately leads to increases in calcium and cAMP that increase anion secretion and decrease sodium absorption.[42,70,92] Inhibiting the effects of prostaglandins on the ENS is a potential method of decreasing the diarrhea associated with *C parvum* without exacerbating the villous atrophy. Specifically, peptide YY, which is naturally found in the intestinal epithelium, is a potent inhibitor of VIP and can abolish the secretory response to PGI_2.[97] Furthermore, if the inhibition caused by prostaglandins can be blocked, the intestine is capable of absorbing NaCl and water despite the villous atrophy, indicating that the transporters are fully functional, even in the immature enterocytes.[85–87]

Treatment and Prevention of Cryptospordium parvum *Diarrhea*

Because of the privileged location of *C parvum*, drug delivery can be difficult. Drugs in the lumen of the intestine may pass through without actually reaching the organism, whereas drugs that penetrate the intestinal epithelial cell would concentrate in the cytoplasm instead of the extracytoplasmic parasitophorous vacuole. Despite these challenges, multiple drugs have been studied as potential treatments with varying degrees of success, and none are currently licensed for calves in North America.[55,57] Halofuginone is licensed for prevention of *C parvum* infection in Europe when administered during the first 7 days of life. Unfortunately, clinical trials have not shown it be consistently effective. When used as directed in a study of 31 bull calves, there was no difference in the incidence of or treatment rates for diarrhea between the treated and control calves. There was a significant delay in shedding of oocysts, but upon withdrawal of the drug, the treated calves began to shed a similar number of organisms. There was no difference in milk intake, weight gain, or age at weaning between the two groups.[98] Another study in which halofuginone treatment was initiated at 7 to 10 days of age saw no difference in the number of calves shedding oocysts or in the incidence of diarrhea. However, the total number of oocysts shed was reduced for the 7 days during treatment as well as the following 7 days. Oocyst shedding then rebounded and was greater than in control animals 21 days after the start of treatment.[99] Other studies have shown more favorable results in which the incidence of diarrhea and excretion of oocysts was reduced. Re-excretion of oocysts after stopping treatment continued to be a problem, but was less if a lower dose was used.[100–102] In an experimental infection, the only difference noted with treatment was a decrease in the number of calves dying. However, calves began excreting oocysts after treatment was discontinued, even though they had been housed individually and reinfection was unlikely. This indicates that halofuginone is cryptosporidiostatic but is unlikely to effectively kill oocysts.[103] Halofuginone appears to be effective at decreasing oocyst shedding only when it is being administered. It may or may not reduce clinical signs in the calf, and has not been consistently shown to be effective as a treatment for *C parvum* diarrhea.

Paromomycin was shown to be effective in one trial of experimental infection as a prophylaxis for *C parvum* infection. The drug was administered 1 day prior to infection and continued for a total of 11 days. Oocyst shedding and diarrhea were decreased, but calves began to shed organisms at the end of the treatment period, and the shedding continued after treatment was stopped.[104] Decoquinate has also been used to control *C parvum* in calves, but trials have not consistently shown it to reduce diarrhea or oocyst shedding in calves.[57,99,105] In a study from Turkey, azithromycin was shown to be effective as a treatment of calves that were know to be shedding *C parvum* when it was administered at a dose of 1,500 mg/calf/day for 7 days. Treatment decreased oocyst shedding and diarrhea, and improved weight gain.[106] However, the cost of azithromycin in the United States would likely prevent its use to treat cryptosporidiosis at this time. In a small study, activated charcoal with wood vinegar liquid was effective in stopping diarrhea and oocyst shedding when administered after the start of experimentally induced *C parvum* diarrhea. This effect was noted 24 hours after addition of this product to the milk replacer.[107] It remains to be seen if this effect can be duplicated in a large-scale field trial.

Similar to chemotherapeutic agents, both active and passive vaccination have not been consistently successful in preventing *C parvum* infection, diarrhea, and oocyst shedding.[108] Vaccination of dry cows with whole organisms[109] or a recombinant protein[110] both reduced oocyst shedding and clinical signs, but neither have been validated under field conditions. An oral vaccine to be given to calves at birth prior to colostrum administration showed promise initially,[111] but was ineffective in a field trial.[112,113]

Because of the questionable benefit of mass medication or vaccination for control, prevention should be focused on decreasing exposure to the organism by appropriate hygiene and husbandry. Because *C parvum* is a zoonotic agent, appropriate personal hygiene is also important for public health and farm employee safety.[112] Specific treatment for *C parvum*–infected calves also cannot be recommended in the United States at this time, although the extralabel use of azithromycin or activated charcoal with wood vinegar appears promising. In general, treatment should be focused on appropriate fluid therapy and supportive care because most calves will recover from cryptosporidiosis if there is not an overwhelming infection or coinfection with another pathogen.

ROTAVIRUS

Rotavirus was one of the first identified viral causes of diarrhea, and was initially known as neonatal calf diarrhea virus. Subsequently, it has been found throughout the world and has been identified as a significant pathogen of children and most other mammals.[114,115] Antibodies to rotavirus can be found in more than 90% of unvaccinated cattle,[116] and the virus was isolated from 94% of dairy calves at a large dairy and calf ranch during the first 2 weeks of life.[117] It has also been isolated from approximately 20% of calf diarrhea samples,[118,119] and from at least one calf on 63% of farms.[120] Calves become infected after ingesting the virus from fecal contamination of the environment, because the virus remains quite stable if the temperature does not get near freezing. The virus typically affects calves less than 3 weeks old, with a peak incidence at 6 days of age. After ingestion of the virus, the incubation period is approximately 24 hours, with resolution of diarrhea in uncomplicated cases in 2 days.[115] Classically, rotavirus diarrhea is thought to be primarily a malabsorptive diarrhea, but recent evidence indicates that there is also a toxin-mediated secretory component as well.

Malabsorptive Diarrhea Caused by Rotavirus

Similar to *C parvum*, rotavirus preferentially targets the mature villous enterocytes and spares the crypts, generally causing moderate villous damage. The virus attaches to these cells via specific receptors and invades through an unknown mechanism. The virus replicates within the cells, leading to enterocyte death. Malabsorption will then occur because of the loss of surface area, and unabsorbed glucose and other carbohydrates create an osmotic load pulling fluid into the lumen. Furthermore, fluid secretion from the crypts increases the amount of fluid in the intestinal lumen relative to villous absorption, which leads to diarrhea.[21,114,115] However, the severity of clinical signs does not always correlate with histologic damage to the villi. This has led to speculation that there may be another mechanism contributing to the diarrhea seen with rotaviral infections, and that enterocyte damage is less critical than previously believed.

In the mid-1990s, a viral enterotoxin was demonstrated to be crucial to the pathogenesis of rotaviral diarrhea.[121] This was the first time an enterotoxin could be identified in a viral diarrheal pathogen, and this changed our fundamental understanding of rotavirus diarrhea.[122] The rotavirus protein, nonstructural glycoprotein 4 (NSP4), was found to induce a dose- and age-dependent diarrhea that is clinically similar to rotavirus diarrhea. Unlike the bacterial enterotoxins, diarrhea due to NSP4 is unrelated to cAMP, cGMP, or CFTR.[123,124] The protein is initially produced during intracellular viral replication and acts on the infected cell. It is secreted or released upon cell death, and acts in a paracrine manner.[125] Exogenous exposure of intestinal epithelial cells to NSP4 allows binding to caveolae, special lipid rafts within the endoplasmic reticulum (ER) and cell membrane. It specifically binds to caveolin-1, a transmembrane, hairpin protein unique to these rafts.[126,127] Binding to caveolin-1 leads to an increase in intracellular calcium concentrations by causing the release of calcium from ER stores and increasing movement across the plasma membrane. This is mediated by phospholipase C (PLC), which increases the level of intracellular inositol 1,4,5-triphosphate (IP_3),[124,128–130] however intracellular NSP4 causes the release of calcium independent of the PLC pathway.[131]

Extracellular and intracellular exposure to NSP4 causes several changes in the movement of nutrients and water across the epithelium (**Fig. 4**). Increases in intracellular calcium inhibit the translocation of disaccharidases from the intracellular vesicles to the luminal surface, decreasing the ability to digest carbohydrates and leading to maldigestion and exacerbation of the diarrhea.[132–134] NSP4 also directly inhibits sodium glucose cotransporter SGLT1, the primary sodium and glucose cotransporter that is critical for effective water absorption, significantly contributing to the pathogenesis of rotaviral diarrhea.[135] The actions of NSP4 better account for the maldigestion and malabsorption that are seen in rotavirus diarrhea, and is are likely more important to the pathogenesis than is histologic damage to the epithelium.

Secretory Diarrhea Caused by Rotavirus

NSP4 has also been implicated in causing secretion of chloride through the increase in intracellular calcium,[124] but the importance of this finding is being increasingly questioned because the increase is relatively mild and only occurs early in the course of diarrhea.[136,137] As previously mentioned, the actions of NSP4 are independent of CFTR, so the ion channel that is important for this chloride movement is unknown, and has been hypothesized to be created by NSP4.[114,124] An alternate mechanism that may explain the chloride secretion occurring in rotaviral diarrhea is activation of the ENS. Pharmacologically inhibiting the ENS dramatically reduces the diarrhea seen with rotavirus infections, although the mechanism by which the virus activates ENS-dependent secretion is unknown.[42,114,138] Prostaglandins and other inflammatory mediators may also play a role in causing secretion by affecting the ENS,[137] similar to other intestinal pathogens such as C parvum.[42,70,92] The ENS appears to play a critical role in rotavirus-induced secretion, but the mechanism responsible for this effect is unclear.

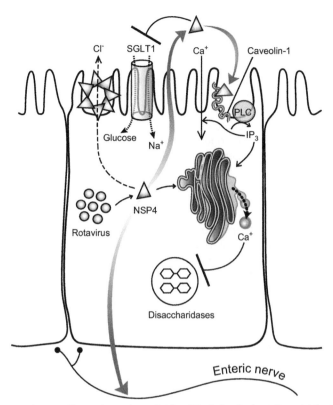

Fig. 4. Once rotavirus replicates in an intestinal epithelial cell, the enterotoxin NSP4 is produced. It has autocrine effects by causing calcium (Ca) release from the endoplasmic reticulum. NSP4 has paracrine effects by being secreted and binding to caveolin-1. This activates PLC, which increases cytoplasmic IP_3. IP_3 increases intracellular calcium by increasing release from the endoplasmic reticulum and increasing calcium movement across the luminal membrane. The increased intracellular calcium inhibits movement of disaccharidases to the luminal surface. NSP4 directly inhibits the SGLT1 which decreases the absorption of sodium (Na) and glucose, and increases chloride (Cl) secretion by an unknown mechanism, but may involve a channel created by NSP4. NSP4 also activates the enteric nervous system by an unknown mechanism.

Treatment and Control of Rotavirus Diarrhea

Treatment of rotavirus diarrhea is focused solely on rehydration because there are no currently available pharmacologic methods of controlling the infection in calves. Whereas the inhibition of SGLT1 and subsequent decrease in sodium and glucose absorption mediated by NSP4 would theoretically make sodium- and glucose-containing oral rehydration solutions less effective, this has not been shown clinically or experimentally. Currently, the Centers for Disease Control and Prevention recommend a low-osmolality rehydration solution that contains sodium and glucose for children with acute gastroenteritis. This recommendation is irrespective of the cause, yet rotavirus is likely involved in a majority of the cases.[139] Similar fluids would be expected to be effective in rehydrating calves with rotaviral diarrhea as well.

Enhancing colostral antibody transfer to the calf from the dam appears to be the most effective method of control for rotaviral diarrhea in calves. First, proper colostrum management is critical to ensure that an adequate IgG mass is delivered to each calf. This can be enhanced by administering vaccines to cows in the dry period to increase the amount of rotavirus-specific antibodies in the colostrum.[140] Experimental evidence has shown these vaccines to be effective at decreasing clinical signs;[141–144] however, some authors feel that the commercial vaccines are not as effective clinically.[145] There appears to be protection initially that is caused by the presence of specific antibodies in the intestinal lumen, but immunity in subsequent weeks is dependent on the resecretion of IgG into the intestine.[142] Oral vaccination of the calves at birth has been found to be less successful, and is not recommended.[145] Similar to other gastrointestinal pathogens, reducing exposure is also critical for control of rotaviral diarrhea in calves. Therefore, appropriate housing, stocking density, and hygiene cannot be ignored.

CORONAVIRUS

The epidemiology and pathophysiology of coronavirus diarrhea in calves overlaps significantly with that caused by rotavirus. Antibodies to coronavirus are ubiquitous in cattle,[146] and the virus is frequently found in both normal and diarrheic feces of calves.[147] Coronavirus typically affects calves with the first 3 weeks of life, and peak incidence occurs between days 7 and 10. The virus is ingested from the environment, which is contaminated by other calves or adult cattle.[115,148] Clinical signs begin approximately 2 days later and continue for 3 to 6 days.[148,149] Diarrhea secondary to coronavirus is mainly caused by intestinal epithelial cell loss and malabsorption. This virus has also been implicated in respiratory disease outbreaks in older calves as well as a diarrheal disease of adult cattle (winter dysentery), but discussion of these syndromes is beyond the scope of this report.

Malabsorptive Diarrhea Caused by Coronavirus

Coronavirus infection begins in the proximal small intestine, but then usually spreads throughout the jejunum, ileum, and colon. Initially, the virus attaches to the enterocyte via the spike and hemagglutinin glycoproteins, which also allow fusion of the viral envelope with the cell membrane or endocytotic vesicles.[148,150–152] Once in the cell, the virus replicates and is released using normal secretory mechanisms and upon cell death.[148,153] Diarrhea begins at the time of virus entry into the cell (before cell death occurs), but it is unknown if this is the result of secretion, malabsorption, or both.[115]

Infected cell loss is significant by 2 days after onset of diarrhea, and villous blunting occurs. The mature villous epithelial cells are the primary target for the virus, but crypt enterocytes are also affected.[154,155] As in rotavirus and C parvum infections, maldigestion and malabsorption lead to diarrhea. Because the crypt enterocytes and the colonocytes can be affected by coronavirus, the clinical signs often have a longer duration.[149,154]

Treatment and Control of Coronavirus Diarrhea

Like rotavirus diarrhea, there are no specific treatment methods for coronavirus infections, and little research has been done to confirm specific control measures for coronavirus in calves. Oral electrolyte solutions should be provided to prevent dehydration and treat acidosis. Methods aimed at controlling rotavirus infections (proper housing and hygiene, good colostrum management, and dry cow vaccination) are believed to be the best measures for control of coronavirus as well. Furthermore, most dry cow vaccinations targeted for neonatal calf diarrhea contain both rotavirus and coronavirus.

OTHER CAUSES OF INFECTIOUS DIARRHEA IN NEONATAL CALVES

Salmonella is the other major infectious cause of diarrhea in calves, but it is discussed in a separate article in this issue. A few other minor causes of diarrhea in calves are worth brief discussion.

Attaching and Effacing E coli

In addition to ETEC, there are several other types of E coli that are potential pathogens in calves, and these fall into the broad category of attaching and effacing E coli. These bacteria are characterized by the presence of the eae gene,[156] which encodes the protein intimin, a key component of the outer membrane that mediates attachment to the intestinal epithelium.[157] If these bacteria do not secrete any enterotoxins, they are classified as enterpathogenic E coli (EPEC).[157] EPEC organisms attach to the epithelium, disrupt the microvilli, and cause malabsorption.[158] They also use a Type III secretory protein to inject effector proteins into the host cell, inducing a secretory response by an undefined mechanism. Furthermore, they disrupt tight junctions between epithelial cells and lead to inflammation; all of which contribute to diarrhea.[159] The importance of EPEC as a pathogen of calves is debatable. It can be found in abnormal fecal samples, but is also frequently found in healthy calves[160] or not found at all.[161]

Enterohemorrhagic E coli (EHEC) are typically defined as expressing the eae gene and Shiga toxin. Strains that lack eae but secrete Shiga toxin are designated STEC.[162] Shiga toxin mediates many of the systemic effects that are seen in humans with E coli O157:H7 infections, and may cause some intestinal damage in some species.[158] Many epidemiological studies have shown that EHEC and STEC are commonly found in calves with normal and abnormal feces, and there is significant interest in these bacteria from the public health standpoint.[160,161,163–166] However, Shiga toxin receptors cannot be found in the intestine of calves or adult cattle, and no diarrhea was seen following experimental infection,[167] calling into question claims that these bacteria are pathogens of calves.

Clostridium difficile

Diarrhea caused by Clostridium difficile appears to be an emerging problem in both humans and veterinary patients. Diarrhea caused by C difficile is mediated by bacterial toxins that lead to epithelial cell death, damage to epithelial cell tight junctions, inflammation of the mucosa and submucosa, and activation of the ENS.[168] C difficile and its toxins can be found in the feces of both normal and diarrheic calves,[169–172] but its role as a pathogen has not been clearly established. Purified toxins will cause epithelial damage and an increase in luminal fluid in a calf intestinal loop model,[169] however experimental infection has not been successful.[172]

Giardia

Giardia organisms can be found in the feces of calves with diarrhea throughout the world, but is also commonly found in the feces of normal calves.[58,59,66,173–182] Some of these studies also found other pathogens along with Giardia, and none were controlled experiments. Only a single study has documented attempted experimental infection of calves with Giardia. In that study, histologic changes were found in only 2 of 12 calves, clinical signs were simply described as not severe, and the incidence of diarrhea was not reported.[183] *Giardia* has been documented to cause villous atrophy in naturally infected calves,[184] and is known to cause a malabsorptive diarrhea in other species.[185,186] Therefore, some have proposed that it may not be a significant cause of disease, but could still negatively impact calf growth.[55] This has also not been experimentally proven. Although *Giardia* is commonly found in the feces of both dairy and beef calves, it is unknown if it is truly a pathogen.

Torovirus

In the early 1980s, an infectious agent similar to coronavirus was identified in a herd of beef cattle in Iowa.[187] It was initially named Breda virus, but has subsequently been renamed torovirus. Since that time, it has been identified in both beef and dairy calves throughout the world, and 94% of adult cattle are seropositive.[188] Torovirus is found in calves with normal and abnormal feces, but is isolated more frequently in diarrheic feces. The incidence in calves with diarrhea ranged from 5% to 35%, while it was never isolated from more than 12% of normal calves. Other pathogens were commonly, but not always, found in conjunction with torovirus, but none appeared to be consistently associated with torovirus infection.[189–193] After ingestion, the virus infects the epithelium of the distal half of the jejunum, the ileum, and colon. Histopathologic lesions in experimental infections include necrosis of the crypt and villous enterocytes and villous atrophy, but infection does not consistently lead to clinical signs or histologic damage.[187,194,195] Although it has not been conclusively shown, these lesions would be expected to lead to a malabsorptive diarrhea. There is no specific information on control of torovirus, but as with other viruses, proper housing, decreasing exposure to adult cattle, and good hygiene are likely important to prevent its spread.

SUMMARY

Pathophysiologic mechanisms of infectious diarrhea in calves can be generally divided into malabsorptive/maldigestive, secretory, or both, and research into these mechanisms at the cellular level may ultimately lead to more specific control and treatment methods. Currently, most information must be extrapolated from other research models because calves are not commonly used. Further elucidation of the mechanisms by which these pathogens affect calves is critical because diarrhea is a significant cause of morbidity and mortality in both dairy and beef cattle.

REFERENCES

1. NAHMS. Reference of 1997 beef cow-calf production management and disease control. USDA survey 1998.
2. NAHMS. Dairy heifer morbidity, mortality, and health management focusing on preweaned heifers. USDA survey 1994.
3. Acres SD. Enterotoxigenic *Escherichia coli* infections in newborn calves: a review. J Dairy Sci 1985;68(1):229–56.
4. Acres SD, Saunders JR, Radostits OM. Acute undifferentiated neonatal diarrhea of beef calves: the prevalence of enterotoxigenic *E. coli*, reo-like (rota) virus and other enteropathogens in cow-calf herds. Can Vet J 1977;18(5):113–21.
5. Sherwood D, Snodgrass DR, Lawson GH. Prevalence of enterotoxigenic *Escherichia coli* in calves in Scotland and northern England. Vet Rec 1983; 113(10):208–12.

6. Myers LL, Guinee PA. Occurrence and characteristics of enterotoxigenic *Escherichia coli* isolated from calves with diarrhea. Infect Immun 1976;13(4): 1117–9.

7. Smith HW. The development of the flora of the alimentary tract in young animals. J Pathol Bacteriol 1965;90(2):495–513.

8. Smith HW. Observations on the flora of the alimentary tract of animals and factors affecting its composition. J Pathol Bacteriol 1965;89:95–122.

9. Hadad JJ, Gyles CL. The role of K antigens of enteropathogenic *Escherichia coli* in colonization of the small intestine of calves. Can J Comp Med 1982;46(1):21–6.

10. Hadad JJ, Gyles CL. Scanning and transmission electron microscopic study of the small intestine of colostrum-fed calves infected with selected strains of *Escherichia coli*. Am J Vet Res 1982;43(1):41–9.

11. Holland RE. Some infectious causes of diarrhea in young farm animals. Clin Microbiol Rev 1990;3(4):345–75.

12. Mainil JG, Bex F, Jacquemin E, et al. Prevalence of four enterotoxin (STaP, STaH, STb, and LT) and four adhesin subunit (K99, K88, 987P, and F41) genes among *Escherichia coli* isolates from cattle. Am J Vet Res 1990;51(2):187–90.

13. Shin SJ, Chang YF, Timour M, et al. Hybridization of clinical *Escherichia coli* isolates from calves and piglets in New York State with gene probes for enterotoxins (STaP, STb, LT), Shiga-like toxins (SLT-1, SLT-II) and adhesion factors (K88, K99, F41, 987P). Vet Microbiol 1994;38(3):217–25.

14. Francis DH, Allen SD, White RD. Influence of bovine intestinal fluid on the expression of K99 pili by *Escherichia coli*. Am J Vet Res 1989;50(6):822–6.

15. Mylrea PJ. Functioning of the digestive tract of young fasted calves. Res Vet Sci 1968;9(1):1–4.

16. Mylrea PJ. Gastro-intestinal disorders and the functioning of the digestive tract of young calves. Res Vet Sci 1968;9(1):14–28.

17. Smith HW. Observations on the aetiology of neonatal diarrhoea (scours) in calves. J Pathol Bacteriol 1962;84:147–68.

18. Constable PD. Pathophysiology of calf diarrhea: new concepts. Presented at the ACVIM Forum Proceedings. Charlotte, NC, June 3–7, 2003.

19. Runnels PL, Moon HW, Schneider RA. Development of resistance with host age to adhesion of K99+ *Escherichia coli* to isolated intestinal epithelial cells. Infect Immun 1980;28(1):298–300.

20. Pearson GR, Logan EF. The pathogenesis of enteric colibacillosis in neonatal unsuckled calves. Vet Rec 1979;105(8):159–64.

21. Argenzio RA. Pathophysiology of neonatal calf diarrhea. Vet Clin North Am Food Anim Pract 1985;1(3):461–9.

22. Field M, Semrad CE. Toxigenic diarrheas, congenital diarrheas, and cystic fibrosis: disorders of intestinal ion transport. Annu Rev Physiol 1993;55:631–55.

23. Mainil JG, Moseley SL, Schneider RA, et al. Hybridization of bovine *Escherichia coli* isolates with gene probes for four enterotoxins (STaP, STaH, STb, LT) and one adhesion factor (K99). Am J Vet Res 1986;47(5):1145–8.

24. Acosta-Martinez F, Gyles CL, Butler DG. *Escherichia coli* heat-stable enterotoxin in feces and intestines of calves with diarrhea. Am J Vet Res 1980;41(7):1143–9.

25. Saeed AM, Magnuson NS, Gay CC, et al. Characterization of heat-stable enterotoxin from a hypertoxigenic *Escherichia coli* strain that is pathogenic for cattle. Infect Immun 1986;53(2):445–7.

26. Giannella RA, Mann EA. *E. coli* heat-stable enterotoxin and guanylyl cyclase C: new functions and unsuspected actions. Trans Am Clin Climatol Assoc 2003; 114:67–85 [discussion: 85–6].

27. Dreyfus LA, Robertson DC. Solubilization and partial characterization of the intestinal receptor for *Escherichia coli* heat-stable enterotoxin. Infect Immun 1984;46(2):537–43.

28. Krause WJ, Cullingford GL, Freeman RH, et al. Distribution of heat-stable enterotoxin/guanylin receptors in the intestinal tract of man and other mammals. J Anat 1994;184(Pt 2):407–17.

29. Al-Majali AM, Asem EK, Lamar CH, et al. Studies on the mechanism of diarrhoea induced by *Escherichia coli* heat-stable enterotoxin (STa) in newborn calves. Vet Res Commun 2000;24(5):327–38.

30. Al-Majali AM, Asem EK, Lamar CH, et al. Characterization of the interaction of *Escherichia coli* heat-stable enterotoxin (STa) with its putative receptor on the intestinal tract of newborn calves. FEMS Immunol Med Microbiol 2000;28(2): 97–104.

31. al-Majali AM, Robinson JP, Asem EK, et al. Age-dependent variation in the density and affinity of *Escherichia coli* heat-stable enterotoxin receptors in mice. Adv Exp Med Biol 1999;473:137–45.

32. Jaso-Friedmann L, Dreyfus LA, Whipp SC, et al. Effect of age on activation of porcine intestinal guanylate cyclase and binding of *Escherichia coli* heat-stable enterotoxin (STa) to porcine intestinal cells and brush border membranes. Am J Vet Res 1992;53(12):2251–8.

33. Golin-Bisello F, Bradbury N, Ameen N, et al. STa and cGMP stimulate translocation to the surface of villus enterocytes in rat jejunum and is regulated by protein kinase G. Am J Physiol, Cell Physiol 2005;289(3):C708–16.

34. Thiagarajah JR, Broadbent T, Hsieh E, et al. Prevention of toxin-induced intestinal ion and fluid secretion by a small-molecule CFTR inhibitor. Gastroenterology 2004;126(2):511–9.

35. Sellers ZM, Childs D, Chow JY, et al. Heat-stable enterotoxin of *Escherichia coli* stimulates a non-CFTR-mediated duodenal bicarbonate secretory pathway. Am J Physiol Gastrointest Liver Physiol 2005;288(4):G654–63.

36. Tantisira MH. Effects of heat-stable *Escherichia coli* enterotoxin on intestinal alkaline secretion and transepithelial potential difference in the rat intestines in vivo. Scand J Gastroenterol 1990;25(1):19–28.

37. Lucas ML, Thom MM, Bradley JM, et al. *Escherichia coli* heat stable (STa) enterotoxin and the upper small intestine: lack of evidence in vivo for net fluid secretion. J Membr Biol 2005;206(1):29–42.

38. Lucas ML. A reconsideration of the evidence for *Escherichia coli* STa (heat stable) enterotoxin-driven fluid secretion: a new view of STa action and a new paradigm for fluid absorption. J Appl Microbiol 2001;90(1):7–26.

39. Mitchell ID, Tame MJ, Kenworthy R. Conditions for the production of *Eschericha coli* enterotoxin in a defined medium. J Med Microbiol 1974;7:395–400.

40. Mourad FH, Nassar CF. Effect of vasoactive intestinal polypeptide (VIP) antagonism on rat jejunal fluid and electrolyte secretion induced by cholera and *Escherichia coli* enterotoxins. Gut 2000;47(3):382–6.

41. Peterson JW, Whipp SC. Comparison of the mechanisms of action of cholera toxin and the heat-stable enterotoxins of *Escherichia coli*. Infect Immun 1995; 63(4):1452–61.

42. Jones SL, Blikslager AT. Role of the enteric nervous system in the pathophysiology of secretory diarrhea. J Vet Intern Med 2002;16(3):222–8.

43. Lucas ML, Duncan NW, O'Reilly NF, et al. Lack of evidence in vivo for a remote effect of *Escherichia coli* heat stable enterotoxin on jejunal fluid absorption. Neurogastroenterol Motil 2008;20(5):532–8.

44. Eklund S. The net fluid secretion caused by cyclic 3'5'-guanosine monophosphate in the rat jejunum in vivo is mediated by a local nervous reflex. Acta Physiol Scand 1986;128(1):57–63.
45. Eklund S. The enteric nervous system participates in the secretory response to the heat stable enterotoxins of *Escherichia coli* in rats and cats. Neuroscience 1985; 14(2):673–81.
46. Rolfe V, Levin RJ. Enterotoxin *Escherichia coli* STa activates a nitric oxide-dependent myenteric plexus secretory reflex in the rat ileum. J Physiol 1994;475(3):531–7.
47. Nzegwu HC, Levin RJ. Role of the enteric nervous system in the maintained hypersecretion induced by enterotoxin STa in the nutritionally deprived intestine. Gut 1994;35(9):1237–43.
48. Nzegwu HC, Levin RJ. Fluid hypersecretion induced by enterotoxin STa in nutritionally deprived rats: jejunal and ileal dynamics in vivo. Exp Physiol 1994; 79(4):547–60.
49. Nzegwu HC, Levin RJ. Neurally maintained hypersecretion in undernourished rat intestine activated by E. coli STa enterotoxin and cyclic nucleotides in vitro. J Physiol 1994;479(Pt 1):159–69.
50. Ahmed AF, Constable PD, Misk NA. Effect of feeding frequency and route of administration on abomasal luminal pH in dairy calves fed milk replacer. J Dairy Sci 2002;85(6):1502–8.
51. Smith HW, Halls S. Observations by the ligated intestinal segment and oral inoculation methods on *Escherichia coli* infections in pigs, calves, lambs and rabbits. J Pathol Bacteriol 1967;93(2):499–529.
52. Constable PD. Antimicrobial use in the treatment of calf diarrhea. J Vet Intern Med 2004;18(1):8–17.
53. Mosier DA, Oberst RD. Cryptosporidiosis. A global challenge. Ann NY Acad Sci 2000;916:102–11.
54. MacKenzie WR, Schell WL, Blair KA, et al. Massive outbreak of waterborne cryptosporidium infection in Milwaukee, Wisconsin: recurrence of illness and risk of secondary transmission. Clin Infect Dis 1995;21(1):57–62.
55. O'Handley RM, Olson ME. Giardiasis and cryptosporidiosis in ruminants. Vet Clin Food Anim 2006;22(3):623–43.
56. Tzipori S, Ward H. Cryptosporidiosis: biology, pathogenesis and disease. Microbes Infect 2002;4(10):1047–58.
57. de Graaf DC, Vanopdenbosch E, Ortega-Mora LM, et al. A review of the importance of cryptosporidiosis in farm animals. Int J Parasitol 1999;29(8):1269–87.
58. O'Handley RM, Cockwill C, McAllister TA, et al. Duration of naturally acquired giardiosis and cryptosporidiosis in dairy calves and their association with diarrhea. J Am Vet Med Assoc 1999;214(3):391–6.
59. Ralston BJ, McAllister TA, Olson MA. Prevalence and infection pattern of naturally acquired giardiasis and cryptosporidiosis in range beef calves and their dams. Vet Parasitol 2003;114(2):113–22.
60. Fayer R, Gasbarre L, Pasquali P, et al. Cryptosporidium parvum infection in bovine neonates: dynamic clinical, parasitic and immunologic patterns. Int J Parasitol 1998;28(1):49–56.
61. Santin M, Trout JM, Xiao L, et al. Prevalence and age-related variation of *Cryptosporidium* species and genotypes in dairy calves. Vet Parasitol 2004; 122(2):103–17.
62. Langkjaer RB, Vigre H, Enemark HL, et al. Molecular and phylogenetic characterization of *Cryptosporidium* and *Giardia* from pigs and cattle in Denmark. Parasitology 2007;134(Pt 3):339–50.

63. Harp JA, Woodmansee DB, Moon HW. Resistance of calves to *Cryptosporidium parvum*: effects of age and previous exposure. Infect Immun 1990;58(7):2237–40.

64. Argenzio RA, Liacos JA, Levy ML, et al. Villous atrophy, crypt hyperplasia, cellular infiltration, and impaired glucose-Na absorption in enteric cryptosporidiosis of pigs. Gastroenterology 1990;98(5 Pt 1):1129–40.

65. Xiao L, Herd RP. Infection pattern of *Cryptosporidium* and *Giardia* in calves. Vet Parasitol 1994;55(3):257–62.

66. Gow S, Waldner C. An examination of the prevalence of and risk factors for shedding of *Cryptosporidium* spp. and *Giardia* spp. in cows and calves from western Canadian cow-calf herds. Vet Parasitol 2006;137(1–2):50–61.

67. Anderson BC. Cryptosporidiosis in bovine and human health. J Dairy Sci 1998; 81(11):3036–41.

68. Tzipori S, Angus KW, Campbell I, et al. Experimental infection of lambs with *Cryptosporidium* isolated from a human patient with diarrhoea. Gut 1982;23(1):71–4.

69. Heine J, Pohlenz JF, Moon HW, et al. Enteric lesions and diarrhea in gnotobiotic calves monoinfected with *Cryptosporidium* species. J Infect Dis 1984;150(5): 768–75.

70. Gookin JL, Nordone SK, Argenzio RA. Host responses to *Cryptosporidium* infection. J Vet Intern Med 2002;16(1):12–21.

71. Moore R, Tzipori S, Griffiths JK, et al. Temporal changes in permeability and structure of piglet ileum after site-specific infection by *Cryptosporidium parvum*. Gastroenterology 1995;108(4):1030–9.

72. Chen XM, Levine SA, Tietz P, et al. *Cryptosporidium parvum* is cytopathic for cultured human biliary epithelia via an apoptotic mechanism. Hepatology 1998;28(4):906–13.

73. Adams RB, Guerrant RL, Zu S, et al. *Cryptosporidium parvum* infection of intestinal epithelium: morphologic and functional studies in an in vitro model. J Infect Dis 1994;169(1):170–7.

74. Laurent F, Eckmann L, Savidge TC, et al. *Cryptosporidium parvum* infection of human intestinal epithelial cells induces the polarized secretion of C-X-C chemokines. Infect Immun 1997;65(12):5067–73.

75. Griffiths JK, Moore R, Dooley S, et al. *Cryptosporidium parvum* infection of Caco-2 cell monolayers induces an apical monolayer defect, selectively increases transmonolayer permeability, and causes epithelial cell death. Infect Immun 1994;62(10):4506–14.

76. Buret AG, Chin AC, Scott KG. Infection of human and bovine epithelial cells with *Cryptosporidium andersoni* induces apoptosis and disrupts tight junctional ZO-1: effects of epidermal growth factor. Int J Parasitol 2003;33(12):1363–71.

77. Chen XM, Gores GJ, Paya CV, et al. *Cryptosporidium parvum* induces apoptosis in biliary epithelia by a Fas/Fas ligand-dependent mechanism. Am J Phys 1999; 277(3 Pt 1):G599–608.

78. Chen XM, Levine SA, Splinter PL, et al. *Cryptosporidium parvum* activates nuclear factor kappaB in biliary epithelia preventing epithelial cell apoptosis. Gastroenterology 2001;120(7):1774–83.

79. McCole DF, Eckmann L, Laurent F, et al. Intestinal epithelial cell apoptosis following *Cryptosporidium parvum* infection. Infect Immun 2000;68(3):1710–3.

80. Ojcius DM, Perfettini JL, Bonnin A, et al. Caspase-dependent apoptosis during infection with *Cryptosporidium parvum*. Microbes Infect 1999;1(14):1163–8.

81. Motta I, Gissot M, Kanellopoulos JM, et al. Absence of weight loss during *Cryptosporidium* infection in susceptible mice deficient in Fas-mediated apoptosis. Microbes Infect 2002;4(8):821–7.

82. Widmer G, Corey EA, Stein B, et al. Host cell apoptosis impairs *Cryptosporidium parvum* development in vitro. J Parasitol 2000;86(5):922–8.
83. Mele R, Gomez Morales MA, Tosini F, et al. *Cryptosporidium parvum* at different developmental stages modulates host cell apoptosis in vitro. Infect Immun 2004; 72(10):6061–7.
84. Argenzio RA, Lecce J, Powell DW. Prostanoids inhibit intestinal NaCl absorption in experimental porcine cryptosporidiosis. Gastroenterology 1993;104(2):440–7.
85. Argenzio RA, Rhoads JM, Armstrong M, et al. Glutamine stimulates prostaglandin-sensitive Na(+)-H+ exchange in experimental porcine cryptosporidiosis. Gastroenterology 1994;106(6):1418–28.
86. Blikslager A, Hunt E, Guerrant R, et al. Glutamine transporter in crypts compensates for loss of villus absorption in bovine cryptosporidiosis. Am J Physiol Gastrointest Liver Physiol 2001;281(3):G645–53.
87. Cole J, Blikslager A, Hunt E, et al. Cyclooxygenase blockade and exogenous glutamine enhance sodium absorption in infected bovine ileum. Am J Physiol Gastrointest Liver Physiol 2003;284(3):G516–24.
88. Topouchian A, Huneau JF, Barbot L, et al. Evidence for the absence of an intestinal adaptive mechanism to compensate for *C. parvum*-induced amino acid malabsorption in suckling rats. Parasitol Res 2003;91(3):197–203.
89. Topouchian A, Kapel N, Huneau JF, et al. Impairment of amino-acid absorption in suckling rats infected with *Cryptosporidium parvum*. Parasitol Res 2001; 87(11):891–6.
90. Klein P, Kleinova T, Volek Z, et al. Effect of *Cryptosporidium parvum* infection on the absorptive capacity and paracellular permeability of the small intestine in neonatal calves. Vet Parasitol 2008;152(1–2):53–9.
91. Holland RE, Herdt TH, Refsal KR. Pulmonary excretion of H_2 in calves with *Cryptosporidium*-induced malabsorption. Dig Dis Sci 1989;34(9):1399–404.
92. Argenzio RA, Armstrong M, Rhoads JM. Role of the enteric nervous system in piglet cryptosporidiosis. J Pharmacol Exp Ther 1996;279(3):1109–15.
93. Kandil HM, Berschneider HM, Argenzio RA. Tumour necrosis factor alpha changes porcine intestinal ion transport through a paracrine mechanism involving prostaglandins. Gut 1994;35(7):934–40.
94. Zadrozny LM, Stauffer SH, Armstrong MU, et al. Neutrophils do not mediate the pathophysiological sequelae of *Cryptosporidium parvum* infection in neonatal piglets. Infect Immun 2006;74(10):5497–505.
95. Gookin JL, Chiang S, Alle J, et al. NF-kappaB-mediated expression of iNOS promotes epithelial defense against infection by *Cryptosporidium parvum* in neonatal piglets. Am J Physiol Gastrointest Liver Physiol 2006;290(1): G164–74.
96. Gookin JL, Foster DM, Coccaro MR, et al. Oral delivery of L-arginine stimulates prostaglandin-dependent secretory diarrhea in *Cryptosporidium parvum*-infected neonatal piglets. J Pediatr Gastroenterol Nutr 2008;46(2):139–46.
97. Argenzio RA, Armstrong M, Blikslager A, et al. Peptide YY inhibits intestinal Cl- secretion in experimental porcine cryptosporidiosis through a prostaglandin-activated neural pathway. J Pharmacol Exp Ther 1997;283(2):692–7.
98. Jarvie BD, Trotz-Williams LA, McKnight DR, et al. Effect of halofuginone lactate on the occurrence of *Cryptosporidium parvum* and growth of neonatal dairy calves. J Dairy Sci 2005;88(5):1801–6.
99. Lallemand M, Villeneuve A, Belda J, et al. Field study of the efficacy of halofuginone and decoquinate in the treatment of cryptosporidiosis in veal calves. Vet Rec 2006;159(20):672–6.

100. Villacorta I, Peeters JE, Vanopdenbosch E, et al. Efficacy of halofuginone lactate against *Cryptosporidium parvum* in calves. Antimicrobial Agents Chemother 1991;35(2):283–7.

101. Peeters JE, Villacorta I, Naciri M, et al. Specific serum and local antibody responses against *Cryptosporidium parvum* during medication of calves with halofuginone lactate. Infect Immun 1993;61(10):4440–5.

102. Lefay D, Naciri M, Poirier P, et al. Efficacy of halofuginone lactate in the prevention of cryptosporidiosis in suckling calves. Vet Rec 2001;148(4):108–12.

103. Naciri M, Mancassola R, Yvore P, et al. The effect of halofuginone lactate on experimental *Cryptosporidium parvum* infections in calves. Vet Parasitol 1993; 45(3–4):199–207.

104. Fayer R, Ellis W. Paromomycin is effective as prophylaxis for cryptosporidiosis in dairy calves. J Parasitol 1993;79(5):771–4.

105. Moore DA, Atwill ER, Kirk JH, et al. Prophylactic use of decoquinate for infections with *Cryptosporidium parvum* in experimentally challenged neonatal calves. J Am Vet Med Assoc 2003;223(6):839–45.

106. Elitok B, Elitok OM, Pulat H. Efficacy of azithromycin dihydrate in treatment of cryptosporidiosis in naturally infected dairy calves. J Vet Intern Med 2005; 19(4):590–3.

107. Watarai S, Tana, Koiwa M. Feeding activated charcoal from bark containing wood vinegar liquid (nekka-rich) is effective as treatment for cryptosporidiosis in calves. J Dairy Sci 2008;91(4):1458–63.

108. de Graaf DC, Spano F, Petry F, et al. Speculation on whether a vaccine against cryptosporidiosis is a reality or fantasy. Int J Parasitol 1999;29(8):1289–306.

109. Fayer R, Andrews C, Ungar BL, et al. Efficacy of hyperimmune bovine colostrum for prophylaxis of cryptosporidiosis in neonatal calves. J Parasitol 1989;75(3):393–7.

110. Perryman LE, Kapil SJ, Jones ML, et al. Protection of calves against cryptosporidiosis with immune bovine colostrum induced by a *Cryptosporidium parvum* recombinant protein. Vaccine 1999;17(17):2142–9.

111. Harp JA, Goff JP. Protection of calves with a vaccine against *Cryptosporidium parvum*. J Parasitol 1995;81(1):54–7.

112. Harp JA, Goff JP. Strategies for the control of *Cryptosporidium parvum* infection in calves. J Dairy Sci 1998;81(1):289–94.

113. Harp JA, Jardon P, Atwill ER, et al. Field testing of prophylactic measures against *Cryptosporidium parvum* infection in calves in a California dairy herd. Am J Vet Res 1996;57(11):1586–8.

114. Ramig RF. Pathogenesis of intestinal and systemic rotavirus infection. J Virol 2004;78(19):10213–20.

115. Torres-Medina A, Schlafer DH, Mebus CA. Rotaviral and coronaviral diarrhea. Vet Clin North Am Food Anim Pract 1985;1(3):471–93.

116. Schlafer DH, Scott FW. Prevalence of neutralizing antibody to the calf rotavirus in New York cattle. Cornell Vet 1979;69(3):262–71.

117. Chinsangaram J, Schore CE, Guterbock W, et al. Prevalence of group A and group B rotaviruses in the feces of neonatal dairy calves from California. Comp Immunol Microbiol Infect Dis 1995;18(2):93–103.

118. Theil KW, McCloskey CM. Molecular epidemiology and subgroup determination of bovine group a rotaviruses associated with diarrhea in dairy and beef calves. J Clin Microbiol 1989;27(1):126–31.

119. Alfieri AA, Parazzi ME, Takiuchi E, et al. Frequency of group A rotavirus in diarrhoeic calves in Brazilian cattle herds, 1998–2002. Trop Anim Health Prod 2006;38(7–8):521–6.

120. Lucchelli A, Lance SE, Bartlett PB, et al. Prevalence of bovine group A rotavirus shedding among dairy calves in Ohio. Am J Vet Res 1992;53(2):169–74.
121. Ball JM, Tian P, Zeng CQ, et al. Age-dependent diarrhea induced by a rotaviral nonstructural glycoprotein. Science 1996;272(5258):101–4.
122. Ciarlet M, Estes MK. Interactions between rotavirus and gastrointestinal cells. Curr Opin Microbiol 2001;4(4):435–41.
123. Morris AP, Estes MK. Microbes and microbial toxins: paradigms for microbial-mucosal interactions. VIII. Pathological consequences of rotavirus infection and its enterotoxin. Am J Physiol Gastrointest Liver Physiol 2001;281(2): G303–10.
124. Morris AP, Scott JK, Ball JM, et al. NSP4 elicits age-dependent diarrhea and Ca(2+)mediated I(-) influx into intestinal crypts of CF mice. Am J Physiol 1999;277(2 Pt 1):G431–44.
125. Zhang M, Zeng CQ, Morris AP, et al. A functional NSP4 enterotoxin peptide secreted from rotavirus-infected cells. J Virol 2000;74(24):11663–70.
126. Parr RD, Storey SM, Mitchell DM, et al. The rotavirus enterotoxin NSP4 directly interacts with the caveolar structural protein caveolin-1. J Virol 2006;80(6): 2842–54.
127. Storey SM, Gibbons TF, Williams CV, et al. Full-length, glycosylated NSP4 is localized to plasma membrane caveolae by a novel raft isolation technique. J Virol 2007;81(11):5472–83.
128. Dong Y, Zeng CQ, Ball JM, et al. The rotavirus enterotoxin NSP4 mobilizes intracellular calcium in human intestinal cells by stimulating phospholipase C–mediated inositol 1,4,5-trisphosphate production. Proc Natl Acad Sci U S A 1997; 94(8):3960–5.
129. Brunet JP, Cotte-Laffitte J, Linxe C, et al. Rotavirus infection induces an increase in intracellular calcium concentration in human intestinal epithelial cells: role in microvillar actin alteration. J Virol 2000;74(5):2323–32.
130. Brunet JP, Jourdan N, Cotte-Laffitte J, et al. Rotavirus infection induces cytoskeleton disorganization in human intestinal epithelial cells: implication of an increase in intracellular calcium concentration. J Virol 2000;74(22):10801–6.
131. Berkova Z, Morris AP, Estes MK. Cytoplasmic calcium measurement in rotavirus enterotoxin-enhanced green fluorescent protein (NSP4-EGFP) expressing cells loaded with Fura-2. Cell Calcium 2003;34(1):55–68.
132. Collins J, Candy DC, Starkey WG, et al. Disaccharidase activities in small intestine of rotavirus-infected suckling mice: a histochemical study. J Pediatr Gastroenterol Nutr 1990;11(3):395–403.
133. Jourdan N, Brunet JP, Sapin C, et al. Rotavirus infection reduces sucrase–isomaltase expression in human intestinal epithelial cells by perturbing protein targeting and organization of microvillar cytoskeleton. J Virol 1998;72(9): 7228–36.
134. Martin-Latil S, Cotte-Laffitte J, Beau I, et al. A cyclic AMP protein kinase A–dependent mechanism by which rotavirus impairs the expression and enzyme activity of brush border–associated sucrase–isomaltase in differentiated intestinal Caco-2 cells. Cell Microbiol 2004;6(8):719–31.
135. Halaihel N, Lievin V, Ball JM, et al. Direct inhibitory effect of rotavirus NSP4(114–135) peptide on the Na(+)-D-glucose symporter of rabbit intestinal brush border membrane. J Virol 2000;74(20):9464–70.
136. Lorrot M, Benhamadouche-Casari H, Vasseur M. Mechanisms of net chloride secretion during rotavirus diarrhea in young rabbits: do intestinal villi secrete chloride? Cell Physiol Biochem 2006;18(1-3):103–12.

137. Lorrot M, Vasseur M. How do the rotavirus NSP4 and bacterial enterotoxins lead differently to diarrhea? Virol J 2007;4:31–7.
138. Lundgren O, Peregrin AT, Persson K, et al. Role of the enteric nervous system in the fluid and electrolyte secretion of rotavirus diarrhea. Science 2000;287(5452):491–5.
139. King CK. Managing acute gastroenteritis among children: oral rehydration, maintenance, and nutritional therapy. MMWR Recomm Rep 2003;52(RR-16):1–16.
140. Kohara J. Enhancement of passive immunity with maternal vaccine against newborn calf diarrhea. J Vet Med Sci 1997;59(11):1023–5.
141. Fernandez FM, Conner ME, Hodgins DC, et al. Passive immunity to bovine rotavirus in newborn calves fed colostrum supplements from cows immunized with recombinant SA11 rotavirus core-like particle (CLP) or virus-like particle (VLP) vaccines. Vaccine 1998;16(5):507–16.
142. Parreno V, Bejar C, Vagnozzi A, et al. Modulation by colostrum-acquired maternal antibodies of systemic and mucosal antibody responses to rotavirus in calves experimentally challenged with bovine rotavirus. Vet Immunol Immunopathol 2004;100(1-2):7–24.
143. Saif LJ, Smith KL. Enteric viral infections of calves and passive immunity. J Dairy Sci 1985;68(1):206–28.
144. Cornaglia EM. Reduction in morbidity due to diarrhea in nursing beef calves by use of an inactivated oil-adjuvanted rotavirus–Escherichia coli vaccine in the dam. Vet Microbiol 1992;30(2-3):191–202.
145. Radostits OM, Gay CC, Blood DC, et al. Viral diarrhea in calves, lambs, kids, piglets, and foals. In: Veterinary medicine: a textbook of the diseases of cattle, sheep, pigs, goats, and horses. 9th edition. New York: WB Saunders and Co, LTD; 1999. p. 1115.
146. Rodak L, Babiuk LA, Acres SD. Detection by radioimmunoassay and enzyme-linked immunosorbent assay of coronavirus antibodies in bovine serum and lacteal secretions. J Clin Microbiol 1982;16(1):34–40.
147. Snodgrass DR, Terzolo HR, Sherwood D, et al. Aetiology of diarrhoea in young calves. Vet Rec 1986;119(2):31–4.
148. Clark MA. Bovine coronavirus. Br Vet J 1993;149(1):51–70.
149. Lewis LD. Pathophysiologic changes due to coronavirus-induced diarrhea in the calf. J Am Vet Med Assoc 1978;173(5 Pt 2):636–42.
150. Schultze B, Gross HJ, Brossmer R, et al. The S protein of bovine coronavirus is a hemagglutinin recognizing 9-O-acetylated sialic acid as a receptor determinant. J Virol 1991;65(11):6232–7.
151. Schultze B, Wahn K, Klenk HD, et al. Isolated HE-protein from hemagglutinating encephalomyelitis virus and bovine coronavirus has receptor-destroying and receptor-binding activity. Virology 1991;180(1):221–8.
152. Payne HR, Storz J, Henk WG. Initial events in bovine coronavirus infection: analysis through immunogold probes and lysosomotropic inhibitors. Arch Virol 1990;114(3-4):175–89.
153. Payne HR, Storz J. Scanning electron microscopic characterization of bovine coronavirus plaques in HRT cells. Zentralbl Veterinarmed B 1990;37(7):501–8.
154. Storz J, Doughri AM, Hajer I. Coronaviral morphogenesis and ultrastructural changes in intestinal infections of calves. J Am Vet Med Assoc 1978;173(5 Pt 2):633–5.
155. Park SJ, Kim GY, Choy HE, et al. Dual enteric and respiratory tropisms of winter dysentery bovine coronavirus in calves. Arch Virol 2007;152(10):1885–900.
156. Moon HW, Whipp SC, Argenzio RA, et al. Attaching and effacing activities of rabbit and human enteropathogenic Escherichia coli in pig and rabbit intestines. Infect Immun 1983;41(3):1340–51.

157. Donnenberg MS, Kaper JB. Enteropathogenic *Escherichia coli*. Infect Immun 1992;60(10):3953–61.
158. Nataro JP, Kaper JB. Diarrheagenic *Escherichia coli*. Clin Microbiol Rev 1998; 11(1):142–201.
159. Hecht G. Microbes and microbial toxins: paradigms for microbial–mucosal interactions. VII. Enteropathogenic *Escherichia coli*: physiological alterations from an extracellular position. Am J Physiol Gastrointest Liver Physiol 2001;281(1):G1–7.
160. Holland RE, Wilson RA, Holland MS, et al. Characterization of eae+ *Escherichia coli* isolated from healthy and diarrheic calves. Vet Microbiol 1999;66(4):251–63.
161. Wieler LH, Sobjinski G, Schlapp T, et al. Longitudinal prevalence study of diarrheagenic *Escherichia coli* in dairy calves. Berl Munch Tierarztl Wochenschr 2007;120(7–8):296–306.
162. Levine MM. *Escherichia coli* that cause diarrhea: enterotoxigenic, enteropathogenic, enteroinvasive, enterohemorrhagic, and enteroadherent. J Infect Dis 1987;155(3):377–89.
163. Leomil L, Aidar-Ugrinovich L, Guth BE, et al. Frequency of shiga toxin–producing *Escherichia coli* (STEC) isolates among diarrheic and non-diarrheic calves in Brazil. Vet Microbiol 2003;97(1–2):103–9.
164. Lee JH, Hur J, Stein BD. Occurrence and characteristics of enterohemorrhagic *Escherichia coli* O26 and O111 in calves associated with diarrhea. Vet J 2008; 176(2):205–9.
165. Kang SJ, Ryu SJ, Chae JS, et al. Occurrence and characteristics of enterohemorrhagic *Escherichia coli* O157 in calves associated with diarrhoea. Vet Microbiol 2004;98(3–4):323–8.
166. Osek J, Gallien P, Protz D. Characterization of shiga toxin–producing *Escherichia coli* strains isolated from calves in Poland. Comp Immunol Microbiol Infect Dis 2000;23(4):267–76.
167. Pruimboom-Brees IM, Morgan TW, Ackermann MR, et al. Cattle lack vascular receptors for *Escherichia coli* O157:H7 Shiga toxins. Proc Natl Acad Sci U S A 2000;97(19):10325–9.
168. Keel MK, Songer JG. The comparative pathology of *Clostridium difficile*–associated disease. Vet Pathol 2006;43(3):225–40.
169. Hammitt MC, Bueschel DM, Keel MK, et al. A possible role for *Clostridium difficile* in the etiology of calf enteritis. Vet Microbiol 2008;127(3–4):343–52.
170. Keel K, Brazier JS, Post KW, et al. Prevalence of PCR ribotypes among *Clostridium difficile* isolates from pigs, calves, and other species. J Clin Microbiol 2007;45(6):1963–4.
171. Rodriguez-Palacios A, Stampfli HR, Duffield T, et al. *Clostridium difficile* PCR ribotypes in calves, Canada. Emerging Infect Dis 2006;12(11):1730–6.
172. Rodriguez-Palacios A, Stampfli HR, Stalker M, et al. Natural and experimental infection of neonatal calves with *Clostridium difficile*. Vet Microbiol 2007; 124(1–2):166–72.
173. Bjorkman C, Svensson C, Christensson B, et al. *Cryptosporidium parvum* and *Giardia intestinalis* in calf diarrhoea in Sweden. Acta Vet Scand 2003;44(3–4):145–52.
174. Huetink RE, van der Giessen JW, Noordhuizen JP, et al. Epidemiology of *Cryptosporidium* spp. and *Giardia duodenalis* on a dairy farm. Vet Parasitol 2001;102(1–2):53–67.
175. Xiao L, Herd RP, Rings DM. Concurrent infections of *Giardia* and *Cryptosporidium* on two Ohio farms with calf diarrhea. Vet Parasitol 1993;51(1–2):41–8.
176. St Jean G, Couture Y, Dubreuil P, et al. Diagnosis of *Giardia* infection in 14 calves. J Am Vet Med Assoc 1987;191(7):831–2.

177. Geurden T, Geldhof P, Levecke B, et al. Mixed *Giardia duodenalis* assemblage A and E infections in calves. Int J Parasitol 2008;38(2):259–64.

178. Mendonca C, Almeida A, Castro A, et al. Molecular characterization of *Cryptosporidium* and *Giardia* isolates from cattle from Portugal. Vet Parasitol 2007; 147(1–2):47–50.

179. Becher KA, Robertson ID, Fraser DM, et al. Molecular epidemiology of *Giardia* and *Cryptosporidium* infections in dairy calves originating from three sources in Western Australia. Vet Parasitol 2004;123(1–2):1–9.

180. Maddox-Hyttel C, Langkjaer RB, Enemark HL, et al. *Cryptosporidium* and *Giardia* in different age groups of Danish cattle and pigs–occurrence and management associated risk factors. Vet Parasitol 2006;141(1–2):48–59.

181. Matsubayashi M, Kimata I, Abe N. Identification of genotypes of *Giardia intestinalis* isolates from a human and calf in Japan. J Vet Med Sci 2005;67(3): 337–40.

182. Smith KE, Stenzel SA, Bender JB, et al. Outbreaks of enteric infections caused by multiple pathogens associated with calves at a farm day camp. Pediatr Infect Dis J 2004;23(12):1098–104.

183. Uehlinger FD, O'Handley RM, Greenwood SJ, et al. Efficacy of vaccination in preventing giardiasis in calves. Vet Parasitol 2007;146(1–2):182–8.

184. Ruest N, Couture Y, Faubert GM, et al. Morphological changes in the jejunum of calves naturally infected with *Giardia* spp. and *Cryptosporidium* spp. Vet Parasitol 1997;69(3–4):177–86.

185. Buret A, Hardin JA, Olson ME, et al. Pathophysiology of small intestinal malabsorption in gerbils infected with *Giardia lamblia*. Gastroenterology 1992; 103(2):506–13.

186. Buret A, Gall DG, Olson ME. Effects of murine giardiasis on growth, intestinal morphology, and disaccharidase activity. J Parasitol 1990;76(3):403–9.

187. Woode GN, Reed DE, Runnels PL, et al. Studies with an unclassified virus isolated from diarrheic calves. Vet Microbiol 1982;7(3):221–40.

188. Koopmans M, van den Boom U, Woode G, et al. Seroepidemiology of Breda virus in cattle using ELISA. Vet Microbiol 1989;19(3):233–43.

189. Duckmanton L, Carman S, Nagy E, et al. Detection of bovine torovirus in fecal specimens of calves with diarrhea from Ontario farms. J Clin Microbiol 1998; 36(5):1266–70.

190. Hoet AE, Nielsen PR, Hasoksuz M, et al. Detection of bovine torovirus and other enteric pathogens in feces from diarrhea cases in cattle. J Vet Diagn Invest 2003;15(3):205–12.

191. Hoet AE, Smiley J, Thomas C, et al. Association of enteric shedding of bovine torovirus (Breda virus) and other enteropathogens with diarrhea in veal calves. Am J Vet Res 2003;64(4):485–90.

192. Kirisawa R, Takeyama A, Koiwa M, et al. Detection of bovine torovirus in fecal specimens of calves with diarrhea in Japan. J Vet Med Sci 2007;69(5):471–6.

193. Haschek B, Klein D, Benetka V, et al. Detection of bovine torovirus in neonatal calf diarrhoea in Lower Austria and Styria (Austria). J Vet Med B Infect Dis Vet Public Health 2006;53(4):160–5.

194. Fagerland JA, Pohlenz JF, Woode GN. A morphological study of the replication of Breda virus (proposed family Toroviridae) in bovine intestinal cells. J Gen Virol 1986;67(Pt 7):1293–304.

195. Pohlenz JF, Cheville NF, Woode GN, et al. Cellular lesions in intestinal mucosa of gnotobiotic calves experimentally infected with a new unclassified bovine virus (Breda virus). Vet Pathol 1984;21(4):407–17.

Salmonella in Calves

Virginia L. Mohler, BS, BVSc, Matthew M. Izzo, BVSc,
John K. House, BVMS, PhD*

KEYWORDS

- Salmonella • Pathophysiology • Diagnosis
- Treatment • Control

Calves may be infected with a diverse array of salmonella serotypes within hours of birth.[1] The subsequent manifestations of disease are variable, reflecting the balance between host immunity, pathogen dose, and virulence. Neonatal disease outbreaks are frequently observed in calves between 4 and 28 days of age.[1] However, older calves may be affected. Clinical signs include fever, dull mentation, loss of appetite, and scours that often contain increased mucus and may contain blood.[2–5] Dehydration, combined with acid–base and electrolyte derangements, contribute to weakness and depressed mentation in acutely infected calves. Calves surviving the acute phase of the disease often go through a cachectic period during recovery. The severity and duration of clinical disease in calves is related to virulence of the strain, challenge dose, calf age, efficiency of passive immunity, nutrition, and degree of environmental stress.

Few clinical signs of disease may be observed in calves that suffer peracute salmonella infections with animals simply found dead. Affected calves may have been noted to be lethargic or inappetent at the previous feeding. Laboratory findings may include leukopenia, neutropenia, hemoconcentration associated with dehydration, metabolic acidosis, and increased blood urea nitrogen.

Inappetence and depressed mentation are typically the first clinical signs observed in acute infections. Pyrexia and diarrhea follow 48 to 72 hours postinfection. Fevers may persist for up to 7 days postinfection.[6,7] The absence of a fever should not rule out the presence of *Salmonella* as the febrile response is transient and calves succumbing to infection are often hypothermic for 12 to 24 hours before death.[6] Fecal consistency ranges from watery, voluminous, and profuse to mucofibrinous and hemorrhagic. Differences are observed between infections with different serovars and potentially between different strains of the same serovar. This is a result of differences in virulence factors that can occur between infecting strains.[6,7] *Salmonella enteritica* serovar Typhimurium is commonly incriminated in outbreaks of enteric disease in calves less than 2 months of age.[2–5,8,9] In contrast, *S enteritica* serovar Dublin is associated with disease of similar frequencies in young and adult cattle.[10] In a longitudinal

Livestock Veterinary Teaching and Research Unit, Faculty of Veterinary Science, University of Sydney, PMB 4, Narellan Delivery Centre, Camden, NSW 2567, Australia
* Corresponding author.
E-mail address: jkhouse@camden.usyd.edu.au (J.K. House).

Vet Clin Food Anim 25 (2009) 37–54
doi:10.1016/j.cvfa.2008.10.009
0749-0720/08/$ – see front matter © 2009 Elsevier Inc. All rights reserved.

vetfood.theclinics.com

surveillance of salmonella shedding by calves, we have observed both high and low mortality associated with high-prevalence salmonella fecal shedding (>80% of calves shedding during the first 10 days of life).[1,11] The increase in mortality corresponded to a shift from isolating a mixture of different salmonella serotypes to a predominance of S Typhimurium.

S Dublin is more invasive than S Typhimurium, and invasive manifestations of disease include meningoencephalitis, septic arthritis, and septic physitis. These may be observed with or without signs of enteric disease. S Dublin also has a propensity to cause respiratory disease in older calves around the time of weaning and occasionally gangrenous necrosis of the distal extremities (**Fig. 1**).[12] An immune-mediated process, known as cold agglutination, has been proposed as the main cause of dry gangrene.[13] A small proportion of calves infected with S Dublin fail to clear the infection and remain chronically infected. These "carrier" animals usually appear normal and go on to shed Salmonella in feces and milk, thus maintaining a source of infection in the herd.[14,15]

PATHOPHYSIOLOGY

Fecal-oral transmission is the primary route of infection. However, other reported routes include the mucosa of the upper respiratory tract and conjunctiva. Following ingestion, salmonellae colonize the intestinal tract and invade through M-cells (which are specialized cells in intestinal lymphoid tissues), enterocytes,[5,16,17] and tonsilar lymphoid tissue.[2] In the lymphoid tissue, salmonellae gain entry into mononuclear phagocytes and are rapidly disseminated throughout the body.[2,16] The capacity of Salmonella to infect calves via the tonsils was demonstrated by experimental challenge studies in esophagectomized calves.[18] In these calves, Salmonella bacteria were isolated from tissues within 3 hours of oral challenge.

The basic virulence mechanisms of Salmonella spp include the ability to invade the intestinal mucosa, to multiply in lymphoid tissues, and to evade host defense systems, leading to systemic disease. The diarrhea associated with salmonellosis is largely believed to be mediated by the inflammatory response to infection. S Typhimurium requires a functional type III secretion system encoded by salmonella pathogenicity islands (SPI1 and SPI5) to cause diarrhea.[8,19,20] The main function of the invasion-associated type III

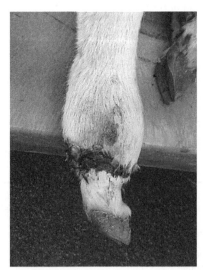

Fig. 1. Gangrenous necrosis of the distal extremity in a calf infected with S Dublin.

secretion system is to translocate effector proteins into the cytosol of a host cell. The resulting cell death is associated with a proinflammatory response and influx of neutrophils into the intestinal mucosa.[5] A positive correlation is seen between the severity of histopathological lesions detected in the ileal mucosa and the volume of fluid secretion.[20] Release of endotoxin, prostaglandins, and proinflammatory cytokines (interleukin 1 and tumor necrosis factor α)[21] also promote vascular permeability and hypersecretion. Sloughing of the intestinal epithelial cells leads to acute hemorrhage, fibrin production, maldigestion, and malabsorption.[5] The resulting hyperosmotic state within the lumen of the intestine draws fluid into the intestinal tract, contributing to a net loss of water, sodium, potassium, and bicarbonate. Mucosal damage also contributes to protein loss and hypoproteinemia.

The bovine host-adapted S Dublin and some strains of S Typhimurium have a virulence plasmid that carries the SpV gene, which promotes the survival of Salmonella in macrophages. The ability to survive intracellularly within the reticuloendothelial cells of liver and spleen, lymph nodes, and macrophages contributes to virulence.[22,23] Other nonadapted serovars may carry the virulence plasmid. However, the virulence plasmid is less common in non-adapted serovars, and their virulence is more variable.

Increased virulence has been observed in some antimicrobial resistant strains of Salmonella. This is reflected by the finding that calves infected with S Typhimurium DT104 are 13 times more likely to die than calves infected with antibiotic-sensitive strains of S Typhimurium.[24] The spread of resistance genes by transformation, transduction, and conjugation is well documented in Salmonella spp and in the Enterobacteriaceae family.[5]

Multidrug-resistant strains of Salmonella are frequently implicated in disease outbreaks in calves and, occasionally, people. During investigations of neonatal salmonellosis, it is prudent to inform farm personnel of the human health risks that Salmonella poses to them and their families. These risks have been highlighted in reports of human salmonellosis caused by the multidrug-resistant S enteritica serovar Newport derived from livestock.[25–27]

GROSS LESIONS

Although pathologists associate salmonellosis with enteric lesions, such as diphtheritic membranes, peracute infections often have few pathologic findings.[2,5] Lesions observed with peracute salmonellosis include pulmonary congestion and submucosal and subserosal petechial hemorrhages of multiple organs, including the intestines and heart.

Acute salmonellosis is typically characterized by diffuse catarrhal hemorrhagic enteritis with diffuse fibrinonecrotic ileotyphlocolitis (**Fig. 2**).[28] The intestinal contents are watery, malodorous, and may contain mucous or whole blood. Inflammation of the gall bladder is common, and histopathological evidence of fibrinous cholecystitis is considered pathognomonic for acute enteric salmonellosis in calves (**Fig. 3**). Enlargement, edema, and hemorrhage are commonly observed in the mesenteric lymph nodes (**Fig. 4**).[28] Abomasal mucosal erosions may be observed, particularly with salmonella dublin infection. Chronic salmonellosis may result in thickening of the intestinal wall with a yellow-gray necrotic material overlying a red mucosal surface (**Fig. 5**).[28]

DIAGNOSIS

There are numerous methods of detecting Salmonella and, at the herd level, it is not difficult to detect or isolate the organism. The diagnostic question more specifically relates to the association between the presence of the organism and the observed disease process. This question arises from the observation that Salmonella may be

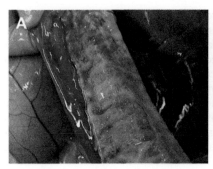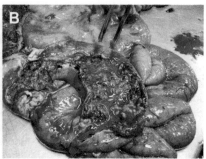

Fig. 2. (*A*) Fibrin deposits in the small intestine of a calf with salmonellosis. (*B*) Catarrhal hemorrhagic enteritis in a calf with salmonellosis.

recovered from the feces of clinically normal calves. During a suspected outbreak of salmonellosis, 10 calves in the affected age group should be sampled to determine the proportion of calves infected with *Salmonella*. While direct culture of feces provides for rapid detection of *Salmonella*, this method of detection is insensitive because of the large number of gram-negative organisms present in feces, which often hinder the isolation *Salmonella* colonies. Diagnostic laboratories use enrichment media, such as selenite or tetrathionate broth, to promote the growth of *Salmonella* and inhibit other fecal flora. Enriched samples are subsequently plated on salmonella-selective media, such as xylose lysine deso-oxycholate or brilliant green agar.[29] Suspect colonies are tested using a series of biochemical tests and serogrouped using serogroup-specific antisera. Serotyping is generally conducted by reference laboratories.

Rapid-detection diagnostic methods include antigen capture ELISA and polymerase chain reactions (PCRs). Preliminary enrichment culture is often employed with both techniques to enhance the sensitivity of detection. ELISAs have a reported sensitivity of 59% and specificity of 97.6% on enrichment cultures.[5,30] Conventional and real-time PCR assays have also been developed to detect the presence of *Salmonella* in feces. PCR is reported to reduce the detection limits and time compared with conventional fecal culture techniques.[31–34]

Outbreaks of neonatal calf diarrhea often involve multiple pathogens. During an outbreak of salmonellosis, it is not uncommon to find 70% to 80% of calves to be

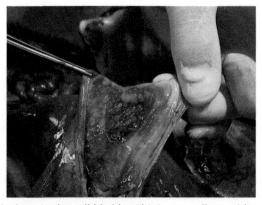

Fig. 3. Ulcerated bile ducts in the gall bladder. This is generally considered to be pathognomonic for acute enteric salmonellosis in calves.

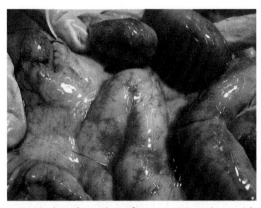

Fig. 4. Enlarged mesenteric lymph nodes often seen in calves with system salmonella infections.

shedding the bacteria.[1] However in experimental challenge and field studies, differences have been observed in the propensity for and persistence of fecal shedding between different salmonella serotypes, with *S* Dublin having a propensity to shed intermittently despite tissue colonization.[6,7,35] A high prevalence of salmonella shedding supports a diagnosis of salmonellosis. Culture techniques are initially preferable to ELISA and PCR detection methods as isolation of the organism provides an opportunity for serotyping and antimicrobial susceptibility testing. *S* Typhimurium and *S* Dublin are commonly associated with disease, so the serotype isolated can provide further indication regarding the likelihood of causal association. Interpretation in this regard may require some local knowledge. For example, in Australia, *S enterica* serovar Bovismorbificans is commonly associated with disease in livestock. However, this same serovar is uncommon in North America.

Calves dying of salmonellosis are often bacteremic. Therefore, isolation of *Salmonella* from systemic sites at necropsy provides robust evidence of causality as well as an isolate relevant for antimicrobial susceptibility testing. If animals are euthanized for necropsy during a herd investigation, it is best to sample calves during the acute stage of the disease. The likelihood of isolating *Salmonella* from cachetic calves recovering from

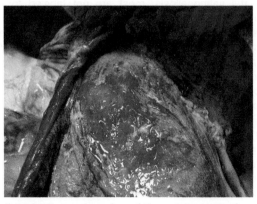

Fig. 5. Abomasal wall thickening and erosion of the mucosa and submucosa, which can be seen with chronic salmonellosis in calves.

salmonellosis is less because survival is associated with clearance of the organism from tissues. Isolation of *Salmonella* from gut contents or mesenteric lymph nodes without demonstrating compatible histologic lesions does not necessarily establish causality.

TREATMENT

Dehydration, electrolyte imbalances, endotoxemia, and bacteremia are common clinical features of salmonella infections in calves. Treatment of salmonellosis in calves is directed at replacing fluid and electrolyte losses, limiting inflammatory cascades through use of nonsteroidal anti-inflammatory drugs (NSAIDs), and the judicious use of antimicrobials.[4,36–38] Provision of a clean, dry, thermoneutral environment and nutritional support improves outcome.

During a herd outbreak, the age of affected calves should be noted and prophylactic electrolyte administration instituted to prevent dehydration and acidosis. The electrolytes are offered between milk feeds. Using electrolyte formulations containing acetate or proprionate as alkalizing agents avoids interfering with milk-clot formation at the subsequent milk feeding. Initiating oral fluid-replacement therapy to calves early in the course of the disease is more effective since the calves still have a suck reflex.

On a herd level, the logistics of treatment becomes more difficult, the cost higher, and the success lower once calves become recumbent. Calves unable to maintain sternal recumbency require intravenous fluid therapy. Saline-based fluids containing alkalinizing agents, such as sodium bicarbonate, are useful in correcting dehydration and acidosis. In the past, field estimation of acid–base status has been based on clinical signs. However, the advent of portable blood-gas and chemistry analyzers (eg, i-STAT; Heska Corp., Loveland, Colorado) has facilitated field assessment and treatment of severely compromised calves. Fluid therapy is fundamental to managing calves with salmonellosis. A detailed approach to fluid therapy is outlined elsewhere in this issue.

There is some controversy surrounding the use of antimicrobials to treat salmonellosis in livestock. Concern relates to selection for antimicrobial resistance and questions regarding the necessity and efficacy, which are largely derived from experience in human medicine where invasive salmonella infections are uncommon and routine use of antimicrobial therapy is not recommended. Bacteremia is a common feature of salmonellosis in calves. Therefore, aggressive treatment with antimicrobials early in the course of infection is recommended.[5,36,37] While a wide range of antimicrobials include a gram-negative spectrum that may appear appropriate for treatment of neonatal salmonellosis, most are not labeled for use in calves at a dose rate that provides therapeutic drug concentrations.

Antimicrobial resistance is common in virulent salmonella serotypes associated with disease outbreaks. Antimicrobial selection ideally should be based on the results of susceptibility testing using a salmonella isolate recovered from the tissues of calves at necropsy. Broad-spectrum antimicrobials are usually employed pending the availability of susceptibility test results.[36–39] Salmonellae show variable resistance patterns to ampicillin, amoxicillin, amoxi-clavulonic acid, ceftiofur, florfenicol, neomycin, sulfonamides, tetracycline, and trimethoprim-sulfa. Salmonellae also show general resistance to penicillin, erythromycin, and tylosin. Because salmonellae are facultative intracellular pathogens, selecting an antimicrobial with good tissue penetration and the ability to attain intracellular therapeutic drug concentrations within macrophages is desirable. A number of experimental studies have evaluated the efficacy of antimicrobial agents in the treatment of salmonellosis in cattle. In a comparative experimental trial, amoxicillin and trimethoprim sulfoxidine were shown to have equivalent efficacy in the treatment of calves with salmonella infections via oral, intravenous, and intramuscular routes when administered at doses based on minimal inhibitory concentration and peak blood levels.[40] Similarly, in an experimental challenge study, extralabel use of ceftiofur at 5 mg/kg was shown to attenuate the severity of clinical disease and reduce fecal shedding of *Salmonella*.[37] Prudent use of antimicrobial drugs is recommended with an emphasis on establishing a herd diagnosis, on susceptibility testing of invasive salmonella serotypes, and on using the narrowest spectrum of antibiotic indicated by the available susceptibility data.[41]

NSAIDs have been used to lessen endotoxin-related symptoms of inflammation in the treatment of calves with bloody diarrhea. NSAIDs inhibit endotoxin-induced inflammation by blocking the arachidonate cyclo-oxygenase pathway, thus reducing the formation of thromboxanes and prostaglandins.[42,43] Because of extensive tissue binding, analgesic and antipyretic effects may persist after serum concentrations have dropped below detection.[44] The therapeutic efficacy of NSAIDs for the treatment of salmonellosis in calves has not been documented. Extralabel use of flunixin meglumine (2.2 mg/kg intravenously) and meloxicam (0.5 mg/kg; intravenously or subcutaneously) have been reported to improve outcome and reduce morbidity in calves with nonspecific diarrhea.[45,46] However, the cause of diarrhea in these studies was not determined. Precautions should be taken when administering NSAIDs to dehydrated calves. Hypotension and reduced renal perfusion increase the risk of NSAID toxicity, so correction and maintenance of hydration are important to avoid potential adverse consequences.[44] Additionally, neonates have immature renal and hepatic systems that are less efficient at metabolizing and excreting some drugs. Currently, flunixin meglumine is the only NSAID approved in the United States for use in cattle for treatment of endotoxemia and pyrexia.[47] However, withdrawal periods have not been established for the use of flunixin meglumine in preruminant calves and this drug is therefore not recommended for use in animals intended for veal. In Europe and Australia, meloxicam, flunixin meglumine, ketoprofen, and tolfenamic acid have been approved for use in cattle with meat-withholding periods of 8, 7, 4, and 7 days, respectively.[47,48]

CONTROL AND PREVENTION

Three principal variables determine the outcome of host-salmonella interactions: host immunity, pathogen dose, and pathogen virulence. Environmental conditions have the potential to influence outcomes by impacting each of these variables. The approach to infectious disease control described by Radostits[49] over 3 decades ago includes (1) removing the source of infection from the calf's environment, (2) removing the calf from the contaminated environment, (3) increasing the nonspecific immunity of the calf, (4) increasing the specific immunity of the calf, and (5) reducing stress. These approaches are still applicable today and represent the core of salmonella control programs. These principles have been adapted in current production animal systems through the uptake of hazard analysis and critical control point programs.

Sources of Infection

Salmonellae may be introduced onto a farm by contaminated feedstuffs, water, fertilizer, livestock, wildlife, insects, people, or equipment. In intensive farming systems, where there is significant exposure to and recycling of effluent, livestock are frequently exposed to *Salmonella*. Management is directed at reducing the risk of adverse health and production consequences through minimizing the challenge dose and promoting host immunity.

While there are numerous potential control points to prevent the introduction of *Salmonella* onto a farm, the direct or opportunity cost of achieving this is often significant and logistically difficult with real effectiveness sometimes limited. Salmonellae are often purchased in the form of commodities and replacement livestock.[1] Dairy farms have an integral association with their water supply for maintenance of dairy facility function and feed supply. Regional dissemination and recycling of salmonellae has been associated with effluent contamination of irrigation water.[1] Salmonellae may also be dispersed and recycled among different types of livestock production systems via water and manure. The use of bovine and poultry manure as fertilizer was identified as a potential risk factor in Virginia and has been responsible for several disease outbreaks in pasture-based dairy systems in Australia.[50–52] The use of poultry manure in particular has led to an increase in the emergence of previously less-common serotypes as causes of neonatal salmonellosis on pasture-based dairies in Australia (Matthew M. Izzo, BVSc, unpublished data, 2007). While it is possible to screen the infection status of introduced animals using fecal culture or ELISA,[14,15] the cost is significant and the reward potentially limited if the animals are subsequently introduced into a contaminated environment. Peak lactation dairy cows can produce 50 kg of manure a day. The herd manure output each day is substantial and ultimately reflects the largest reservoir of *Salmonella* on the farm. The number of salmonellae in this reservoir is also dynamic as bacteria may proliferate when the availability of substrates, moisture, and temperature are favorable.[53]

Strategies to mitigate the potential adverse consequences of introduced and endemic *Salmonella* come back to good feed management and implementation of good husbandry practices that avoid compromised herd immunity. Important areas include waste management, forage preparation and storage, and commodity sourcing and storage, as well as nutritional, environmental, and reproductive management. The interactions between different aspects of management are complex with the consequences of failure having broad ramifications. For example, poor reproductive performance can lead to prolonged lactations, excessive body condition in late lactation, and increased risk of metabolic disease at calving, which may subsequently increase the risk of salmonellosis in postpartum cows and calves.

In regards to feed management, the risk posed by forages irrigated with salmonella-contaminated effluent can be reduced by ensuring effective ensilage.[1] Salmonellae are eliminated when the pH drops below 5, and ensilage failure is associated with persistence of the organism. Rodent control in commodity barns is also recommended to prevent dissemination and amplification of contamination in the feed storage area. Wildlife and insects may also play a role in the introduction or dispersal of salmonellae on a farm.[54–57] Over the last 5 years, there has been renewed interest in waste management as public concern mounts regarding environmental impacts and carbon emissions. Another potential positive aspect of modern waste management systems is more effective and consistent pathogen reduction.[58,59]

Maternity Pen Risks and Management

Calves have numerous opportunities to become infected with *Salmonella*. On dairy farms experiencing problems with neonatal salmonellosis, it is not uncommon to find evidence of disease and a high prevalence of salmonella fecal shedding in postpartum cows.[1] Calves may be exposed to *Salmonella* by fecal material from the dam during birth when the calf contacts the environment, or when calves contact the underside of the cow attempting to nurse. Salmonellae may also proliferate in organic bedding material used in calving pens. The presence of moisture in the environment favors salmonella proliferation and can result in environmental loads of 10^7 salmonellae per gram.[53] It is important to appreciate that significant pathogen exposure can occur within the first few hours of life. In a longitudinal study, 65% of calves were determined to be shedding salmonellae in feces within 24 hours of birth.[11]

Control points in maternity pens are directed at minimizing contamination (time cows spend in the pen, choice of bedding material, and frequency of bedding changes) and exposure risk (time calves spend in the maternity pen).

Colostrum

While cows chronically infected with Salmonella may shed the organism in colostrum and milk, most cows do not. Despite this, several studies have identified contaminated colostrum as a significant source of infection.[60] When we aseptically collected colostrum from cows on a large endemically infected dairy farm, 0.5% (1 out of 200) of cows were found to be shedding salmonellae in colostrum, and 3.33% (5 out of 150) of colostrum bottles cultured positive, indicating contamination associated with harvest and storage. Pooling colostrum increases the risk of salmonella infection by disseminating the organism in a larger colostral volume and subsequently infecting a larger number of calves.[61] Pooling colostrum also reduces the efficiency of colostral transfer and subsequently compromises calf immunity. A paradoxical increase in the incidence of salmonellosis and an earlier onset of clinical signs following increased volume of colostrum administration to newborn calves is consistent with salmonella contamination of colostrum. The concept of infectious disease transmission is often missed on farms when they use the same esophageal feeder to give electrolytes to sick calves and colostrum to newborn calves.

Steps for reducing the risk of disease transmission associated with the feeding of colostrum include (1) effective cleaning of equipment used in the harvest and storage of colostrum (if you wipe your finger on the inside of a container and there is a milk fat residue, it is not clean), (2) ensuring that colostrum does not pool, (3) verifying that refrigeration units used for storing colostrum are working, (4) limiting the volume of colostrum to 2 L per bottle to achieve rapid cooling, (5) recording dates of collection on refrigerated colostrum and discarding after 2 days, and (6) maintaining dedicated equipment for administering colostrum. Measures to reduce the pathogen load in colostrum include the use of potassium sorbate,[62] the use of on farm pasteurization,[63] and the use of colostrum replacer products. Colostrum should be pasteurized at a temperature of 60°C for 30 minutes. This ensures adequate destruction of common pathogens, such as Salmonella and Mycoplasma spp, without significantly denaturing immunoglobulins.[55,63,64] Plating 10 μL of colostrum onto a blood plate and incubating at 37°C overnight provides a simple crude assessment of microbial contamination of colostrum being fed to calves. In the event that bacteria counts are elevated, the same technique can be used to identify the origin of the process failure. Fresh colostrum fed to calves should contain less than 100,000 colony forming units per milliliter total bacteria count and less than 10,000 coliforms/mL.[65]

Bottlenecks

To evaluate the risk of calf exposure to Salmonella, it is necessary to trace the path from the place calves are born to the location where they are housed. Bottlenecks that have the potential to concentrate pathogen exposure (eg, calf warmers, temporary holding pens, and trailers used for transporting calves) should be avoided when possible and regularly disinfected when they must be used. Salmonella is susceptible to most disinfectants when they are used according to their directions. Primary removal of organic material reflects 99% of the cleaning process and is important to avoid neutralization of the disinfectant. Scheduling cleaning activities to specific days and times of the week helps to establish a consistent routine that ultimately gets done. Salmonella is susceptible to ultraviolet radiation, so it is a good idea to leave hutches upside down between calves during summer months to help reduce pathogen load.

Housing

Ideally, calves should be placed in a clean, dry, comfortable environment in an area that has good drainage and is not exposed to manure from adult cattle or to dairy effluent. In Australia, we experienced an outbreak of neonatal salmonellosis associated with runoff from a pasture where cows had been infected by contaminated hay. Individual calf hutches provide an effective means of minimizing calf-to-calf pathogen transfer. To avoid pathogen buildup, hutches should be moved to clean ground before they are reused. A disadvantage of this system is that calves are spread over a larger area, increasing the time and labor required for feeding. Calf sheds and crates represent alternative housing systems. Group housing provides efficient use of space and, when calves are healthy, reduces labor requirements. On farms that calve cows in groups, these systems can be quite effective as calves of similar ages move through periods of susceptibility together. The age range of calves in group housing should be kept as tight as possible. Mixing age groups increases the risk of pathogen exposure in young calves and can compromise their access to milk at feed time. Group housing is more difficult to manage in year-round calving systems where there is a propensity for pathogen buildup to occur over time. Attempts should be made to rodent-proof calf barns to minimize the role of wildlife and rodents in environmental contamination.

In regards to calf comfort, if calves get wet and are exposed to cold and windy conditions, energy reserves are rapidly depleted and sick calves rapidly succumb to disease. Placing straw in the hutches of newborn calves helps to keep them warm and dry. Calves housed on grating off the ground are particularly prone to cold wet conditions. In hot climates, calves can be subjected to extremely warm temperatures, and it becomes increasingly important to provide continuous access to fresh water. The design of calf hutches is important to avoid drafts in the winter and heat stress in the summer. The temperature in hutches can be extreme during summer months. One way of avoiding this problem is to tether calves to hutches (**Fig. 6**) so they can get out of the hutch and use it for shade by moving around the outside during the course of the day.

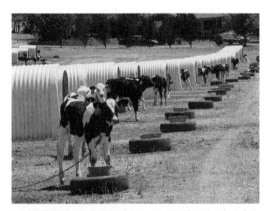

Fig. 6. Tethering calves to hutches allows them to use the shade of the hutch during hot weather. In the hutches shown, temperatures can reach 50°C (125°F) when the ambient temperature is 40°C (100°F).

Nutrition

Adequate calf nutrition is critical for host immunity, and energy-deprived calves are more likely to succumb to disease. When assessing nutritional requirements, it is important to factor in seasonal conditions that increase the calf's energy demands. In an epidemiologic study, feeding medicated milk replacer and hay to calves from 24 hours of age to weaning was associated with a reduced risk of salmonella shedding.[66] The finding regarding the use of medicated milk replacer contradicts experimental studies in which feeding chlortetracycline in milk replacer increased the severity of disease as well as the rate and duration of shedding.[67]

The microbial quality of milk fed to calves is important. On a farm feeding milk collected from recently calved and "hospital" cows, we isolated *Salmonella* from 26.9% (31 of 115) of the calf milk bottles. Salmonella contamination and proliferation in calf milk can be a problem when makeshift tanks are used to store and transport milk. Problems encountered relate to the difficulties associated with cleaning and lack of refrigeration. These systems often use non–dairy grade fittings that are difficult or impossible to effectively clean. Lack of refrigeration carries significant risk when residual milk from one feeding is kept for subsequent feedings. This is particularly important during hot weather when proliferation of salmonellae is increased. Designing calf-milk storage and delivery systems to conform to safe food standards reduces the risk of disease transmission. Pasteurization is also effective at eliminating salmonella contamination and, when implemented professionally, provides robust risk management. Inclusion of quality-control monitors is important to detect failures in the pasteurization process. Pasteurizers can also be difficult to clean, so it is appropriate to implement routine bacterial (total plate) counts for calf milk (after pasteurization) to verify that the system is functioning according to expectations. Feeding utensils and personnel often play a significant role in transmitting *Salmonella* to calves.[68] *Salmonella* infects the salivary glands and is shed in saliva and nasal secretions, contaminating nipples, bottles, buckets, and esophageal feeders.[69,70] Adequate cleaning and disinfection of feeding utensils is necessary to remove salmonella contamination.

Sick Calf Management

Sick calves can shed 10^9 salmonellae per gram of feces, thus amplifying bacterial numbers in the environment as well as contaminating equipment and personnel. There are contrasting philosophies regarding the management of calves with salmonellosis. One school of thought advocates the rapid removal of infected calves into a "sick" pen for treatment. The objective is to minimize contamination of the environment and subsequently the challenge to other calves in the area. A high prevalence of salmonella shedding has been observed in calves at 24 hours of age with disease manifesting at 4 to 7 days of age, so salmonella exposure may have been significant by the time sick calves were removed.[11] A potential risk associated with using a sick calf pen is that it can be a source of mixed pathogen infection if strict quarantine and appropriate management procedures are not maintained.[71]

An alternative philosophy is based on the observation that, by the time infected calves are identified, the other calves in the group have already been exposed. Therefore, movement of calves may be contraindicated because of the potential for dissemination of salmonella contamination. The decision to move calves depends on the number of affected calves and space constraints. In the face of a disease outbreak, it is desirable to be able to break the infection cycle by avoiding the placement of newborn calves in a contaminated environment. Prior to moving sick calves, consideration should be given to clean space availability. If clean space is limited, it is better to preserve these areas for newborns.

Environmental Control

While it is feasible to reduce the number of salmonellae in the environment, it is unrealistic to expect elimination of the organism. It is desirable to clean calf sheds between groups of calves. Calf pens should be scraped and scrubbed to remove organic material before disinfection between groups. Bedding material should be maintained to keep calves clean and dry. Feed and water buckets/bottles are positioned to reduce the risk of fecal contamination and should be cleaned daily (**Fig. 7**). Equipment used to handle milk products should be washed with warm water and a detergent of commercial dairy plant chemicals to remove milk residue, which will support the growth of salmonella. Alkaline compounds have been used in pasture-based systems for decontamination and control of *Salmonella* in outdoor areas. Calcium oxide and calcium hydroxide are reported to decrease pathogen load. However, to what degree is not clear.[72]

Vaccines

There are three general classes of salmonella vaccines: killed whole cell (bacterin), bacterial fractions (subunit), and attenuated modified live. Most commercial salmonella vaccines are bacterins. Reports regarding the efficacy of salmonella bacterins in cattle are conflicting. Experimental studies have produced equivocal results.[11,73] Salmonella bacterins have several perceived limitations. For example, salmonella bacterins fail to present antigens expressed in vivo, and also fail to induce cellular and mucosal immunity.[11,23,73,74] Under field conditions, neonatal exposure often occurs during the first few days of life, limiting the opportunity to stimulate acquired immune mechanisms through vaccination of calves.[11] Passive immunity acquired from maternal salmonella bacterin vaccination and colostral transfer is limited. However, partial protection has been reported in some experimental challenge trials.[75,76] Adverse reactions in the form of anaphylactic reactions are occasionally reported in cattle vaccinated with salmonella bacterins. The cause of these reactions is unknown but has been suggested to be associated with the high content in these products of the endotoxin lipopolysaccharide. Injection of sublethal doses of lipopolysaccharide induces a transient tolerance to endotoxin that appears as early as 24 hours after injection

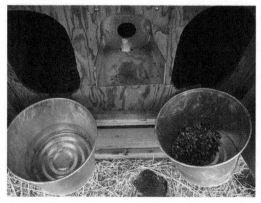

Fig. 7. Calves should be provided with clean water and calf starter. Positioning the buckets outside the pen reduces the amount of fecal contamination.

and lasts for several days.[77–79] Generally, salmonella vaccines are used in salmonella-infected herds where it is likely that some animals may have been recently infected with *Salmonella*. Following sublethal salmonella infections, the sensitivity of animals to the lethal activity of lipopolysaccharide increases exponentially.[80]

Subunit vaccines are composed of bacterial fractions or surface antigens. The salmonella Newport bacterial extract vaccine (SRP; Agri Laboratories, St. Joseph, Missouri) is a relatively new subunit cattle vaccine composed of purified extracts of siderophore receptors and porins.[81] These proteins are common to all strains of *Salmonella* and offer the potential to induce immunity to homologous and heterologous salmonella serovars. We were unable to find any controlled clinical trials documenting the efficacy of this product at preventing salmonellosis in cattle.

The observation that calves exposed to low doses of virulent *Salmonella* were protected against subsequent high-dose challenge suggested that prevention of salmonellosis with the use of live vaccines was possible.[23,73,82] Modified live attenuated vaccines induce a broad immune response via stimulation of cellular, humoral, and mucosal immunity, similar to the response after natural infection.[23,83] An aromatic amino acid (aro) auxotroph salmonella dublin vaccine (Entervene-d; Fort Dodge Animal Health, Fort Dodge, Iowa) is available in the United States. Experimental studies with aro minus salmonella vaccines in calves demonstrated protective immunity to homologous and heterologous salmonella serovars when calves were challenged within 3 weeks of vaccination.[84,85] The heterologous protection is afforded by transitory T-cell–independent, nonspecific protection. This disappears about 1 month after immunization following clearance of the organisms from the reticuloendothelial system. Thereafter, longer protection is limited to homologous challenge with recall of immunity, presumably involving specific antigen recognition.[86,87]

SUMMARY

Salmonellae are endemic on most large intensive farms and salmonellosis is a common cause of neonatal morbidity and mortality. Disease and mortality usually reflect a variety of management events and environmental stressors that contribute to compromised host immunity and increased pathogen exposure. The diversity of salmonella serovars present on farms, and the potential for different serovars to possess different virulence factors, requires the implementation of broad prophylactic strategies that are efficacious for all salmonellae. Calf immunity is optimized by good colostrum management and provision of adequate nutrition and a comfortable environment. salmonella serotype–specific immunity can also be enhanced through vaccination. Environmental management requires a focus on minimizing the bacterial challenge to neonates via contaminated colostrum, milk, equipment, personnel, and feces. Strategies to promote host immunity and minimize pathogen exposure at the farm level reflect an exercise in risk management. The benefits include a reduction in disease incidence and mortality, reduced drug and labor costs, and improved growth rates.

REFERENCES

1. Anderson RJ, House JK, Smith BP, et al. Epidemiologic and biological characteristics of salmonellosis in three dairy herds. J Am Vet Med Assoc 2001;219: 310–22.
2. Gelberg HB. Alimentary system 1. In: McGavin MD, Carlton WW, Zachary JF, editors. Thomson's special veterinary pathology. 3rd edition. St. Louis (MO): Mosby, Inc.; 2001. p. 1–79.

3. Quinn PJ, Markey BK, Carter ME, et al. Enterobacteriaceae. In: Veterinary micro-biology and microbiology disease. Carlton (Victoria, Australia): Blackwell Science Ltd.; 2002. p. 106–23.

4. Smith BP. Diseases of the alimentary tract. Salmonellosis in ruminants. In: Smith BP, editor. Large animal internal medicine. 3rd edition. St. Louis (MO): Mosby, Inc.; 2002. p. 775–9.

5. Wray C, Davies R. Salmonella infections in cattle. In: Wray C, Wray W, editors. Sal-monella in domestic animals. New York: CABI Publishing; 2000. p. 169–90.

6. Mohler VL, Heithoff DM, Mahan MJ, et al. Cross-protective immunity in calves conferred by a DNA adenine methylase deficient Salmonella enterica serovar Typhimurium vaccine. Vaccine 2006;24:1339–45.

7. Mohler VL, Heithoff DM, Mahan MJ, et al. Cross-protective immunity conferred by a DNA adenine methylase deficient *Salmonella enterica* serovar Typhimurium vac-cine in calves challenged with *Salmonella* serovar Newport. Vaccine 2008;26:1751–8.

8. Tsolis RM, Adams LG, Ficht TA, et al. Contribution of *Salmonella typhimurium* vir-ulence factors to diarrheal disease in calves. Infect Immun 1999;67:4879–85.

9. Wray C, Todd N, Hinton MH. The epidemiology of *Salmonella typhimurium* infec-tion in calves: excretion of *S. typhimurium* in faeces of calves in different manage-ment systems. Vet Rec 1987;121:293–6.

10. Sojka WJ, Field HI. Salmonellosis in England and Wales 1958–1967. Vet Bull 1970;40:515–31.

11. House JK, Ontiveros MM, Blackmer NM, et al. Evaluation of an autogenous *Sal-monella* bacterin and a modified live *Salmonella* serotype Choleraesuis vaccine on a commercial dairy farm. Am J Vet Res 2001;62:1897–902.

12. Mee JF. Terminal gangrene and ostitis in calves attributed to Salmonella-Dublin infection. Ir Vet J 1995;48:22–8.

13. Loeb E, Toussaint MJM, Rutten VPMG, et al. Dry gangrene of the extremities in calves associated with Salmonella Dublin infection; a possible immune-mediated reaction. J Comp Pathol 2006;134:366–9.

14. House JK, Smith BP, Dilling GW, et al. Enzyme-linked immunosorbent assay for serologic detection of *Salmonella* Dublin carriers on a large dairy. Am J Vet Res 1993;54:1391–9.

15. Smith BP, Oliver DG, Singh P, et al. Detection of *Salmonella* Dublin mammary gland infection in carrier cows, using an enzyme-linked immunosorbent assay for antibody in milk or serum. Am J Vet Res 1989;50:1352–60.

16. Holt P. Host susceptibility, resistance and immunity to Salmonella in animals. In: Wray C, Wray W, editors. *Salmonella* in domestic animals. New York: CABI Pub-lishing; 2000.

17. Reis BP, Zhang SP, Tsolis RM, et al. The attenuated sopB mutant of *Salmonella en-terica* serovar Typhimurium has the same tissue distribution and host chemokine re-sponse as the wild type in bovine Peyer's patches. Vet Microbiol 2003;97:269–77.

18. De Jong H, Ekdahl MO. Salmonellosis in calves—the effect of dose rate and other factors on the transmission. N Z Vet J 1965;13:59–64.

19. Zhang SP, Kingsley RA, Santos RL, et al. Molecular pathogenesis of *Salmonella enterica* serotype typhimurium–induced diarrhea. Infect Immun 2003;71:1–12.

20. Zhang SP, Santos RL, Tsolis RM, et al. The Salmonella enterica serotype typhimu-rium effector proteins SipA, SopA, SopB, SopD, and SopE2 act in concert to in-duce diarrhea in calves. Infect Immun 2002;70:3843–55.

21. Tizard IR. Veterinary immunology: an introduction. 6th edition. Philadelphia: W.B. Saunders Company; 2000.

22. Baumler AJ, Tsolis RM, Heffron F. Virulence mechanism of Salmonella and their genetic basis. In: Wray C, Wray W, editors. Salmonella in domestic animals. New York: CABI Publishing; 2000. p. 57–72.
23. Mastroeni P, Chabalgoity JA, Dustan SJ, et al. *Salmonella*: immune responses and vaccines. Vet J 2000;162:132–64.
24. Evans S, Davies R. Case control study of multiple-resistant *Salmonella typhimurium* DT104 infection of cattle in Great Britain. Vet Rec 1996;139:557–8.
25. CDC. Outbreak of multidrug-resistant Salmonella Newport-United States, January-April 2002. Available at: http://www.cdc.gov/mmwr/preview/mmwrhtml/mm5125a1.htm. Accessed June 28, 2002.
26. Devasia RA, Varma JK, Whichard J, et al. Antimicrobial use and outcomes in patients with multidrug-resistant and pansusceptible Salmonella Newport infections, 2002–2003. Microb Drug Resist 2005;11:371–7.
27. Varma JK, Marcus R, Stenzel SA, et al. Highly resistant Salmonella Newport-MDRAmpC transmitted through the domestic US food supply: a FoodNet case-control study of sporadic Salmonella Newport infections, 2002–2003. J Infect Dis 2006;194:222–30.
28. McGavin M, Carlton W, Zachary J. Thompsons special veterinary pathology. 3rd edition. Mosby Inc.; 2001.
29. Waltman WD. Methods for the cultural isolation of Salmonella. In: Wray C, Wray A, editors. Salmonella in domestic animals. Wallingford (UK): CABI Publishing; 2000. p. 355–72.
30. Poppe C, Duncan CL. Comparison of detection of Salmonella by the Tecra(R) Unique(TM) Salmonella test and the modified Rappaport Vassiliadis medium. Food Microbiol 1996;13:75–81.
31. Boraychuk VM, Gensler GE, McFall ME, et al. A real-time PCR assay for the detection of Salmonella in a wide variety of food and food-animal matrices. J Food Prot 2007;70:1080–7.
32. Eriksson E, Aspan A. Comparison of culture, ELISA and PCR techniques for Salmonella detection in faecal samples for cattle, pig and poultry. BMC Vet Res 2007;3:21.
33. Zahraei Salehi T, Mahzounieh MR, Vatankhah J. Identification and diagnosis of Salmonella serotypes in cow's faecal samples by polymerase chain reaction (PCR). University of Tehran. Journal of the Faculty of Veterinary Medicine 2006; 61:243–7.
34. Zahraei Salehi T, Tadjbakhsh TH, Atashparvar N, et al. Detection and identification of Salmonella Typhimurium in bovine diarrhoeic fecal samples by immunomagnetic separation and multiplex PCR assay. Zoonoses Public Health 2007; 54:231–6.
35. Dueger EL, House JK, Heithoff DM, et al. Salmonella DNA adenine methylase mutants elicit early and late onset protective immune responses in calves. Vaccine 2003;21:3249–58.
36. Constable P. Antimicrobial use in the treatment of calf diarrhea. J Vet Intern Med 2004;18:8–17.
37. Fecteau M, House JK, Kotarski SF, et al. Efficacy of ceftiofur for treatment of experimental salmonellosis in neonatal calves. Am J Vet Res 2003;64:918–25.
38. McGuirk S. Disease management of dairy calves and heifers. Vet Clin Food Anim 2008;24:139–54.
39. Bell SM, Gatus BJ, Pham JN, et al. Performance of the CDS test. In: Antibiotic susceptibility testing by the CDS method: a manual for medical and veterinary

laboratories 2004. 3rd edition. Randwick NSW (Australia): South Eastern Area Laboratory Services; 2004. p. 12–20.

40. Groothuis DG, van Miert AS. Salmonellosis in veal calves: some therapeutic aspects. Vet Q 1987;9:91–6.

41. Helmuth R. Antibiotic resistance in Salmonella. In: Wray C, Wray W, editors. Salmonella in domestic animals. New York: CABI Publishing; 2000. p. 89–106.

42. MacKay RJ. Diseases of the alimentary tract: endotoxemia. In: Smith BP, editor. Large animal internal medicine. 3rd edition. St. Louis (MO): Mosby, Inc; 2002. p. 633–41.

43. Rang HP, Dale MM, Ritter JM. Anti-inflammatory and immunosuppressant drugs. In: Pharmacology. 4th edition. London: Churchill Livingstone; 2001. p. 229.

44. George LW. Pain control in food animals. In: Steffey EP, editor. Recent advances in anesthetic management of large domestic animals. Ithaca (NY): International Veterinary Information Service; 2003.

45. Barnett SC, Sischo WM, Moore DA, et al. Evaluation of flunixin meglumine as an adjunct treatment for diarrhea in dairy calves. J Am Vet Med Assoc 2003;223: 1329–33.

46. Todd CG, McKnight DR, Millman ST, et al. An evaluation of meloxicam (Metacam (R)) as an adjunctive therapy for calves with neonatal calf diarrhea complex. J Anim Sci 2007;85:369 [abstract].

47. Smith GW, Davis JL, Tell LA, et al. FARAD digest—extralabel use of nonsteroidal anti-inflammatory drugs in cattle. J Am Vet Med Assoc 2008;232:697–701.

48. MIMS. 2007 IVS annual. 17th edition. Singapore: Kyodo Printing Company; 2007.

49. Radostits OM, Acres SD. The prevention and control of epidemics of acute undifferentiated diarrhea of beef calves in Western Canada. Can Vet J 1980;21:243–9.

50. Hutchison ML, Walters LD, Avery SM, et al. Analyses of livestock production, waste storage, and pathogen levels and prevalences in farm manures. Appl Environ Microbiol 2005;71:1231–6.

51. Vanselow BA, Hum S, Hornitzky MA, et al. Salmonella Typhimurium persistence in a Hunter Valley dairy herd. Aust Vet J 2007;85:446–50.

52. Warnick LD, Crofton LM, Pelzer KD, et al. Risk factors for clinical salmonellosis in Virginia, USA, cattle herds. Prev Vet Med 2001;49:259–75.

53. Murray CJ. Environmental aspects of Salmonella. In: Wray C, Wray A, editors. Salmonella in domestic animals. Wallingford (Oxon, UK): CABI Publishing; 2000. p. 265–83.

54. Bidawid SP, Edeson JF, Ibrahim J, et al. The role of non-biting flies in the transmission of enteric pathogens (Salmonella species and Shigella species) in Beirut, Lebanon. Ann Trop Med Parasitol 1978;72:117–21.

55. Johnston WS, MacLachlan GK, Hopkins GF. The possible involvement of seagulls (Larus sp) in the transmission of salmonella in dairy cattle. Vet Rec 1979;105:526–7.

56. Klowden MJ, Greenberg B. Salmonella in the American cockroach: evaluation of vector potential through dosed feeding experiments. J Hyg (Lond) 1976;77:105–11.

57. Smith-Palmer A, Stewart WC, Mather H, et al. Epidemiology of Salmonella enterica serovars Enteritidis and Typhimurium in animals and people in Scotland between 1990 and 2001. Vet Rec 2003;153:517–20.

58. Effenberger M, Bachmaier J, Garces G, et al. Mesophilic-thermophilic-mesophilic anaerobic digestion of liquid dairy cattle manure. Water Sci Technol 2006;53: 253–61.

59. Goodrich PR, Schmidt D, Haubenschild D. Anaerobic digestion for energy and pollution control. Manuscript EE 03. 001. Agricultural Engineering International 2005;7.

60. Giles N, Hopper SA, Wray C. Persistence of *S. typhimurium* in a large dairy herd. Epidemiol Infect 1998;103:235–41.
61. Veling J, Wilpshaar H, Frankena K, et al. Risk factors for clinical Salmonella enterica subsp. enterica serovar Typhimurium infection on Dutch dairy farms. Prev Vet Med 2002;54:157–68.
62. Stewart S, Godden S, Bey R, et al. Preventing bacterial contamination and proliferation during the harvest, storage, and feeding of fresh bovine colostrum. J Dairy Sci 2005;88:2571–8.
63. Godden S, McMartin S, Feirtag J. Heat-treatment of bovine colostrum II: effects of heating duration on pathogen viability and immunoglobulin G. J Dairy Sci 2006; 89:3476–83.
64. McMartin S, Godden S, Metzger L, et al. Heat treatment of bovine colostrum. I: effects of temperature on viscosity and immunoglobulin G level. J Dairy Sci 2006;89:2110–8.
65. McGuirk SM, Collins M. Managing the production, storage, and delivery of colostrum. Vet Clin Food Anim 2004;20:593–603.
66. Losinger WC, Wells SJ, Garber LP, et al. Management factors related to Salmonella shedding by dairy heifers. J Dairy Sci 1995;78:2464–72.
67. Dey BP, Blenden DC, Burton GC, et al. Influence of chlortetracycline feeding on salmonellosis in calves. I. Rate and duration of shedding. II. Severity of illness. Int J Zoonoses 1978;5:97–110.
68. Hardman PM, Wathes CM, Wray C. Transmission of salmonellae among calves penned individually. Vet Rec 1991;129:327–9.
69. Nolan LK, Giddings CW, Boland EW, et al. Detection and characterization of Salmonella typhimurium from a dairy herd in North Dakota. Vet Res Commun 1995; 19:3–8.
70. Richardson A, Fawcett AR. Salmonella Dublin infection in calves: the value of rectal swabs in diagnosis and epidemiological studies. Br Vet J 1973;129(2):151–6.
71. Fossler C, Wells S, Kaneene J, et al. Herd-level factors associated with isolation of *Salmonella* in a multi-state study of conventional and organic farms II. *Salmonella* shedding in calves. Prev Vet Med 2005;70:279–91.
72. Oliver DM, Heathwaite LA, Hodgson CJ, et al. Mitigation and current management attempts to limit pathogen survival and movement within farmed grassland. Advances in Agronomy 2007;93:95–140.
73. Curtiss R, Kelly SM, Hassan JO. Live oral avirulent *Salmonella* vaccines. Vet Microbiol 1993;37:397–405.
74. Robertsson JA, Lindberg AA, Hoiseth S, et al. *Salmonella typhimurium* infection in calves: protection and survival of virulent challenge bacteria after immunization with live or inactivated vaccines. Infect Immun 1983;41:742–50.
75. Jones PW, Collins P, Aitken MM. Passive protection of calves against experimental infection with *Salmonella typhimurium*. Vet Rec 1988;123:536–41.
76. Mortola ME, Pennimpede PE, Arauz PM, et al. Calf salmonellosis: prophylaxis by maternal immunization. Avances en Ciencias Veterinarias 1992;7:203–8.
77. Fahmi H, Chaby R. Desensitization of macrophages to endotoxin effects is not correlated with a down-regulation of lipopolysaccharide-binding sites. Cell Immunol 1993;150:219–29.
78. Gupta JD, Reed CE. Amount, class and specificity of antibody to the lipopolysaccharide of Salmonella enteritidis after immunization by various schedules. Int Arch Allergy Appl Immunol 1971;40:256–63.

79. Randow F, Syrbe U, Meisel C, et al. Mechanism of endotoxin desensitization: involvement of interleukin 10 and transforming growth factor beta. J Exp Med 1995; 181:1887–92.

80. Matsuura M, Galanos C. Induction of hypersensitivity to endotoxin and tumor necrosis factor by sublethal infection with *Salmonella typhimurium*. Infect Immun 1990;58:935–7.

81. Emery D, Straub D, Slinden L, et al. Effect of a novel Salmonella vaccine on performance in a large expansion dairy. In: Proceedings of the American Association of Bovine Practitioners Annual Conference, Stillwater, 2002. p. 185 [abstract].

82. Barrow PA, Wallis TS. Vaccination against Salmonella infections in food animals: rationale, theoretical basis and practical application. In: Wray C, Wray W, editors. Salmonella in domestic animals. New York: CABI Publishing; 2000. p. 323.

83. Villarreal-Ramos B, Manser J, Collins R, et al. Susceptibility of calves to challenge with *Salmonella typhimurium 4/74* and derivatives harbouring mutations in *htrA or purE*. Microbiol SGM 2006;146:2775–83.

84. Rankin JD, Newman G, Taylor RJ. The protection of calves against infection with *Salmonella typhimurium* by means of *Salmonella dublin* (strain 51) vaccine. Vet Rec 1967;78:720–6.

85. Smith BP, Reina-Guerra M, Hoiseth SK, et al. Aromatic-dependent *Salmonella typhimurium* as modified live vaccines for calves. Am J Vet Res 1984;45:59–66.

86. Collins FM. Vaccines and cell-mediated immunity. Bacteriol Rev 1974;38: 371–402.

87. Hormaeche CE, Joysey HS, Desilva L, et al. Immunity conferred by Aro-Salmonella live vaccines. Microb Pathog 1991;10:149–58.

Treatment of Calf Diarrhea: Oral Fluid Therapy

Geof W. Smith, DVM, MS, PhD

KEYWORDS

• Calf diarrhea • Acid-base • Fluid therapy • Neonatology
• Acidosis • Dehydration • Oral electrolyte

Neonatal diarrhea remains the most common cause of death in beef and dairy calves. Despite significant progress in understanding the pathophysiology of neonatal diarrhea, it continues to be a major cause of economic loss to the cattle industry. According to the World Health Organization (WHO), the development of oral rehydration therapy was one of the most significant advances in human medicine of twentieth century. Oral rehydration also continues to serve as the backbone of treatment protocols for diarrhea in neonatal calves. This article provides an overview of oral electrolyte therapy in calves, emphasizing when they should be used, how they should be used, and what practitioners should be looking for when choosing a product.

A complete review of the pathophysiology of diarrhea is beyond the scope of this article and is covered elsewhere in this issue. Some pathogens cause secretory diarrhea, causing small intestinal enterocytes to switch from net absorption of fluid to net secretion of chloride, sodium, and water into the intestinal lumen. This increase in secretion overwhelms the absorptive capacity of the large intestine resulting in diarrhea. Other pathogens damage the small intestinal villi, which results in failure to absorb electrolytes and water (malabsorptive diarrhea). Regardless of the pathogen or the mechanism involved, diarrhea increases the loss of electrolytes and water in the feces of calves and decreases milk intake. This process results in dehydration, strong ion acidosis, electrolyte abnormalities (usually decreased sodium and increased or decreased potassium), increased D-lactate concentrations, and a negative energy balance (from anorexia and malabsorption of nutrients). Diarrhea is by far the most common indication for fluid therapy in neonatal calves. Oral electrolyte solutions have classically been used to replace fluid losses, correct acid–base and electrolyte abnormalities, and provide nutritional support, because they are cheap and easy to administer on-farm.

The goals of oral fluid therapy are to replace fluid, acid–base, and electrolyte deficits and to provide nutritional support. They are indicated in any diarrheic calf that has at

Department of Population Health and Pathobiology, College of Veterinary Medicine, North Carolina State University, 4700 Hillsborough Street, Raleigh, NC 27606, USA
E-mail address: geoffrey_smith@ncsu.edu

Vet Clin Food Anim 25 (2009) 55–72
doi:10.1016/j.cvfa.2008.10.006
0749-0720/08/$ – see front matter © 2009 Elsevier Inc. All rights reserved.

least a partially functional gastrointestinal tract. If oral electrolytes are administered to a calf that has ileus, the fluid pools in the rumen resulting in bloat and rumen acidosis. In general, a calf that has any sort of suckle reflex or that demonstrates any "chewing" action can be considered to safely tolerate oral fluids.

ASSESSING DEHYDRATION IN CALVES

Dehydration in calves that have diarrhea is accompanied by large decreases in extracellular fluid volumes along with small increases in intracellular fluid volumes.[1-3] The intestinal loss of electrolytes in these calves results in hypoosmotic extracellular (plasma and interstitial) fluid, which causes free water to move from the extracellular fluid (ECF) to the intracellular fluid (ICF) space (thereby increasing ICF space). The practitioner must therefore attempt to clinically estimate the degree of ECF loss in dehydrated calves during physical examination.

Attempts to estimate dehydration based on physical examination findings have been around for more than 40 years. In 1965, Watt[4] evaluated hydration status by assessing the attitude of the calf, eyeball position, skin elasticity, mucous membrane appearance, capillary refill time, and urine production and classified dehydration as mild, moderate, or severe. It was later recognized, however, that these guidelines were certainly subject to error.[5] One of the more accurate predictors of acute dehydration is monitoring change in body weight. Using this principle, Bywater[6] took the three established categories of severity and assigned weight losses of 1% to 5% for mild dehydration, 6% to 8% for moderate dehydration, and 9% to 11% for severe dehydration. These categories were likely developed based on data that indicated most calf deaths occurred when weight loss was between 12.7% and 13.4% of body weight.[7,8]

A study by Constable and colleagues[1] has provided more accurate data for estimating hydration status in calves in the field. This study used an experimental model that produced severe, acute diarrhea.[9] Several clinical and laboratory parameters were monitored throughout the duration of the study and compared with actual percent dehydration of each calf. The results of this study indicated that the most accurate methods for assessing dehydration in calves are eyeball recession into orbit (degree of enophthalmos), skin tent duration in the neck region, and plasma protein concentration. All other methods of assessment are inferior to these. The degree of enophthalmos is estimated by gently everting the lower eyelid and estimating the recession of the globe into the orbit (**Fig. 1**). Skin elasticity is best measured on the lateral side of the midcervical area by pinching a fold of skin, rotating it 90 degrees, and measuring the time for the skinfold to disappear. The data from this study provide

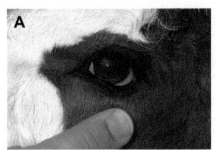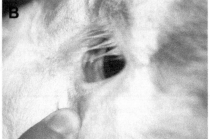

Fig. 1. Calf on the left (A) has a normal hydration status. There is no space between the eyelid and the eyeball. The calf on the right (B) is severely dehydrated. The eye is sunken at least 7 to 8 mm into the orbit. (*Courtesy of* Peter Constable, BVSc, MS, PhD, MRCVS, West Lafayette, IN.)

the most practical and accurate method for predicting hydration status in calves that have diarrhea (**Table 1**).

Eyeball recession may not be as accurate in chronic cachexia. Because the position of the eye depends partially on body fat stores, it is possible that eyeball recession is of limited value to predict hydration status in calves that have chronic diarrhea. In these calves it is likely that skin elasticity over the neck region or thorax may be a better indicator.[1] Using these clinical parameters can be somewhat subjective and initial assessments may occasionally be inaccurate. Eyeball recession and skin tent duration in the neck region provide more accurate clinical indicators of dehydration than any other parameter that can be easily measured during the physical examination process.

CHOOSING AN ORAL ELECTROLYTE PRODUCT

Oral electrolyte solutions were originally developed in human medicine for treatment of diarrhea associated with cholera infection and have been credited as being one of the most significant medical advances of the twentieth century. The original WHO electrolyte formulation was based on the following main principles:[10]

It was an isotonic solution that contained an approximately equimolar mixture of sodium (90 mmol/L) and glucose (2%).
It contained potassium because of the severe potassium depletion associated with diarrhea and anorexia.
It contained glycine to facilitate absorption of sodium, glucose, and water.
It contained bicarbonate to correct the metabolic acidosis associated with diarrhea.

Although much research has been done on oral fluid therapy since that time, we have not moved far from the original principles of the 1960s.

Considerable variability exists in the quality of commercial oral electrolyte solutions available today and practitioners must put some thought into the product they choose to use in practice (**Table 2**). As was eloquently stated in a previous article by Dr. Robert Michell,[11] simply recommending oral electrolyte rehydration in this decade is as imprecise as advocating antibiotics without considering the drug or condition being treated. There are several important factors to consider when deciding on a product. Current knowledge indicates that an oral electrolyte solution must satisfy the following four requirements: (1) supply sufficient sodium to normalize the ECF volume; (2) provide agents (glucose, citrate, acetate, propionate, or glycine) that facilitate absorption of sodium and water from the intestine; (3) provide an alkalinizing agent (acetate, propionate, or bicarbonate) to correct the metabolic acidosis usually present in calves that have diarrhea; and (4) provide energy, because most calves that have diarrhea

Table 1			
Guidelines for assessment of hydration status in calves with diarrhea			
Dehydration	Demeanor	Eyeball Recession	Skin Tent Duration (s)
<5%	Normal	None	<1
6%–8% (mild)	Slightly depressed	2–4 mm	1–2
8%–10% (moderate)	Depressed	4–6 mm	2–5
10%–12% (severe)	Comatose	6–8 mm	5–10
>12%	Comatose/dead	8–12 mm	>10

Table 2
Comparison of oral electrolyte products available in North America

	Sodium (mmol/L)	Potassium (mmol/L)	Chloride (mmol/L)	Strong Ion Difference	Alkalinizing Agent	Total Osmolality (mOsm/L)
Advance Arrest (MS Specialty Nutrition)[a]	46	7	30	23	Bicarbonate (12 mmol/L)	245
Biolyte (Pfizer)	142	24	80	86	Bicarbonate (86 mmol/L)	732
Bounce Back (Manna Pro)[a]	136	10	112	34	Bicarbonate (48 mmol/L)	
Blue Ribbon Calf Electrolytes (Merrick)[a]	144	20	75	89	None	390
Bovine Bluelite C (Techmix)	59	24	56	27	None	269
Calf-Lyte II (Vetoquinol)	112	15	43	84	Acetate (80 mmol/L)	428
Calf-Lyte II HE (Vetoquinol)	112	15	43	84	Acetate (80 mmol/L)	726
Calf Quencher (Vedco)	142	24	80	86	Bicarbonate (86 mmol/L)	731
Deliver (Agri-Labs)[a]	67	16	49	34	Bicarbonate (36 mmol/L)	305
Diaque (Boehringer Ingelheim)	90	15	55	50	Bicarbonate (25 mmol/L) and acetate (12 mmol/L)	377
Entrolyte HE (Pfizer)	106	26	51	81	Bicarbonate (80 mmol/L)	739
Epic calf electrolyte (Bioniche)	92	30	45	77	Acetate (52 mmol/L)	360
Hydrafeed (A&L Laboratories)	110	10	40	80	Bicarbonate (80 mmol/L)	380
Hydralyte (Vet-A-Mix)	90	30	45	75	Acetate (60 mmol/L)	614
Hysorb (Bimeda)	120	10	70	60	Bicarbonate (40 mmol/L)	360
OneBetter calf electrolyte (Felton)	124	24	63	85	Bicarbonate (12 mmol/L)	440
Resorb (Pfizer)	75	25	80	20	None	315
Revibe (Wyeth)	120	20	50	90	Acetate (80 mmol/L)	466
Revitilyte (Vets Plus Inc.)	110	50	20	140	Bicarbonate (90 mmol/L)	577
VitaLyte (Vita Plus Corp.)	150	31	45	136	Bicarbonate (80 mmol/L)	527

This listing does not include every product available in North America. No discrimination or specific endorsement of any product is intended.
[a] Signifies data were calculated from product label instead of provided by the manufacturer. In some cases there was insufficient information on the label to provide an exact calculation so values may not be completely accurate.

are in a state of negative energy balance.[12] Factors to consider when choosing an oral electrolyte solution include the following.

Sodium Concentration

Sodium is the osmotic skeleton of the extracellular fluid and therefore of plasma. Because sodium is the principal determinant of the ECF volume, it must be present in an oral electrolyte solution to rapidly correct the losses that have occurred with dehydration and diarrhea. The ideal sodium concentration for oral rehydration therapy in calves is not completely known; however, most research would suggest it should be between 90 and 130 mmol/L. Products containing sodium at lower concentrations are not able to adequately correct dehydration. For example, one study compared the ability of three different commercially available oral electrolyte solutions to resuscitate calves using an enterotoxigenic *Escherichia coli* diarrhea model.[11] The three electrolyte products had sodium concentrations of 120, 73, and 50 mmol/L. Results of this study showed that the product containing sodium at 120 mmol/L was able to restore extracellular fluid volume and correct dehydration, whereas the other two products containing lower sodium concentrations were not. Oral electrolyte products with very high sodium concentrations might be expected to cause hypernatremia; however, there is not a lot of research to demonstrate what sodium concentration would be too much. Results from studies that have fed oral electrolyte products for multiple days containing either 120 or 134 mmol/L of sodium have not resulted in hypernatremia;[11,13] however, in the author's opinion, products with sodium concentrations much higher than 130 mmol/L should be avoided. Very high sodium concentrations have also been shown to delay abomasal emptying rates because of increased osmolality and may cause ileus, thus predisposing to abomasal bloat and other gastrointestinal disorders.[14]

Chloride Concentration

Although calves lose chloride during diarrhea, this loss does not occur nearly to the same degree as sodium.[15] A general guideline has been that oral electrolyte products should contain chloride in concentrations between 40 and 80 mEq/L. When considering the importance of strong ion difference (SID) in correcting metabolic acidosis (see more thorough discussion later under alkalinizing agents), it may be advisable to use products with chloride concentrations toward the low end of the above range to increase the SID (see later discussion).

Potassium Concentration

Like sodium and chloride, potassium is lost in the feces of calves that have diarrhea. All calves that have diarrhea therefore have a total body deficit of potassium.[8] In acute cases of diarrhea, however, calves may have elevated blood potassium concentrations (hyperkalemia). This paradoxical situation arises in response to metabolic acidosis. The Na^+-K^+-ATPase pump functions optimally at physiologic pH ranges. During acidemia, the pump starts to fail, causing intracellular Na^+ ions to increase (they are not pumped out of the cell) and extracellular K^+ ions to increase. The ECF (which usually contains only about 5% of the total body potassium) therefore has greater-than-normal potassium concentrations, which can result in hyperkalemia. Because of increased fecal loss, however, ICF and total body potassium concentrations are decreased.

With dehydration, aldosterone is released from the pituitary gland. Aldosterone acts on the kidney to conserve sodium and water at the expense of increased potassium losses. In chronic cases of diarrhea, therefore, calves can have profound depletion of body potassium stores and generally have low serum concentrations of K^+. Clinical signs of hypokalemia include profound muscular weakness, which is often present in calves with chronic diarrhea. General recommendations are that oral electrolyte products used in calves that have diarrhea contain potassium concentrations between 10 and 30 mmol/L. Higher K^+ concentrations might theoretically be beneficial in calves with chronic diarrhea that have extreme depletion of total body potassium; however, there is no research available to support this recommendation nor is the author aware of any commercially available products contain levels of K^+ significantly higher than 30 mmol/L.

Sodium Absorption

Sodium absorption by the small intestine is a passive process and is linked to the movement of actively absorbed or secreted solutes. If sodium is present in the lumen of the small intestine without either glucose or amino acid, there is either a small net absorption or no net sodium movement across the jejunum.[16] One of the earliest mechanisms of intestinal sodium absorption discovered was linked with sugar.[17] Glucose can be co-transported with sodium from the intestinal lumen to the inside of the enterocyte at the brush border membrane. At the basolateral membrane, the Na^+-K^+-ATPase actively pumps Na^+ ions out of the cell thus raising the intercellular osmolality.[16] Any increase in sodium influx at the brush border must be compensated for by an increase in sodium efflux from the enterocyte at the base of the cell. This increase in intercellular osmolality then draws more water from the intestinal lumen through the tight junctions between cells, thus expanding extracellular fluid volume and rehydrating the calf. Because this mechanism was well understood by the 1960s, almost all early oral electrolyte formulations were mixtures of sodium and glucose.

Neutral amino acids, such as glycine, alanine, or glutamine, can also facilitate sodium absorption in the small intestine by a mechanism similar to glucose.[16] Whether amino acids are needed in addition to glucose in oral electrolyte solutions is not well understood; however, the addition of glycine does seem to further improve water absorption in the intestine. In addition, volatile fatty acids, such as acetate or propionate, have been shown to facilitate sodium absorption in the gut.[18,19] In studies using isolated loops of small intestine from calves, electrolyte solutions containing acetate showed markedly enhanced sodium absorption when compared with formulations with other solutes.[18] The mechanism by which volatile fatty acids stimulate sodium absorption in the intestine seems to be different from that of glucose or amino acids. Acetate therefore seems to have an additive effect to glucose and amino acids, meaning you can expect a significant increase in intestinal sodium absorption in electrolyte products containing volatile fatty acids, even when they already contain high concentrations of glucose or glycine.

Glucose-To-Sodium Ratio

Glucose is present in various concentrations in virtually all commercially available oral electrolyte solutions. It is necessary to facilitate sodium absorption and to provide an energy source for the calf. The ratio of glucose to sodium present in an oral electrolyte solution should also be considered, however. This ratio can be calculated by adding the mmol/L of dextrose in a product (along with glycine if present) and dividing by the mmol/L concentration of sodium. This ratio should fall somewhere between 1:1 and 3:1.[20] Products that have a glucose-to-sodium ratio less than 1:1 do not contain adequate solute to facilitate sodium absorption (unless perhaps the product also contained significant levels of acetate or propionate). Conversely, products that have a glucose-to-sodium ratio greater than 3:1 are likely to increase the risk for osmotic diarrhea.

Osmolality

Commercially available oral electrolyte products in North America can range from isotonic (280–300 mOsm/L) to extremely hypertonic (700–800 mOsm/L). The primary difference in most of these products is the amount of glucose that is added. Because of a countercurrent exchange mechanism in the small intestine, the effective osmolality at the tip of the intestinal villus is about 600 mOsm/L.[21] We can therefore take advantage of hypertonic solutions that have higher energy levels. On the other hand, low osmolality fluids (<350 mOsm/L) generally have inadequate energy content because they have insufficient glucose. Hypertonic solutions provide greater nutritional support to calves relative to isotonic products and have not been shown to cause detrimental effects, particularly in relation to maintaining hydration status, intestinal osmolality, serum glucose concentrations, and intestinal flow rate.[22] Research has demonstrated that milk replacer is better able to maintain normal serum glucose concentration than either hypertonic or isotonic oral electrolyte solutions.[12] As expected, however, oral electrolyte solutions rehydrated calves and prevented the development of metabolic acidosis more effectively than did milk replacer because they have a much higher sodium concentration.[12] Multiple studies have demonstrated that hypertonic oral electrolyte solutions maintain higher serum glucose and lower β-OH butyrate (ketone) concentrations when compared with isotonic electrolyte solutions.[12,23] Previous research has also shown that when calves were deprived of milk, those fed isotonic oral electrolyte solutions had significantly greater weight loss as compared with calves fed hypertonic oral electrolytes.[24]

With the principle that hypertonic oral electrolytes supply more energy to calves as compared with isotonic products, the next question becomes at what osmolality might we start to see deleterious effects? The physiologic effect of higher-than-normal intestinal glucose concentrations in calves that have diarrhea is not completely understood; however, the addition of glucose to facilitate intestinal sodium and water absorption increases the risk for osmotic diarrhea if the glucose is not absorbed. Although the research available to date does not provide a good answer to that question, there are certainly indications that electrolyte solutions with extremely high osmolalities (>700–750 mOsm/L) and glucose concentrations might cause problems. To begin with, a product with an osmolality greater than what is already present in the intestinal lumen could worsen diarrhea. Most calves that have enteric pathogens already have hypersecretion of electrolytes and water into the small intestinal lumen, which could be exacerbated with the feeding of extremely hypertonic solutions (electrolyte or milk replacer). Raising the intraluminal tonicity would serve to increase the secretion of water and electrolytes into the intestine, thus increasing the severity of diarrhea. This effect would likely be magnified with severe villus damage, which is often present in diarrheic calves.

The primary energy source in an oral electrolyte solution is glucose, which is provided in most oral electrolyte solutions between 2 to 3 g of glucose per kg of body weight. The small intestine of the healthy calf has been shown to absorb all glucose when fed at 2.5 g/kg of body weight.[22] In anesthetized calves, glucose was absorbed in both healthy and diarrheic calves at a rate of 2.4 to 7.2 mg/cm of small intestinal segment per hour.[25] Based on a mean small intestinal length of 15.8 to 18.6 m in 1- to 2-week-old Holstein calves,[26] the total glucose absorption rate in the small intestine is estimated to range from 3.8 to 13.4 g per hour.[14] Assuming twice a day feeding, calves should be able to absorb up to 161 g of glucose per feeding. This calculation suggests that for a 45-kg calf that has normal plasma glucose concentration and gastrointestinal motility, the upper limit of glucose in an oral electrolyte solution should about 3.6 g/kg.[14] Higher concentrations may allow unabsorbed glucose to carry over into the large intestine, where it may be fermented to short-chain volatile fatty acids, exacerbate fecal water loss, and worsen diarrhea.

Hypertonic oral electrolyte solutions have also been shown to slow abomasal emptying rates as compared with isotonic products.[14,27] Calves fed an oral electrolyte solution with a total osmolality of 360 mOsm/L had a significantly faster abomasal emptying rate as compared with calves fed a solution with an osmolality of 717 mOsm/L.[27] This finding suggests that electrolyte products with a high osmolality (or high glucose concentrations) would be likely to induce abomasal ileus, thus increasing the risk for bloat or abomasitis. Abomasal bloat is a syndrome in young calves characterized by anorexia, abdominal distension, bloat, and often death in 6 to 48 hours. This condition occurs most commonly in dairy calves and seems to have a sporadic occurrence with some farms having multiple outbreaks at times. Recently the abomasal bloat syndrome was experimentally reproduced by drenching young Holstein calves with a carbohydrate mixture containing milk replacer, corn starch, and glucose mixed in water.[28] The authors of this study proposed that the pathophysiology of abomasal bloat is primarily excess fermentation of high-energy gastrointestinal contents. Gas-producing bacteria, such as *Clostridium perfringens*, *Sarcina ventriculi*, or *Lactobacillus* species have also been believed to play a role in this syndrome.[28,29] Although the exact pathogenesis of abomasal bloat is not completely understood, the disease is likely to be multifactorial in origin. Having large amounts of fermentable carbohydrate present in the abomasum (from milk, milk replacer, or high-energy oral electrolyte solutions) along with the presence of fermentative enzymes (produced by bacteria) would likely lead to gas production and bloat. This process would be exacerbated by anything that slowed abomasal emptying or caused gastrointestinal ileus. In fact, feeding high-osmolality electrolyte products or milk replacers has been noted to be a risk factor on some farms for the development of abomasal bloat in calves (Geof W. Smith, DVM, MS, PhD, unpublished data, 2008).

Although the ideal osmolality of an oral electrolyte solution for calves is not completely understood, a hypertonic oral electrolyte solution (500–600 mOsm/L) would be ideal in dairy calves or in beef calves that have been separated from the dam. Certainly if milk were to be withheld for any length of time, a hypertonic oral electrolyte solution would be indicated to provide energy to the calf. Isotonic solutions might still be appropriate, however, for beef calves that are still suckling or in conjunction with milk replacer in dairy calves that maintain a good appetite. The author recommends avoiding extremely hypertonic oral electrolyte product (>700 mOsm/L) for the reasons stated previously.

Alkalinizing Ability

Acidemia and metabolic acidosis occur in almost all cases of calf diarrhea. This finding was originally attributed to bicarbonate loss in the feces along with a decrease glomerular filtration rate in response to severe dehydration.[7,15,30] More recent data have indicated that metabolic acidosis in calves that have diarrhea actually results from differences in strong ion balance (described in more detail later).[15] We must therefore attempt to correct this strong ion acidosis when using oral fluid therapy. Research examining intravenous fluid therapy protocols has indicated that severely acidemic calves are unable to correct their metabolic acidosis, even when rehydrated with non-alkalinizing fluids.[31] It is imperative, therefore, that either oral or intravenous fluid therapy protocols be able to increase blood pH. Classically this has been done by adding alkalinizing agents (ie, bicarbonate, acetate, or propionate) to oral electrolyte mixtures. More recently, there has been growing interest in looking at the SID of electrolytes as they relate to the efficacy of a different product to promote alkalinization. In reality, both (having an alkalinizing agent and a high SID) are likely important and warrant discussion.

Alkalinizing agents

Acetate, propionate, and bicarbonate are all considered alkalinizing agents and are frequently present in commercial oral electrolyte solutions. Bicarbonate-containing fluids are effective at correcting a severe acidosis, because bicarbonate reacts directly with H^+ ions to form CO_2 and H_2O. Acetate and propionate are also alkalinizing agents and have been shown to have alkalinizing effects similar to bicarbonate.[32–34] Acetate and propionate are only effective alkalinizing agents when they are metabolized by the liver; a process that forms water and creates hydrogen ions. This metabolic process seems to still function efficiently in calves that have severe diarrhea because the alkalinizing ability of the acetate has been shown to be as effective as bicarbonate.[33] Acetate and propionate have several advantages over bicarbonate:

- Acetate and propionate facilitate sodium and water absorption in the calf small intestine, whereas bicarbonate does not.
- Acetate and propionate produce energy when metabolized, whereas bicarbonate does not.
- Acetate and propionate do not alkalinize the abomasum, whereas bicarbonate does; low abomasal pH is a natural defense mechanism against bacterial proliferation.
- Acetate and propionate do not interfere with milk clotting in calves, whereas bicarbonate may potentially cause some disturbance of the normal digestive process.

Alkalinization of the abomasum Gastric acidity is a well-accepted barrier to colonization and infection of the gastrointestinal tract by bacteria, and is a primary defense mechanism against pathogens that are ingested orally.[35] Bacteria, such as E coli and Salmonella, are killed at gastric pH between 2.5 and 3.0, whereas they multiply at pH greater than 5.0.[36,37] Maintaining a low abomasal pH is therefore critical to avoid colonization of the intestinal tract with pathogenic bacteria in calves. An example of the importance of abomasal acidity is provided by enterotoxigenic E coli (ETEC). ETEC is an important cause of diarrhea in calves 1 to 2 days of age, but does not cause disease in older calves. In colostrum-fed calves older than 24 hours of age, oral administration of $NaHCO_3$ (4–10 g in 60–150 mL of water), followed immediately by an inoculum of viable ETEC bacteria, can produce clinical disease. Alkalinization of the abomasum with bicarbonate is thus necessary to produce ETEC in older calves. This modified protocol has been successful in producing an experimental model of diarrhea in calves up to 14 days of age.[7,25,38,39] Oral administration of the bacteria without $NaHCO_3$ does not produce any clinical diarrhea, however.

The feeding of oral electrolyte products containing bicarbonate has been shown to alkalinize the abomasum in calves.[40–43] Suckling of bicarbonate-containing oral electrolyte solutions can cause a large and sustained increase in abomasal pH (**Fig. 2**). A similar effect is not seen with acetate-based products.[41,42] Abomasal acidity provides a natural barrier to ingested bacteria, and maintaining a low abomasal pH decreases the number of viable coliform bacteria that reach the small intestine. This process increases nonspecific resistance to intestinal colonization. The increase in abomasal pH

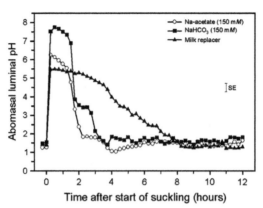

Fig. 2. Mean 12-hour abomasal luminal pH (least square mean ± SEM values) in five Holstein calves fed 2 L of milk replacer or 150 mmol/L solutions of sodium acetate or sodium bicarbonate. (*Courtesy of* Peter Constable, BVSc, MS, PhD, MRCVS, West Lafayette, IN; and *Modified from* Marshall TS, Constable PD, Crochik SS, et al. Effect of suckling an isotonic solution of sodium acetate, sodium bicarbonate, or sodium chloride on abomasal emptying rate and luminal pH in calves. Am J Vet Res 2008;69:824–31; with permission.)

seen with electrolyte products that contain high concentrations of bicarbonate may therefore facilitate growth of bacterial diarrheal pathogens and thus increase the severity, duration, and mortality rate associated with diarrhea in calves.

Interference with normal digestion During the normal digestion process, milk clots in the abomasum as casein coagulates under the influence of renin and pepsin. The whey fraction then passes quickly into the small intestine, whereas digestion of the abomasal clot continues for up to 12 hours.[44] In the early 1990s, in vitro experiments demonstrated that bicarbonate-containing oral electrolyte products inhibited the clotting of milk in the abomasum.[45] A further study examining 50 different commercially available oral electrolyte products formulated for calf oral rehydration therapy showed that those that contained bicarbonate consistently inhibited milk clotting, whereas those that contained acetate or propionate did not.[46] The conclusion of this research was that bicarbonate-based oral electrolyte solutions would upset the normal digestive process if fed together with milk or milk replacer. The recommendation to separate the feeding of milk and electrolytes by 2 to 4 hours has been common for the last 15 years. In fact, the labels of many electrolyte products still contain statements warning against concurrent feeding with milk for this reason. A more recent study demonstrated that an oral electrolyte product containing low concentrations of bicarbonate (25 mmol/L) and citrate (12 mmol/L) did not inhibit clot formation in calves.[47]

The importance of abomasal clot formation in milk digestion has since been questioned. Early milk replacers in the United States were formulated with casein-containing protein sources. Currently the milk replacer industry uses protein sources that are nonclotting, such as whey and soy protein, to formulate milk replacers.[48] Although first judged as inferior to casein, many of these nonclotting milk replacers can produce growth rates far superior to products that were originally used. Eventually it was determined that factors other than clot formation were responsible for calf performance and this process may not be as important as was originally believed.[48] Although the significance of bicarbonate inhibiting abomasal clot formation is not well understood, it is possible that these products do somehow interfere with the normal digestive process. It has been shown that electrolyte solutions containing bicarbonate reduce growth rates in calves when fed simultaneously with milk.[49] Although the exact cause or clinical importance of this reduction in growth rate is not well understood, some experts still recommend that bicarbonate-based oral electrolytes not be fed together with milk or milk replacer. Products containing acetate or propionate as an alkalinizing agent would not have similar concerns and are well tolerated when fed with milk.

Strong ion difference

Strong ion theory is a different approach to looking at acid–base abnormalities. Traditionally, veterinarians have been taught to use the Henderson-Hasselbalch equation that uses measured pH and pCO_2 values along with calculated HCO_3 concentrations to characterize acid–base disturbances. This approach has several limitations that make it less than ideal for clinical use in sick animals.[50,51] The strong ion model reduces chemical reactions in plasma to that of simple ions in solution.[50] Strong ions are nonbuffer ions, meaning they are fully dissociated at physiologic pH values and do not participate in chemical reactions, yet exert an electrical effect. According to the strong ion model, the plasma SID is the primary determinant of acid–base balance in vivo. The primary strong cations are sodium (Na^+) and potassium (K^+) with minor contributions from calcium (Ca^{2+}) and magnesium (Mg^{2+}), and the primary strong anions are chloride (Cl^-), D- and L-lactate, and organic acids. Using the strong ion approach, the relationship between these ions becomes the primary factor that determines the acid–base status of an animal. Calves that have diarrhea have a tremendous loss of cations (Na^+ and K^+) relative to normal or increased strong anion concentrations, which creates a strong ion (metabolic) acidosis.[15] A significant part of the increase in strong anions is from D-lactic acid, which comes from bacterial fermentation of malabsorbed nutrients in calves that have diarrhea.[52] Calves that have diarrhea have a significantly higher serum concentration of D-lactic acid as compared with normal calves[52,53] and intravenous administration of D-lactate to normal calves has been demonstrated to induce many of the adverse clinical signs traditionally associated with metabolic acidosis.[54]

Based on strong ion theory, it is not necessarily imperative that an electrolyte solution contain an alkalinizing agent to correct metabolic acidosis; rather, the product must deliver an excess of strong cations (Na^+) relative to the concentration of strong anions (Cl^-). It has therefore been advocated to consider the SID of an oral electrolyte solution when choosing a product.[55] The SID can be calculated as follows: [Na^+] + [K^+] − [Cl^-] = SID. Although there has not been any definite research to determine the optimal or minimum SID that an oral electrolyte product should contain, a minimum SID of 60 to 80 mEq/L would be recommended in a calf that has diarrhea. A case example may provide a better understanding of this concept. Suppose you are treating a calf that has diarrhea that can still stand but is lethargic and has a weak suckle reflex. We can assume this calf has a moderate metabolic acidosis with a base deficit somewhere around 8 mmol/L. Assuming the calf weighs 40 kg we can calculate a total base deficit as follows:

$$40 \text{ kg} \times 8 \text{mmol/L} \times 0.6 \text{ (\%ECF)} = 192 \text{ mmol}$$

If we then administer 2 L of an oral electrolyte solution that has an SID of 80 we have corrected 160 mmol of this calf's base deficit. The metabolic acidosis would not be fully resolved; however, the pH would move much closer to the normal range. In contrast, if we fed 2 L of an oral electrolyte product that has an SID of 30, we have only corrected the base deficit by 60 mmol and the calf will continue to have a significant metabolic acidosis. This acidosis is likely to increase in severity as the calf has ongoing electrolyte losses associated with diarrhea. From this example the practitioner can appreciate the importance of administering a solution rich in strong cations (high SID value) in calves that have diarrhea. Another important point is that oral fluid therapy in calves that have severe metabolic acidosis is not practical. These calves often have base deficit values greater than 20 mmol/L and much larger total body deficits (40 kg calf × 20 mmol/L × 0.6 = 480 mmol). Even with good quality electrolyte products, it becomes impractical or impossible to correct a deficit this severe with oral fluid therapy.

There are two different ways of thinking about alkalinizing ability when considering oral electrolyte products in calves. Is it more important to choose a product with an alkalinizing agent, or one with a high SID? In reality there is not a good answer to this question; however, to achieve optimal results, both factors are important. Studies with intravenous fluid therapy have demonstrated that the metabolic acidosis in calves does not resolve just by rehydrating the animal.[31] Several studies in diarrheic calves have shown that oral electrolytes without alkalinizing agents do not correct metabolic acidosis; in fact, they can have a mild acidifying effect.[11,33,34,56] Recovery rates are always higher and mortality always lower in studies that compare an oral electrolyte solution with an alkalinizing agent to one without.[33,56,57] It has generally been accepted, therefore, that oral electrolyte products should contain 50 to 80 mmol/L of an alkalinizing agent.[44]

When thinking about the strong ion approach, it would certainly be possible to correct metabolic acidosis in a calf without an alkalinizing agent by choosing a product with a high SID. Studies comparing different oral electrolyte solutions that do not contain any alkalinizing agent consistently show that products with higher SIDs have a greater alkalinizing effect than products with lower SIDs.[11,38] To achieve maximum alkalinizing ability out of an oral electrolyte product, however, the author believes that both elements are important. For example, one study showed there was no difference in the alkalinizing ability of an electrolyte solution that contained 80 mmol/L of acetate and had an SID of 90 when compared with a product that contained 80 mmol/L of bicarbonate and had an SID of 88.[33] Both products were far superior to an oral electrolyte solution that contained no alkalinizing agent and had an SID of 15, however. The ideal electrolyte solution for use in calves that have diarrhea should contain at least 50 mmol/L of an alkalinizing agent (preferably acetate or propionate) and have a SID of at least 60 to 80. Unfortunately, products without alkalinizing agents and with low SIDs are commonly available in North America and should be avoided in calves that have diarrhea.

Psyllium

It has been hypothesized that adding dietary fiber (mucilage) in the form of psyllium to oral electrolyte solutions would enhance nutrient absorption from the digestive tract and improve glucose absorption by slowing gastric emptying.[58] In addition, fiber may help reduce the severity of diarrhea. It is able to pass undigested through the gastrointestinal tract and give a more formed appearance to the feces, which some practitioners and producers have correlated with increased efficacy of the oral electrolyte product. This improvement in fecal consistency is due to the gelling of liquid and should not be mistaken for a real improvement in the calf's overall condition. Research from multiple clinical trials has shown that the addition of psyllium to oral electrolyte solutions does not improve glucose absorption in calves that have diarrhea.[59,60] In fact, one study showed that calves fed oral electrolytes containing psyllium had significantly lower glucose concentrations after feeding as compared with the same oral electrolyte formulation without psyllium.[59] Although supplemental dietary fiber may generate slight improvements in fecal consistency, it seems to impair glucose absorption in the small intestine and is not recommended for inclusion in oral electrolyte products intended for calves.

ADMINISTRATION OF ORAL ELECTROLYTES

In general, oral electrolytes should be fed as an extra meal to calves that have diarrhea. For example, if calves are normally being fed twice a day (morning and evening), then oral electrolytes can be fed in the middle of the day. If the additional labor required for the extra feeding is not available, then electrolytes can be fed along with milk (particularly those products that contain acetate or very low concentrations of bicarbonate). Some farms prefer to offer diarrheic calves constant access to low-osmolality electrolytes throughout the day. Regardless of the feeding schedule for electrolytes, it is best to continue milk or milk replacer in these calves.

Some experts have recommended a "rest the gut" approach to treating calf diarrhea, suggesting that continued milk feeding worsens the diarrhea. This concept is based on the principle that milk supplies nutrients in the intestines that the bacteria could use as an energy source. This process would lead to further maldigestion of nutrients and increased excretion of fluids (thus more diarrhea). Other arguments for withholding milk in calves that have diarrhea include a faster healing of the intestines, less opportunity for overgrowth of the intestines with harmful bacteria, and impaired digestion and use of milk or milk replacer. Despite these ideas, research has shown milk feeding does not prolong or worsen diarrhea, nor does it speed healing of the intestines. In a study by Garthwaite and colleagues,[61] 42 calves that had naturally occurring diarrhea were divided into three groups. In one group milk was withheld and calves were fed only oral electrolytes, followed by a gradual return to milk after 2 days. In the second group there was partial removal of milk; calves were fed only a small amount (2.5% of body weight for 2 days followed by 5% of body weight for 2 days) along with oral electrolytes. In the third group calves were continued on their full allotment of milk (10% of body weight per day) along with electrolytes. There was no difference in the severity or duration of diarrhea between any of the groups during the study. The calves that had diarrhea that were fed both milk and oral electrolytes gained more weight than did calves from which milk was withheld for 1 to 2 days. The calves that continued to receive milk actually gained weight during the study period, whereas calves in the other two groups lost weight. Weight loss in calves limited to only oral electrolyte solutions has been reported in other studies also.[24]

Another study used an experimentally induced model of diarrhea in calves fed either milk (2 L every 12 hours), an isotonic oral electrolyte solution (85 mmol glucose), or a hypertonic oral electrolyte solution (330 mmol glucose) over a 48-hour period. Serum glucose concentrations were unchanged over the 48-hour period in the calves fed milk, but steadily declined throughout the study in both groups fed only oral electrolytes.[12] Calves fed only electrolytes developed significant increases in β-OH butyrate and nonesterified fatty acid concentrations over the 48-hour period, indicating these calves were in a profound negative energy balance (**Fig. 3**). These studies indicate that even hypertonic oral electrolyte products with very high glucose concentrations do not provide significant energy to meet the maintenance and growth requirements of a calf. The recommendation to temporarily discontinue milk feeding in calves that have diarrhea is therefore inappropriate. Calves should be maintained on their full milk diet plus oral electrolytes when possible. If calves are depressed and refuse to suckle, milk can be withheld for one feeding (12 hours) and a hypertonic oral electrolyte product substituted. Milk feeding should always be resumed within 12 hours.

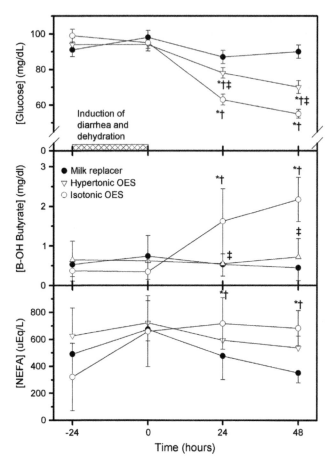

Fig. 3. Serum glucose, β-OH butyrate, and nonesterified fatty acid concentrations in neonatal calves that had experimentally induced diarrhea and dehydration. Calves were administered milk replacer, hypertonic oral electrolyte solution, or isotonic oral electrolyte solution. Values are expressed as mean ± SD. *$P<.05$; compared with time = 0 value; †$P<.05$ compared with milk replacer group at the same time interval; ‡$P<.05$ compared with the isotonic group at the same time interval. (*Modified from* Constable PD, Thomas E, Boisrame B. Comparison of two oral electrolyte solutions for the treatment of dehydrated calves with experimentally-induced diarrhea. Vet J 2001;162:129–40; with permission.)

SUMMARY

In summary, oral electrolytes continue to be the hallmark of routine therapy for treating neonatal calf diarrhea. It is important that practitioners are able to assess dehydration accurately and understand how and when to use oral electrolyte products. There are tremendous differences in the formulation of commercially available electrolyte products found in North America and around the world. All products are not created equally and choosing which of these products to use in practice is an important decision. Practitioners should focus on selecting oral electrolyte solutions that satisfy the following four requirements: (1) supply sufficient sodium to normalize the ECF volume, (2) provide agents that facilitate absorption of sodium and water from the intestine,

(3) correct the metabolic acidosis usually present in calves with diarrhea, and (4) provide energy. Additionally, the oral electrolyte should not cause any deleterious effects (such as abomasal bloat). Because veterinarians are often not directly involved with the administration of oral electrolytes to calves, it is important that they examine the electrolyte product being used in their clients' herds and make recommendations when appropriate.

REFERENCES

1. Constable PD, Walker PG, Morin DE, et al. Clinical and laboratory assessment of hydration status in neonatal calves with diarrhea. J Am Vet Med Assoc 1998;212: 991–6.
2. Fayet JC. Plasma and faecal osmolality, water kinetics and body fluid compartments in neonatal calves with diarrhoea. Br Vet J 1971;127:37–43.
3. Phillips RW, Lewis LD, Knox KL. Alterations in body water turnover and distribution in neonatal calves with acute diarrhea. Ann N Y Acad Sci 1971;176:231–43.
4. Watt JG. The use of fluid replacement in the treatment of neonatal diseases in calves. Vet Rec 1965;77:1474–82.
5. Buntain BJ, Selman IE. Controlled studies of various treatments for neonatal calf diarrhoea in calves of known immunoglobulin levels. Vet Rec 1980;107:245–8.
6. Bywater RJ. Diarrhoea treatments – fluid replacement and alternatives. Ann Rech Vét 1983;14:556–60.
7. Groutides CP, Michell AR. Changes in plasma composition in calves surviving or dying from diarrhoea. Br Vet J 1990;146:205–10.
8. Lewis LD, Phillips RW. Water and electrolyte losses in neonatal calves with acute diarrhea. A complete balance study. Cornell Vet 1972;62:596–607.
9. Walker PG, Constable PD, Morin DE, et al. A reliable, practical, and economical protocol for inducing diarrhea and severe dehydration in the neonatal calf. Can J Vet Res 1998;62:205–13.
10. Michell AR. Drips, drinks and drenches: what matters in fluid therapy. Ir Vet J 1988;42:17–22.
11. Michell AR, Brooks HW, White DG, et al. The comparative effectiveness of three commercial oral solutions in correcting fluid, electrolyte and acid-base disturbances caused by calf diarrhoea. Br Vet J 1992;148:507–22.
12. Constable PD, Thomas E, Boisrame B. Comparison of two oral electrolyte solutions for the treatment of dehydrated calves with experimentally-induced diarrhea. Vet J 2001;162:129–40.
13. Jones R, Phillips RW, Cleek JL. Hyperosmotic oral replacement fluid for diarrheic calves. J Am Vet Med Assoc 1984;184:1501–5.
14. Sen I, Constable PD, Marshall TS. Effect of suckling isotonic or hypertonic solutions of sodium bicarbonate or glucose on abomasal emptying rate in calves. Am J Vet Res 2006;67:1377–84.
15. Constable PD, Stämpfli HR, Navetat H, et al. Use of a quantitative strong ion approach to determine the mechanism for acid-base abnormalities in sick calves with or without diarrhea. J Vet Intern Med 2005;19:581–9.
16. Desjeux JF, Tannenbaum C, Tai YH, et al. Effects of sugars and amino acids on sodium movement across small intestine. Am J Dis Child 1977;131:331–40.
17. Fisher RB. The absorption of water and some small solute molecules from the isolated small intestine of the rat. J Physiol 1955;130:655–64.
18. Deminge C, Remesy C, Chartier F, et al. Effect of acetate or chloride anions on intestinal absorption of water and solutes in the calf. Am J Vet Res 1981;42:1356–9.

19. Demigne C, Remesy C, Chartier F, et al. Utilization of volatile fatty acids and improvement of fluid therapy for treatment of dehydration in diarrheic calves. Ann Rech Vét 1983;14:541–7.

20. Avery ME, Snyder JD. Oral therapy for acute diarrhea. N Engl J Med 1990;323: 891–4.

21. Jodal M, Lundgren O. Countercurrent mechanisms in the mammalian intestinal tract. Gastroenterology 1986;91:225–41.

22. Levy M, Marritt AM, Levy LC. Comparison of the effects of an isosmolar and hyperosmolar oral rehydrating solution on the hydration status, glycemia and ileal content composition of healthy neonatal calves. Cornell Vet 1990;80: 143–51.

23. Brooks HW, White DG, Wagstaff AJ, et al. Evaluation of a nutritive oral rehydration solution for the treatment of calf diarrhoea. Br Vet J 1996;152:699–708.

24. Fettman MJ, Brooks PA, Burrows KP, et al. Evaluation of commercial oral replacement formulas in healthy neonatal calves. J Am Vet Med Assoc 1986;188: 397–401.

25. Bywater RJ. Evaluation of an oral glucose-glycine-electrolyte formulation and amoxicillin for treatment of diarrhea in calves. Am J Vet Res 1977;38:1983–7.

26. Naylor JM, Leibel T, Middleton DM. Effect of glutamine or glycine containing oral electrolyte solutions on mucosal morphology, clinical and biochemical findings, in calves with viral induced diarrhea. Can J Vet Res 1997;61:43–8.

27. Nouri M, Constable PD. Comparison of two oral electrolyte solutions and route of administration on the abomasal emptying rate of Holstein-Friesian calves. J Vet Intern Med 2006;20:620–6.

28. Panciera RJ, Boileau MJ, Step DL. Tympany, acidosis, and mural emphysema of the stomach in calves: report of cases and experimental induction. J Vet Diagn Invest 2007;19:392–5.

29. Songer JG, Miskimins DW. Clostridial abomasitis in calves: case report and review of the literature. Anaerobe 2005;11:290–4.

30. Tennant B, Harrold D, Reina-Guerra M. Physiologic and metabolic factors in the pathogenesis of neonatal enteric infections in calves. J Am Vet Med Assoc 1972; 161:993–1007.

31. Kasari TR, Naylor JM. Clinical evaluation of sodium bicarbonate, sodium L-lactate, and sodium acetate for the treatment of acidosis in diarrheic calves. J Am Vet Med Assoc 1985;187:392–7.

32. Naylor JM. Alkalinizing abilities of calf oral electrolyte solutions. In: Proceedings of the XIV World Congress on Diseases of Cattle. Dublin; 1986. p. 362–7.

33. Naylor JM, Petrie L, Rodriguez MI, et al. A comparison of three oral electrolyte solutions in the treatment of diarrheic calves. Can Vet J 1990;31:753–60.

34. Naylor JM, Forsyth GW. The alkalinizing effects of metabolizable bases in the healthy calf. Can J Vet Res 1986;50:509–16.

35. Martinsen TC, Bergh K, Waldum HL. Gastric juice: a barrier against infectious diseases. Basic Clin Pharmacol Toxicol 2005;96:94–102.

36. Wray C, Callow RJ. Studies on the survival of Salmonella dublin, S. typhimurium, and E. coli in stored bovine colostrum. Vet Rec 1974;94:407–12.

37. Zhu H, Hart CA, Sales D, et al. Bacterial killing in gastric juice – effect of pH and pepsin on Escherichia coli and Helicobacter pylori. J Med Microbiol 2006;55: 1265–70.

38. Dupe RJ, Goddard ME, Bywater RJ. A comparison of two oral rehydration solutions in experimental models of dehydration and diarrhoea in calves. Vet Rec 1989;125:620–4.

39. White DG, Johnson CK, Cracknell V. Comparison of danofloxacin with baquilo-prim/sulphadimidine for the treatment of experimentally induced *Escherichia coli* diarrhoea in calves. Vet Rec 1998;143:273–6.
40. Bachmann L, Reinhold S, Hartmann H. Effect of milk, milk replacer and oral rehydration solutions on abomasal luminal conditions and on the acid-base status in dairy calves. In: Proceedings of the 13th International Conference on Production Diseases in Farm Animals. Leipzig, Germany; 2007. p. 334.
41. Constable PD, Ahmed AF, Misk NA. Effect of oral electrolyte solution formulation on abomasal luminal pH in suckling dairy calves. J Vet Intern Med 2003;17:391 [abstract].
42. Marshall TS, Constable PD, Crochik SS, et al. Effect of suckling an isotonic solution of sodium acetate, sodium bicarbonate, or sodium chloride on abomasal emptying rate and luminal pH in calves. Am J Vet Res 2008;69:824–31.
43. Reinhold S, Hertsch BW, Höppner S, et al. Wirkung von Milch und Diättränken mit und ohne HCO_3-Ionen auf den inraluminalen pH-Wert im Labmagen und den systemischen Säuren-Basen-Status beim Kalb. Tierärztl Prax 2006;34(G):368–76.
44. Nappert G, Zello GA, Naylor JM. Oral rehydration therapy for diarrheic calves. Compend Contin Educ Pract Vet 1997;19:S181–9.
45. Naylor JM. Effects of electrolyte solutions for oral administration on clotting of milk. J Am Vet Med Assoc 1992;201:1026–9.
46. Nappert G, Spennick H. Effects of neonatal calf oral rehydration therapy solutions on milk clotting time. Cattle Practice 2003;11:285–8.
47. Constable PD, Grünberg W, Carstensen L. Effect of suckling Diakur® Plus in cow's milk on milk clotting, luminal pH, and abomasal emptying rates in Holstein-Friesian calves. In: Proceedings of the XXV World Buiatrics Congress. Budapest: Hungarian Vet J 2008; (Suppl 2) p. 227.
48. Longenbach JI, Heinrichs AJ. A review of the importance and physiological role of curd formation in the abomasum of young calves. Anim Feed Sci Technol 1998;73:85–97.
49. Heath SE, Naylor JM, Guedo BL, et al. The effect of feeding milk to diarrheic calves supplemented with oral electrolytes. Can J Vet Res 1989;53:477–85.
50. Constable PD. Clinical assessment of acid-base status: strong ion theory difference. Vet Clin Food Anim Pract 1999;15:447–71.
51. Constable PD. Clinical assessment of acid-base status: comparison of the Henderson-Hasselbalch and strong ion approaches. Vet Clin Pathol 2000;29:115–28.
52. Omole OO, Nappert G, Naylor JM, et al. Both L- and D-lactate contribute to metabolic acidosis in diarrheic calves. J Nutr 2001;131:2128–31.
53. Lorenz I. Influence of D-lactate on metabolic acidosis and on prognosis in neonatal calves with diarrhea. J Vet Med A 2004;51:425–8.
54. Lorenz I, Gentile A, Klee W. Investigations of D-lactate metabolism and the clinical signs of D-lactataemia in calves. Vet Rec 2005;156:412–5.
55. Stämpfli HR, Pringle JH, Lumsden JH, et al. Experimental evaluation of a novel oral electrolyte solution in the treatment of natural occurring neonatal calf diarrhoea. In: Proceedings of the XIX World Buiatrics Congress. Edinburgh; 1996. p. 98–101.
56. Booth AJ, Naylor JM. Correction of metabolic acidosis in diarrheal calves by oral administration of electrolyte solutions with or without bicarbonate. J Am Vet Med Assoc 1987;191:62–8.
57. Naylor JM. Oral fluid therapy in neonatal ruminants and swine. Vet Clin Food Anim Pract 1990;6:51–67.

58. Fettman MJ. Potential benefits of psyllium mucilloid supplementation of oral replacement formulas for neonatal calf scours. Compend Contin Educ Pract Vet 1992;14:247–54.
59. Cebra ML, Garry FB, Cebra CK, et al. Treatment of neonatal calf diarrhea with an oral electrolyte solution supplemented with psyllium mucilloid. J Vet Intern Med 1998;12:449–55.
60. Naylor JM, Liebel T. Effect of psyllium on plasma concentration of glucose, breath hydrogen concentration, and fecal composition in calves with diarrhea treated orally with electrolyte solutions. Am J Vet Res 1995;56:56–9.
61. Garthwaite BD, Drackley JK, McCoy GC, et al. Whole milk and oral rehydration solution for calves with diarrhea of spontaneous origin. J Dairy Sci 1994;77: 835–43.

Treatment of Calf Diarrhea: Intravenous Fluid Therapy

Joachim Berchtold, Dr Med Vet

KEYWORDS

• Calves • Diarrhea • Dehydration • Acidosis
• Intravenous fluid therapy

One of the most important factors in decreasing mortality associated with diarrhea in calves is the proper use of oral and intravenous (IV) fluid therapy. Sick calves without significant dehydration, as seen in other diseases (eg, persistent anorexia, septicemia, ruminal acidosis from ruminal drinking, severe pneumonia, and hypothermia) also may benefit from administration of IV fluids. The recommendations for type, amount, route, and rate of administration of solutions for IV fluid therapy in calves vary and often are too complicated or not suitable for use in field practice. This article presents a simplified protocol for administration of IV fluids and a simple technique for on-farm IV fluid therapy by ear vein catheterization in calves. Recent insights in the development of metabolic acidosis in calves and studies on IV fluid therapy are reviewed.

Diarrhea in neonatal calves remains the leading cause of morbidity and mortality in North America and Europe,[1,2] with no change in mortality rates between 1995 and 2001 in dairy heifer calves in the United States.[1] Neonatal calf diarrhea is a complex disease that occurs predominantly during the first 4 weeks of life. Calves with diarrhea have an increased chance of fecal isolation of one or more viral (rotavirus, coronavirus), bacterial (*Escherichia coli*, *Salmonella* sp.), or protozoal (*Cryptosporidium parvum*, *Eimeria* sp.) pathogens than healthy control calves.[3] Regardless of the origin, most calves with diarrhea have increased numbers of coliform bacteria in their small intestine (bacterial overgrowth), which contributes to morphologic damage of the intestinal mucosa and may result in increased susceptibility to bacteremia.[4] Metabolic acidosis is a frequent consequence of gastrointestinal disease and is found in calves with dehydration and in clinically sick calves with minimal or no signs of dehydration, the so-called "acidosis-without-dehydration-syndrome."[5]

The importance of bacterial overgrowth in the intestines of calves with diarrhea gained more attention when the role of D-lactate (the anion of D-lactic acid) in the development of metabolic acidosis was discovered. Production of D-lactic acid results from bacterial fermentation of carbohydrates in the gastrointestinal tract of

Veterinary Practice, Drs. Prechtl and Berchtold, Haiming 4, 83119 Obing, Germany
E-mail address: joachim@altental.de

Vet Clin Food Anim 25 (2009) 73–99
doi:10.1016/j.cvfa.2008.10.001   vetfood.theclinics.com
0749-0720/08/$ – see front matter © 2009 Elsevier Inc. All rights reserved.

milk-fed calves and is a common finding in sick calves with and without diarrhea. Studies have demonstrated that D-lactate is a major component of the metabolic acidosis generally present in calves with diarrhea, in calves with the "acidosis-without-dehydration-syndrome," and in calves with ruminal acidosis from drinking milk into the rumen (ruminal drinking).[6-15] D-lactate also has been identified as the major component of metabolic acidosis in the floppy kid syndrome of young goat kids.[16] Clinical signs of impaired central nervous system (CNS) function, including ataxia and coma in sick calves, have been historically attributed to metabolic acidosis; however, recent findings indicated that many of the clinical signs formerly attributed to acidosis are caused by an increase in D-lactate concentrations.[17,18] The pathophysiology of D-lactate accumulation is important for bovine practitioners to understand and is discussed in more detail in the next section.

INDICATIONS FOR INTRAVENOUS FLUID THERAPY
Dehydration and Electrolyte Imbalances

The pathophysiology of diarrhea includes increased intestinal secretion and decreased intestinal absorption of fluids along with increased passage of intestinal contents. Severe dehydration caused by fecal loss of fluids and electrolytes is a frequent complication of diarrhea and the primary indication for oral and intravenous fluid therapy. A higher total body water content (approximately 75% body weight) and a higher extracellular fluid volume content (approximately 45% body weight) in newborn calves make them more sensitive to fluid losses compared with adult cattle. The higher proportional water content does not serve as a water reservoir and has no protective effect against dehydration.[19] Fecal fluid loss in calves with severe watery diarrhea can reach 13% to 18% of body weight per day and is probably underestimated in most cases.[20] The highest fecal fluid loss reported was in a calf that lost 21% of its body weight over 24 hours, although ad libitum oral fluids were provided.[20] The kidneys compensate for increased fluid loss in diarrhea by decreasing urine production; however, if losses exceed fluid intake, dehydration follows.[21]

Fecal losses of water occur in combination with losses of electrolytes, primarily sodium and potassium. Serum electrolyte concentrations are also affected by a reduced dietary (milk) intake and can be masked by hemoconcentration.[22] The decrease in extracellular fluid volume decreases plasma volume and venous return, which results in extracellular dehydration and total body loss of water and electrolytes. Fluid and electrolyte losses in the early stages of calf diarrhea are primarily of secretory origin and—to a much lesser extent—of osmotic origin.[23]

Blood electrolyte concentrations can vary considerably in calves with diarrhea because most calves generally have been treated with oral fluids before presentation.[20,24-26] Mixing errors of oral electrolyte solutions often occur, and many calves do not have access to fresh water.[26] In dehydrated calves with diarrhea, decreased serum concentrations of glucose, sodium, potassium, and chloride have been reported.[27] Hyponatremia is generally present as a result of increased fecal loss (secretory diarrhea);[22,27-29] however, hypernatremia also may be present. This is particularly true in calves that have been treated or overtreated with oral electrolyte solutions and do not have access to fresh water[26] or calves to which an electrolyte solution with excessive sodium concentration was fed (> 140 mEq/L). Total body potassium concentrations decrease in diarrhea; however, hyperkalemia is often present in calves with diarrhea with severe acidosis.[22,27] Hyperkalemia is thought to result from translocation of potassium from the intracellular to the extracellular compartment.[19] An impaired renal excretion of potassium also may play a role in this not-fully-understood mechanism of hyperkalemia involving hyponatremia, hypo-osmolality, acidemia, and cellular hypoxia.[5] Calcium concentrations are often low, and magnesium concentrations vary in calves with diarrhea.[22,30] Electrolyte imbalances (sodium, total calcium, magnesium) have been found to be present even 10 days after completion of therapy in calves that were successfully treated for diarrhea.[30]

Diarrhea in young calves causes a hypo-osmotic extracellular dehydration with decreased extracellular fluid volume (plasma and interstitial) and a small increase in intracellular fluid volume.[31–33] In calves with chronic diarrhea or shortly before death, hyperosmotic dehydration may be present.[21,34] Electrolyte disturbances and type of dehydration (iso-, hypo-, or hyperosmotic) vary among individual cases and cannot be predicted from clinical findings without laboratory analysis. Scouring calves may be in poor body condition when they have not been fed milk for several days and were treated only with oral fluids.[20,35] Hypothermia is also a logical consequence in the pathophysiology of dehydration, and a decreased rectal temperature is frequently observed in calves with diarrhea.[36–38]

The traditional recommendation for IV fluid therapy is predominantly based on the degree of dehydration. A decrease of more than 8% body weight is believed to require IV fluid administration rather than only oral fluids for successful rehydration. Under field conditions, the indications for IV fluid therapy in calves may be extended to non-dehydrated sick calves with gastrointestinal or other diseases.[39–41] Calves with less severe dehydration may benefit from IV fluids if they show signs of severe depression or coma, are recumbent or severely depressed, or do not have a suckle reflex. In the authors' opinion, the indication for IV fluid therapy should be extended to some calves that may be less than 8% dehydrated. Regardless of the degree of clinical dehydration, when calves show signs of severe CNS depression or weakness, are comatose, are unable to stand, do not suckle for more than 24 hours, or have a rectal temperature of less than 100°F (38 °C) (in newborn calves), IV fluid therapy is indicated. The authors recommend IV fluid therapy for other diseases or syndromes in sick calves without diarrhea, including diseases that cause a decrease in oral fluid intake because of abdominal pain or an inability to suckle, which can be seen with severe respiratory distress.

Metabolic Acidosis and D-Lactate

Development of strong ion (metabolic) acidosis is common in calves with diarrhea and other gastrointestinal diseases. Our understanding of the pathophysiology of this acidosis has increased tremendously during the past decade, primarily because of discoveries by researchers in Europe and Canada on the significance of D-lactate in calves with gastrointestinal disorders. The importance of D-lactate in the pathophysiology of gastrointestinal diseases in calves has been elucidated in several clinical and experimental studies. Two thorough review articles were published recently on this subject;[8,11] however, a brief discussion is still warranted here. We have known for years that adult ruminants with acute rumen acidosis develop D-lactic acidosis after grain overfeeding.[42] Only recently, however, were increased D-lactate concentrations identified to be responsible for most of the systemic acidemia that occurs in calves with the "acidosis-without-dehydration syndrome"[12,14] and for a major portion of the acidemia seen in calves with diarrhea.[6,7,9,10,13,43] In calves with ruminal acidosis after drinking or drenching of whole milk into the rumen, acidemia may follow after absorption of sufficient amounts of D-lactate from the gastrointestinal tract.[15,44]

D- and L-lactate are end products of organic acids normally produced in the gastrointestinal tract by bacterial metabolism of carbohydrates without any deleterious consequences to the animal.[45] In adult cattle with grain overload, fermentation of larger amounts of carbohydrates induces an increased concentration of organic acids that leads to a decrease in intraruminal pH. This decrease in pH favors the overgrowth of bacteria (mainly *Lactobacillus* spp.) that are able to produce D- and L-lactate in high quantities.[8] In calves with diarrhea, the increased production of D- and probably L-lactate is thought to result from villous atrophy, with subsequent malabsorption and fermentation of nutrients by intestinal bacteria.[8,11] Both the L- and D-isomers of lactic acid can be absorbed from the gastrointestinal tract; however, the hepatic metabolism and renal excretion of D-lactate are significantly slower in ruminants compared with L-lactate. With increased production and absorption of L- and D-lactate, the metabolic acidosis that develops is primarily caused by increases in D-lactate concentrations.[8]

Development of metabolic acidosis in calves with diarrhea has long been attributed to (1) loss of bicarbonate ions (HCO_3^-) in the feces, (2) decreased renal excretion of hydrogen ions (H^+) associated with dehydration and decreased renal blood flow, and (3) the presence of unidentified organic acids in plasma.[46–50] In the late 1980s, Naylor[51] found that metabolic acidosis is based at least in part on the presence of increased L-lactate concentrations in the serum of calves with diarrhea younger than 8 days. Compared with the recent findings of elevated D-lactate concentrations in the blood, however, the small increases in L-lactate concentrations seen in earlier studies do not explain the high anion-gap ($AG = ([Na^+] + [K^+]) - ([Cl^-] + [HCO_3^-])$) often found in calves with diarrhea.[6,13,48,52] An increase in the anion gap is the result of an increased concentration of strong anions in blood, mainly from organic acids (eg, lactic acid). Experimental induction of severe dehydration (at least 14% body weight) produced only a mild L-lactic acidosis.[53] The discovery of D-lactate ended speculation of which unidentified anion or anions might be most responsible for the increase in the anion gap. It is clear that increased D-lactate concentrations explain most of the acidemia and elevated anion gaps present in calves with diarrhea and in clinically sick calves without diarrhea and dehydration ("acidosis without dehydration syndrome").

The first two reports of D-lactic acidosis from France found a mean D-lactate concentration between 10 and 13 mmol/L in the plasma of clinically sick Charolais calves without signs of dehydration or diarrhea and a mean D-lactate concentration of 5 mmol/L in calves with simple diarrhea. This finding was compared with healthy control calves that had D-lactate concentrations between 1 and 2 mmol/L.[12,14] The mean L-lactate concentrations seen in acidotic calves (1–2.5 mmol/L) were much lower than the reported D-lactate levels. Subsequent studies from Canada and Germany showed that hyper-D-lactatemia is often present in calves with more severe diarrhea and dehydration. A blood D-lactate concentration above 3 mmol/L was found in 55% of 300 calves with neonatal diarrhea.[9] Median D-lactate concentration was 4.1 mmol/L and ranged from 0 to 17.8 mmol/L. The correlation between D-lactate concentration and base deficit was statistically significant but not linear, and the degree to which D-lactate contributed to metabolic acidosis varied from calf to calf (**Fig. 1**). Calves with a severe metabolic acidosis (base deficit > 25 mmol/L) always had increased D-lactate concentrations, whereas calves with a less severe acidosis (base deficit between 10 and 25 mmol/L) had D-lactate concentrations that varied from 0 to 17.8 mmol/L.[9,10]

The concentration of D-lactate and L-lactate accounted for 64% of the elevated anion gap in one study,[13] and significant correlations between D-lactate concentration and the anion gap were found in subsequent studies.[6,9] Ewaschuk and colleagues[7] measured D- and L-lactate in rumen, blood, fecal, and urine samples in calves with diarrhea and in healthy control calves. Despite a markedly higher L-lactate concentration in rumen and fecal samples of diarrheic calves as compared with control calves, the L-lactate concentrations were not high enough to induce a systemic acidosis. The

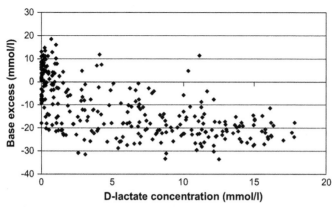

Fig. 1. Blood base excess and serum D-lactate concentrations in 300 calves with neonatal diarrhea. (*From* Lorenz I. Influence of D-lactate on metabolic acidosis and on prognosis in neonatal calves with diarrhoea. J Vet Med A 2004;51:425–8; with permission.)

calves with diarrhea in that study had significantly higher values for D-lactate in all four samples (rumen, feces, blood, urine) than healthy control calves.[7] The mean values for D-lactate were highest in the feces (25.4 mmol/L), followed by urine (19.2 mmol/L), rumen (17 mmol/L), and serum (13.9 mmol/L). The authors concluded that D-lactate production and absorption in the colon were more likely to have contributed to the systemic acidosis than other possible sites of absorption (rumen). Accumulated D-lactate may be effectively eliminated by the kidneys in nondehydrated calves.[54] The role of IV fluid therapy to restore or maintain hydration status in sick calves is also important to speed elimination of D-lactate; however, kinetic studies of D-lactate elimination in calves are not currently available.

D-Lactate in Ruminal Drinker Calves

The role of D- and L-lactate in the pathophysiology of ruminal acidosis in adult cattle with grain overload was identified more than 40 years ago.[42] Briefly, overfeeding with highly fermentable concentrates results in excessive bacterial fermentation of carbohydrates by the anaerobic bacteria of the rumen. Grain overload leads to production of short chain fatty acids and large amounts of D- and L-lactate.[8] Because the ruminant liver is not efficient in metabolizing D-lactate, it begins to accumulate in the blood and systemic acidemia often follows. The same absorptive mechanisms for D-lactate in ruminating cattle may be responsible for systemic accumulation of D-lactate in preruminating calves with persistent ruminal acidosis from spilling milk into the rumen (ruminal drinking).[15] Experimentally induced rumen acidosis in calves after repeated intraruminal force feeding of whole milk resulted in D-lactic acidosis. Calves developed hyper-D-lactatemia with concentrations between 6.8 and 11.1 mmol/L, generally in conjunction with metabolic acidosis, dehydration, severe depression, and lack of appetite or reduced suckle reflex.[15] Calves that suffered from spontaneous diarrhea and concurrent ruminal acidosis (rumen pH < 6.0) had a higher mean D-lactate concentration (6.6 ± 5.2 mmol/L) in blood as compared with calves with a normal rumen pH (5.3 ± 5.4 mmol/L).[9] The author stated that her study could not clarify whether the ruminal acidosis was a cause or a consequence of systemic D-lactic acidosis.

In summary, recent research has demonstrated that D-lactate is responsible for a major portion of the acidemia that generally accompanies diarrhea in calves suckling their dam or fed whole milk. D-lactic acidosis occurs after sufficient amounts of D-lactate have been absorbed from the gastrointestinal tract (primarily colon) and neutralization of the accumulated D-lactate by buffer mechanisms in the body becomes inadequate. Reports of D-lactate concentrations in calves with diarrhea that are being fed milk-replacer diets with or without antimicrobials are unavailable, so it is unknown whether these calves develop D-lactic acidosis to the same degree as calves on whole milk diets.

Metabolic Acidosis in Newly Born Calves With Asphyxia

A further indication for IV fluid therapy in calves is mixed respiratory and metabolic acidosis resulting from birth asphyxia.[55] In calves that suffer from severely depressed uteroplacental gas exchange, the partial pressure of oxygen (pO_2) decreases, which indicates hypoxia, and the partial pressure of CO_2 (pCO_2) increases, which indicates hypercapnia. The resulting mixed respiratory and metabolic acidosis is associated with increased mortality rates when venous blood pH falls below 7.2.[56,57] These calves benefit from IV fluid therapy with sodium bicarbonate solutions to increase blood pH.

Bacteremia, Sepsis, and Endotoxemia

Calves with neonatal diarrhea often have increased numbers of coliform bacteria in their small intestine.[4] This bacterial overgrowth is associated with altered intestinal function, morphologic damage, and increased susceptibility to bacteremia. Studies have documented that bacteremia is a frequent complication of diarrhea in calves.[58,59] Fluid therapy is important for maintaining fluid and electrolyte balance in these calves; however, specific therapy of bacteremia focuses on administration of antibiotics (see the article by Constable found elsewhere in this issue.)

ASSESSING THE NEED FOR INTRAVENOUS FLUID THERAPY

Food animal practitioners generally decide if IV fluid therapy is necessary in sick calves based on clinical examination rather than on laboratory values. Important clinical parameters to guide decision making on fluid therapy are obtained from the evaluation of hydration status and CNS function. Degree of enophthalmus is the best predictor of dehydration in calves, followed by skin elasticity determined on the neck and thorax.[60] More detailed information on the clinical assessment of hydration status in calves is presented in the article by Smith on oral fluid therapy found elsewhere in this issue. In clinically sick calves, it is important to evaluate hydration status along with other clinical signs, including the ability of the calf to suckle, severity of CNS depression, and whether the calf can stand (degree of weakness). These factors in combination are used to determine whether IV fluid therapy is indicated.

Laboratory Tests to Aid the Assessment of Strong Ion Acidosis

Blood-gas and acid-base status can be determined in practice with a portable blood gas analyzer, such as the I-Stat unit (Heska Corporation, Fribourg, Switzerland). These laboratory analyzers are expensive, however, and are not used in most practices. Other less expensive methods for determination of acid-base status use a portable pH meter (Cardy Twin pH meter, Spectrum Technologies, Inc., Plainfield, IL)[61] or the Harleco-System to determine total carbon dioxide concentration.[24,51] To the authors' knowledge, these methods are not widely used in bovine practice. A more detailed presentation of tools for laboratory assessment of acid-base status in bovine field practice is discussed elsewhere.[62]

The concentration of stereospecific D-lactate is determined by high-performance liquid chromatography or via enzymatic measurements.[63] D-lactate has been determined in experimental studies and in teaching hospitals. Portable lactate analyzers for use in practice do exist, but they measure only L-lactate.[62] Determination of D-lactate is not performed in most diagnostic laboratories, and simple assays for use in practice are not available.

Clinical Assessment of Metabolic Acidosis

Assessing and diagnosing metabolic acidosis on the basis of clinical signs are common practice. The predictive accuracy of the degree of metabolic acidosis on the basis of clinical signs has varied among studies. The clinical signs of neurologic depression (weakness, ataxia, and decreased menace, suckle, and panniculus reflex) correlated highly with the severity of metabolic acidosis in calves without dehydration.[52] Also in calves with diarrhea, signs of CNS depression, ability to stand, and suckling force all correlated well with metabolic acidosis.[36,51,64,65] The degree of enophthalmos and peripheral skin temperature are important and obvious signs that determine whether IV fluid therapy is indicated; however, they do not correlate with the degree of metabolic acidosis.[10,24,28,36,51,52]

An important discovery was that metabolic acidosis in calves with diarrhea varies during the first weeks of life. Naylor discovered that metabolic acidosis is less severe during the first week of life than in calves with diarrhea older than 8 days.[36,51] The base deficit in calves with diarrhea that were older than 1 week was almost twice as high as in calves that presented with diarrhea during the first week of life. Subsequent studies confirmed that calves with diarrhea older than 1 week of age usually exhibit a higher base deficit.[24,25,50,66,67] On the basis of his findings, Naylor[68] developed a chart for predicting the severity of metabolic acidosis based on body position, strength of suckle reflex, and age of the calf, with corresponding values for base deficit and bicarbonate requirements for the treatment of metabolic acidosis in calves with diarrhea younger or older than 8 days. This protocol became a popular approach to guide diagnosis and treatment of acidosis in calves with diarrhea and is presented in common veterinary medical textbooks. An even more simplified approach to fluid therapy in the field is presented later in this article.

Another study estimated the base deficit from suckling force or ability to stand without dividing calves into age groups.[69] Data from 65 calves with diarrhea showed that when suckle reflex was strong, weak, or absent, the calves had a mean base deficit of 4.2 mEq/L, 11.4 mEq/L, or 21.5 mEq/L, respectively. The calves standing strongly, weakly, or unable to stand had a mean base deficit of 5.2 mEq/L, 7.8 mEq/L, and 19.1 mEq/L, respectively.[69] Newer studies focusing on the clinical signs associated with D-lactic acidosis have reported only minor differences for the base deficit between calves standing securely compared with calves with diarrhea with a wobbly posture or not able to stand.[10,43] Severe metabolic acidosis from accumulation of D-lactate is likely present in depressed, wobbly, or recumbent calves with no or minimal diarrhea and dehydration.[10,12,14,24,43,52,70]

Clinical Assessment of D-Lactic Acidosis

The recent discovery that D-lactate is responsible for most of the acidemia present in calves with diarrhea with and without dehydration was accompanied by the discovery that D-lactate is also responsible for most of the CNS depression that was formerly been attributed to metabolic acidosis.[10,17,18,43] Practitioners have commonly used depression scores to predict the degree of metabolic acidosis in calves with diarrhea; however, a recent study questioned if the degree of acidosis can be predicted based on the severity of clinical signs, because administration of hydrochloric acid induced severe hyperchloremic metabolic acidosis but no abnormal clinical behavior.[71] Other studies suggested that currently, D-lactate is the most important factor responsible for the clinical signs of weakness and CNS depression in calves with diarrhea.

The first descriptions of D-lactate suggested that it was the major cause of metabolic acidosis in nondehydrated calves without significant diarrhea, a syndrome that is characterized by CNS depression, ataxia, recumbency, and coma.[12,14] A D-lactate concentration up to 2 mmol/L is considered normal;[44] however, values consistently associated with abnormal clinical signs have not been established. Markedly elevated D-lactate concentrations in calves with diarrhea are found when calves show a wobbly posture or cannot stand, exhibit a tired, listless, or comatose behavior, and have a delayed, incomplete, or completely absent palpebral reflex.[10,11,43] The mean D-lactate concentration (between 10 and 11 mmol/L) was approximately four times higher in calves with diarrhea showing these abnormal signs compared with calves with normal posture (secure standing), alert behavior, or a prompt and complete palpebral reflex.[10] Mean D-lactate concentration was 11.0 ± 3.6 mmol/L in calves with diarrhea that were unable to rise or had a wobbly posture; calves that were able to stand without difficulty had a mean D-lactate of 2.4 ± 2.1 mmol/L.[10] Only minor differences were noted for the corresponding base deficit values (18.9 ± 3.9 mEq/L in wobbly or recumbent calves and 16.1 ± 3.5 mEq/L in calves standing securely).

A staggering and drunken appearance also has been described and is often found in calves with diarrhea and ruminal drinking in the authors' experience. D-lactic acidosis in experimentally induced ruminal acidosis was characterized by depression, reduced or absent suckle reflex, dehydration, and recumbency.[15] The degree of dehydration does not correlate well with the degree of acidosis[10,64,72] or D-lactate concentration.[9] A negative correlation between D-lactate concentration in blood and dehydration was described in one study, however.[9] Higher D-lactate concentrations were present in calves with a normal or slightly sunken position of the eyeballs than in calves with clearly sunken eyeballs.[10] The author speculated that this finding may be explained by the preselection of severely sick calves admitted to a teaching hospital.

Increased D-lactate concentrations in blood and cerebrospinal fluid (CSF) are associated with signs of dysfunction of the CNS because D-lactic acid has been identified as a neurotoxic agent.[18] Two studies clearly demonstrated that impaired neurologic function in healthy calves can be reproduced by administration of hypertonic sodium-D-lactate or isotonic DL-lactic acid.[17,18] Calves given D-lactate showed a delayed palpebral reflex, appeared tired and closed their eyes, and had a staggering (ataxic) gait, and some lay down with one foreleg extended backward parallel to the body (a sign seen in some weak calves requiring IV fluid therapy in the authors' experience).[17] The suckle reflex was not depressed in a study that experimentally induced a short-term (2 hours) D-lactic acidosis;[17] nor was it depressed after a short-term (2 hours) hyperchloremic metabolic acidosis after the administration of hydrochloric acid to healthy calves.[71] The infusion of isotonic DL-lactic acid, L-lactic acid, and hydrochloric acid over 6 hours in another study did result in depression of the suckle reflex, however.[18] The weak suckle reflex was more strongly correlated with CSF bicarbonate concentration, base excess values, and blood pH than it was with CSF D-lactate concentrations.[18] It seems that increases in D-lactate alone do not impair the suckle reflex and that a decrease in CSF pH is needed to reduce a calf's suckling ability.[17,18,71] Researchers do not completely understand how the decrease in suckling behavior develops in calves with diarrhea.

In summary, the age of a calf needs to be taken into consideration when assessing the severity of metabolic acidosis and determining bicarbonate requirements of calves with diarrhea.[51] Calves with diarrhea and dehydration during their first week of life are less acidotic than older calves and require less sodium bicarbonate to correct their acidemia. Calves that are unable to stand or have a weak or absent suckle reflex have a more severe acidosis and require intravenous sodium bicarbonate to correct their acidemia. D-lactic acidosis may be present in sick calves with or without diarrhea and dehydration that are recumbent or wobbly, tired, listless or comatose, and have a delayed, incomplete, or absent palpebral reflex. If the suckle reflex is absent or weak or the calf chews irregularly instead of suckling normally, D-lactic acidosis may be the underlying disease state. Clinical assessment for weakness and ability to stand is performed by careful manipulation to help calves stand up (not performed in comatose calves), for duration of anorexia by obtaining history and determining suckle reflex, and for hypothermia by palpation of extremities and recording rectal temperature.

INDICATIONS FOR INTRAVENOUS FLUID THERAPY

The major indications for IV fluid therapy in neonatal calves are (1) dehydration, (2) severe depression, weakness, or inability to stand, (3) anorexia for more than 24 hours, and (4) hypothermia (temperature < 100°F [38.0 °C]) in newborn calves. An estimated dehydration of more than 8% of the calf's body weight is the most widely accepted indication for IV fluid administration,[73] although experimental evidence supporting this as the most appropriate intervention point is currently unavailable. One study demonstrated that calves dehydrated more than 8% required at least 24 hours to be adequately rehydrated with orally administered electrolyte solutions.[74] Calves that are recumbent, severely depressed, or comatose and calves without a suckle reflex also need IV fluid therapy. Calves with rapidly progressing dehydration and consistent profuse watery diarrhea should be treated intravenously rather than rehydrated by ororuminal intubation. If treatment with oral fluids is not successful and only a weak suckle reflex is present, initial IV restoration of fluid and electrolyte deficits is preferred. Collapsed dehydrated calves in severe hypovolemic shock are not able to rapidly resorb sufficient amounts of oral or subcutaneously administered fluids and should receive IV rehydration.[74] Resuscitation by IV fluid administration restores oxygen delivery and removes the metabolic products of poorly perfused tissues.[60]

IV fluids are also recommended in sick calves that show signs of CNS depression and other underlying diseases.[39–41] Severely depressed calves with suspected acidemia (most likely D-lactic acidosis) but without clinical signs of dehydration need IV alkalinizing fluids to restore a normal acid-base status.[14,52,70] Severely depressed calves with acidemia need IV alkalinizing fluids to help to decrease D-lactate concentrations.[5,14] The authors also recommend IV fluid therapy for other diseases or syndromes in sick calves without diarrhea but with a decrease in oral fluid intake from pain or inability to suckle caused by severe respiratory distress. Finally, IV fluid therapy is needed for resuscitation of newly born calves that suffer from asphyxia and mixed respiratory-metabolic acidosis.[56,57]

GOALS OF INTRAVENOUS FLUID THERAPY

In a previous edition of this article, the goals of IV fluid therapy in calves were defined as (1) correcting extracellular dehydration and restoring circulating blood volume, (2) correcting metabolic acidosis (increase blood pH >7.20), (3) correcting mental depression and restoring the suckle reflex, (4) correcting electrolyte abnormalities, (5) correcting the energy deficit, and (6) facilitating repair of damaged intestinal surface.[73] Because of the importance of D-lactate in sick calves with gastrointestinal disease, another goal of fluid therapy in calves is to decrease the concentration of D-lactate. This goal was defined by Naylor and colleagues[5] after D-lactate was identified as an important factor of metabolic acidosis that acts as a neurotoxic agent. The reduction of D-lactate helps to correct depression and restore the suckle reflex. Current research efforts concentrate on the development and evaluation of efficient strategies to decrease D-lactate concentrations.[43,54,75] The administration of IV fluids may speed renal elimination of D-lactate and removal from body compartments such as the brain and CSF.[54]

Administration of IV sodium bicarbonate in calves with D-lactic acidosis had no significant effect on blood D-lactate concentrations 4 hours after starting buffer therapy and did not correct the base deficit in 53% of calves, despite correct calculation of bicarbonate requirements.[43] After 24 hours, the mean D-lactate concentration decreased from 10 mmol/L before therapy to 5.4 mmol/L with administration of sodium bicarbonate followed by isotonic saline. Whether IV fluid therapy alone is sufficient to reduce the D-lactate levels found in acidotic calves with diarrhea is questionable. Administration of oral electrolyte solutions with a high strong ion difference for at least 2 days may help hasten the renal excretion of D-lactate and avoid relapses. A Canadian study reported significant reductions of D-lactate concentrations within 24 hours after starting a treatment protocol with a combination of IV fluids, oral electrolytes, and antibiotics.[75] This study examined the effects of orally administered *Lactobacillus rhamnosus* GG, a probiotic bacteria that does not produce D-lactate. Unfortunately, the probiotic had no effect on D-lactate levels in serum and feces. The exact treatment plan was not presented in this study; however, combining IV buffer therapy and oral electrolytes with antibiotics seems logical for the treating D-lactic acidosis in calves with diarrhea and preventing relapses by controlling bacterial D-lactate production in the gastrointestinal tract with antimicrobials. A study from France suggested milk withdrawal for a short period combined with administration of antibiotics for the treatment of D-lactic acidosis in addition to administration of sodium bicarbonate.[14] Further studies are desperately needed to evaluate the efficacy of various treatment protocols in calves with D-lactic acidosis.

Correcting the energy deficit by adding dextrose seems like a logical indication for IV fluid therapy in calves with diarrhea, but it should be used cautiously. A recent study found that the addition of 100 or 400 g of dextrose to 10 L of isotonic saline and sodium bicarbonate solution for the treatment of calves with diarrhea was associated with a decrease in voluntary milk intake as compared with calves that did not receive dextrose.[76] Another deleterious effect of dextrose administration in adult cattle was a decrease in serum phosphorus concentration.[77] A dextrose-enriched solution seems to be beneficial in newborn calves for the treatment of severe hypothermia during the first 24 hours of life.

SOLUTIONS FOR INTRAVENOUS ADMINISTRATION

Food animal practitioners need only a few crystalloid solutions for effective IV fluid therapy in calves, including isotonic and hypertonic saline (NaCl), isotonic and hypertonic sodium bicarbonate ($NaHCO_3$), acetated or lactated Ringer's solution, and concentrated solutions of dextrose. These solutions are commercially available in most countries and come in plastic bags or bottles that are convenient to use and easily attachable in the environment of single-housed or tied (tethered) calves. If solutions are not commercially available or too expensive for routine use in calves, preparation of homemade, nonsterile solutions with clean tap water has been recommended[78] and is presented elsewhere.[79] This approach is questioned if approved products for use in food animals are available at reasonable costs.

Types of Solutions

Solutions for IV application are classified as crystalloid or colloid and—according to their osmolarity—as hypotonic, isotonic, or hypertonic.[80] Balanced crystalloid solutions have a composition similar to extracellular fluid (ie, lactated Ringer's solution), whereas unbalanced solutions differ from extracellular fluid (ie, 0.9% NaCl). The solutes of crystalloid solutions form a true solution, can be crystallized, and are distributed throughout the extracellular fluid space into all body fluid compartments. Compounds of crystalloid solutions are electrolytes, mainly based on sodium and chloride, and organic compounds like dextrose or lactate. Sodium is the backbone of the extracellular fluid, and solutions based on sodium are always indicated in hypovolemia.[80] To increase or maintain the extracellular volume, isotonic solutions (approximately 300 mOsm/L) must contain a sodium concentration of at least 140 mEq/L. Solutions that contain less sodium do not resuscitate dehydrated calves as effectively as isotonic saline that has a sodium concentration of 154 mEq/L.[81] Sodium-containing solutions should not be used in calves with severe hypoalbuminemia because they decrease plasma albumin concentration and oncotic pressure, which forces fluid movement into the interstitial space and exacerbates tissue edema.[80] Calves known to have hypoalbuminemia before the start of IV fluid therapy benefit from the administration of colloid solutions or blood transfusion.

Colloids are substances with a high molecular weight that are too large to pass through a semipermeable membrane. Colloid substances are restricted to the plasma compartment and provide sustained plasma volume expansion. Examples of colloid solutions are whole blood, blood substitutes, plasma, and high molecular glucose polymers such as dextran preparations (dextran-70) and hydroxyethyl starch preparations (hetastarch and pentastarch). The basics and the use of colloid solutions in cattle were discussed in the November 2003 issue of *Veterinary Clinics of North America: Food Animal Practice*.[80]

Alkalinizing Solutions

Because acidemia is common in calves with gastrointestinal disease requiring IV fluid therapy, these patients need administration of alkalinizing substances.[82] Sodium bicarbonate is the alkalinizing agent of choice and is often recommended as a 1.3% isotonic solution (13 g NaHCO$_3$/L).[66,73,80,83–85] Isotonic sodium bicarbonate has an effective strong ion difference of 155 mEq/L and is alkalinizing because it buffers hydrogen ions and increases the strong ion difference in blood. Many studies have documented that sodium bicarbonate is the most important buffer for the treatment of acidemia in calves with and without dehydration. Available hypertonic preparations of sodium bicarbonate include 4.2%, 5%, and 8.4% solutions with a theoretic osmolality of 1000 mOsm/L, 1190 mOsm/L, and 2000 mOsm/L, respectively. Hypertonic formulations of sodium bicarbonate are ideal for adding to larger quantities of isotonic saline to create a mildly hypertonic solution containing volume-expanding fluid and buffer.[39,66,78] Sodium bicarbonate (NaHCO$_3$) is available in 100-mL or 250-mL glass bottles as 4.2% or 8.4% hypertonic formulations, which provides for easy calculation of the volumes for buffer requirements because 1 mL of 8.4% sodium bicarbonate provides 1 mEq of buffer (HCO$_3^-$). One or two (250 mL) bottles of 8.4% sodium bicarbonate can easily be added to a 5 L bag of isotonic saline with a large syringe and mixed on the farm just before administration to avoid potential contamination.[39,66] In North America, 500-mL bottles of 5% sodium bicarbonate are widely available and contain 0.6 mEq of HCO$_3^-$ per milliliter (298 mEq per bottle). Administration of undiluted 4.2% or 2.1% sodium bicarbonate has been recommended at a dosage of 500 mL to 1000 mL for resuscitation of comatose or severely acidotic calves before starting a volume-expanding or replacement solution.[35]

Administration of undiluted 8.4% hypertonic sodium bicarbonate solution should be used with caution, especially in dehydrated calves that are unable to suckle. Potential adverse effects of hypertonic sodium bicarbonate include hyperosmolality of extracellular fluid, hypokalemia, hypernatremia, hypocalcemia, and paradoxic intracellular and CSF acidosis. A recent study administered 8.4% hypertonic sodium bicarbonate (10 mL/kg over 8 minutes) or 5.85% hypertonic saline solution (5 mL/kg over 4 minutes) followed by oral electrolytes to dehydrated calves with diarrhea and severe acidosis.[67] Administration of 8.4% hypertonic sodium bicarbonate resulted in greater cure rates as compared with hypertonic saline. Although no significant clinical side effects were observed, the authors warned against using hypertonic (high sodium) solutions in calves with hypernatremia.[67] Hypertonic sodium bicarbonate should not be used in calves with diarrhea that have concurrent respiratory disease, because they may not be able to effectively exhale the excess CO_2 generated in buffer reactions.

There are conflicting data on the ability of 8.4% hypertonic sodium bicarbonate solution to induce a paradoxic intracellular and CSF acidosis in normovolemic calves. The administration of 5 mL/kg of 8.4% $NaHCO_3$ over 5 minutes to nondehydrated calves with an experimentally induced respiratory and metabolic acidosis did not result in a paradoxic acidosis of CSF in one study,[55] whereas in another study a paradoxic CSF acidosis was reported in calves after treatment of an induced strong ion acidosis with sodium bicarbonate (formulation of solution not given).[86] A 5% hypertonic sodium bicarbonate formulation has been used for the treatment of newborn calves with asphyxia accompanied by a mixed (respiratory and metabolic) acidosis.[56,57] The dose of sodium bicarbonate was determined on the basis of the base deficit and body weight. These two studies did not report significant side effects, and there was no increase in the partial pressure of carbon dioxide (pCO_2) of blood to indicate the development of a paradoxic acidosis in blood.

Lactate and acetate are metabolizable bases and are included in popular polyionic solutions (lactated Ringer's and acetated Ringer's). Both substances produce an alkalinizing effect because they are metabolized predominantly to bicarbonate (HCO_3^-); however, they do not alkalinize as rapidly as sodium bicarbonate.[80] Sodium-L-lactate showed a delayed effect in increasing blood pH when compared with sodium bicarbonate.[64] A theoretic disadvantage of commercially available lactated Ringer's solution is that the lactate is a racemic equimolar mixture of L-lactate and D-lactate, and it should be avoided in severely acidemic calves with a blood pH of less than 7.2 because D-lactate concentrations already may be increased.[11,14,80] Acetated Ringer's solution is theoretically superior to lactated Ringer's solution because acetate is metabolized faster and alkalinization is more rapid. Acetate would not exacerbate D- and L-lactic acidosis.[64] A disadvantage of commercially available acetated Ringer's solutions is that it contains gluconate, which is slowly metabolized by neonatal calves.[87] Despite these concerns, lactated Ringer's solution is popular and still widely used by practitioners. In general, acetated or lactated Ringer's solution is preferred to correct a less severe acidemia (pH > 7.20 or base deficit < 10 mEq/L), and sodium bicarbonate should be used for the treatment of severe acidemia in sick calves.

Nonalkalinizing Solutions

Nonalkalinizing solutions are more frequently used in fluid therapy for adult cattle because they tend to get alkalemic instead of acidemic.[82] Besides isotonic saline solution (0.9% NaCl), the classic balanced polyionic and isotonic crystalloid fluid for adult ruminants is Ringer's solution, which contains physiologic concentrations of sodium, potassium, calcium, and chloride. The addition of dextrose to IV fluid solutions is popular to provide energy during cold weather and counteract negative energy balance in calves with diarrhea. This practice should be questioned because of a recent study that showed that the addition of either 100 or 400 g of dextrose to 10 L of saline and sodium bicarbonate IV fluids (given over 24 hours) resulted in decreased milk intake as compared with calves that received the same fluids but without dextrose.[76] In that study, adding dextrose to the fluids was also accompanied by an increase in the amount of sodium bicarbonate that was necessary to correct the base deficit.

Administration of crystalloid solutions that do not contain an alkalinizing agent have a strong ion difference of zero (ie, isotonic saline or Ringer's solution) and are acidifying because they decrease the normal strong ion difference in calves.[80] Solutions without an alkalinizing agent induce a strong ion acidosis and should be used cautiously in calves with acidemia.[74,80] Several studies documented that isotonic saline or small amounts of hypertonic saline solutions do not significantly alter base deficits in healthy or acidemic calves.[64,67,74,87,88]

In summary, alkalinizing fluids are the appropriate choice for the IV rehydration of calves with diarrhea and dehydration (**Fig. 2**). Currently, isotonic sodium bicarbonate (1.3% = 13 g of $NaHCO_3$/L = 155 mEq HCO_3^-/L + 155 mEq Na^+/L) at a dose of 1 to 4 L is the recommended solution for IV treatment of calves with diarrhea. Isotonic sodium bicarbonate rapidly corrects acidosis and dehydration and restores normal cellular function. When a calf's suckle reflex is re-established, further treatment can be given orally. Undiluted 8.4% hypertonic sodium bicarbonate solutions should be used with caution in severely dehydrated calves with diarrhea but are ideal for adding to larger quantities of isotonic saline. Correcting dehydration with rapid administration of small volumes of hypertonic saline solution (4–5 mL/kg body weight, 7.2% NaCl or 7.2% NaCl in 6% dextran-70) successfully resuscitates dehydrated calves but does not correct metabolic acidosis. Administration of hypertonic saline solutions should be accompanied by IV sodium bicarbonate in severely acidemic calves or by oral alkalinizing agents (acetate, propionate) in mildly to moderately acidemic calves.[67] For additional information, a detailed review of solutions used for fluid and electrolyte therapy in ruminants was published in the November 2003 issue of *Veterinary Clinics of North America: Food Animal Practice*.[80]

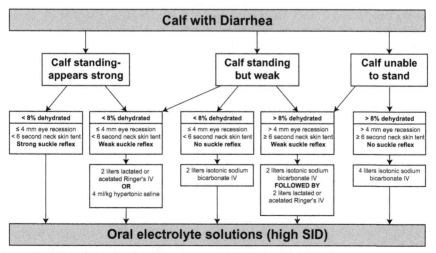

Fig. 2. Algorithm for initial fluid therapy of dehydrated calves with diarrhea.

AURICULAR VEIN CATHETERIZATION IN CALVES

The focus of this section is on catheterization of the auricular vein in calves. Catheterization of the jugular vein is still widely used for fluid therapy in calves and adult cattle.[35,78] Other routes for administration of fluids in cattle have been presented but are not considered in this article. Schmid and Rüsse[89] were the first to describe the technique of auricular vein catheterization in neonatal calves using a small flexible catheter, and the method quickly became popular among practitioners in Germany and other countries.[90–92] Even in severely dehydrated calves, ear vein catheterization is possible, and a surgical cutdown of the jugular vein (which is often performed in severely dehydrated calves) can be avoided. Ear catheters allow the administration of adequate volumes of fluids by continuous drip infusion to calves.[73,91,93,94] Despite the lack of studies comparing the use of ear vein catheters with other approaches in calves, this technique is believed to result in fewer complications compared with jugular catheters.[95] In pigs, long-term ear vein catheterization for 7 to 14 days was superior to jugular catheterization.[96] In this study, jugular vein catheters occluded more often and caused thrombophlebitis, whereas ear catheters showed no reactions. A study that evaluated the use of auricular vein catheters in adult cattle stated that this technique is easy to perform, safe, and less expensive because fewer catheters need to be discarded.[91]

The ear vein approach initially should be practiced in calves with minimal or no dehydration before trying to catheterize severely dehydrated calves. Initially, it may be difficult to place a catheter into the ear of a severely dehydrated calf with a collapsed and small auricular vein. Blocking the vein with a tourniquet becomes essential for proper placement of the catheter. Small rubber bands are recommended and usually fit well around the base of the ear. To achieve better distention and visualization of the ear vein, gauze soaked with warm water can be applied to the ear for a short period of time to increase regional blood flow. The catheterization site needs to be shaved or clipped and prepared aseptically with iodine or alcohol before catheter insertion. The alcohol or iodine solution also acts as a lubricant and aids the advancement of the catheter into the ear. Lidocaine anesthesia of the venipuncture site is not necessary and is not recommended for ear vein catheterization. Subcutaneous administration of lidocaine creates a fluid bubble, which makes the vein difficult to visualize. Mild sedation with xylazine is occasionally necessary in vigorous calves that do not have any CNS depression; however, xylazine is not needed and should be avoided in severely dehydrated calves with hypovolemic shock because it further decreases blood pressure and causes the ear vein to collapse.

Current recommendations for ear vein catheterization in neonatal calves are to use a 22 gauge, 1-in (0.9 × 25 mm) over-the-needle catheter (ie, Vasocan Braunüle, B. Braun Melsungen AG, Melsungen, Germany) with a butterfly-shaped wing. Other suitable catheters for ear vein catheterization should incorporate a guide wire needle to facilitate easier placement. Older calves and adult cattle require larger gauge sizes for increased flow rates. A disadvantage of the over-the-needle catheters is that they may fray or splinter at the tip during insertion and then must be discarded. Advancing an already frayed catheter should be avoided because it damages the internal wall of the vein and increases the risk of thrombosis.[97]

The anatomy of the ear veins may differ slightly among calves. Normally there are one or two cranial, one medial, and one caudal ear vein that are large enough for catheterization. Identification of the ear vessels is important to avoid arterial puncture or placement of the catheter into the auricular artery. This artery is located between the cranial ear vein and the medial ear vein. It is usually more prominent than the ear veins and is visible even before applying a tourniquet. Identification of the auricular artery by palpating for a pulse is difficult; however, the artery feels harder than the veins and can be rolled under the skin. The author prefers the cranial ear vein for catheterization (**Fig. 3**A) followed by the medial vein. The cranial vein runs dorsally across the auricular pinna, which is flatter and more rigid than the caudal part of the ear. Catheterization should begin as far distally as possible to allow for repeated attempts more proximally if the first attempt is not successful. If the tip of the catheter lies too close to the base of the ear, the fluid flow rate may be slow.

Procedure for Auricular Vein Catheterization

The following steps are used to proceed with auricular vein catheterization:

1. First prepare all materials needed, including fluids, 22-gauge catheter, infusion line, tourniquet (rubber bands), razor, iodine or alcohol solution spray, scissors, tape, bandage, and a light source (**Figs. 3** and **4**).
2. Warm all fluids during cold weather.
3. Prepare four strips of tape 12 to 15 in (30–40 cm) long and attach them loose nearby.
4. Use right ear if right handed and left ear if left handed.
5. Place rubber band as a tourniquet around the base of the ear to distend veins (see **Fig. 3**A).
6. Spray the area for catheter placement, preferably the cranial third of the ear, vigorously with iodine and alcohol.
7. Shave dorsal pinna of the ear carefully with a single razor.

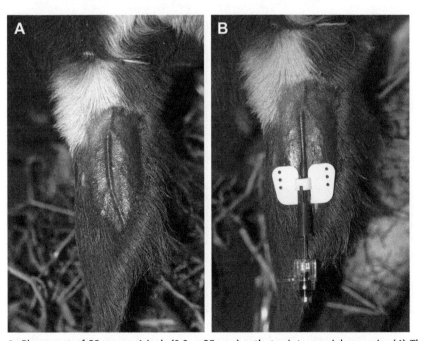

Fig. 3. Placement of 22 gauge 1-inch (0.9 × 25 mm) catheter into cranial ear vein. (*A*) The vein is blocked with a rubber band at the base of the ear. The venipuncture site is shaved and sprayed with alcohol. (*B*) The catheter is advanced into the vein at least 0.5 in (1 cm) at once. The guide wire steel needle is then retracted slightly before the catheter is fully advanced into the ear vein. Confirm correct catheter position by checking for blood in the catheter hub and then withdraw guide wire needle completely.

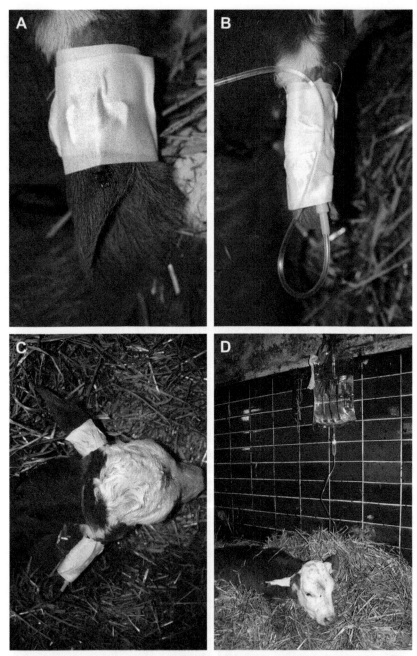

Fig. 4. (*A*) Fixation of the ear vein catheter with one strip of adhesive tape after removing rubber band. Press adhesive tape firmly to the ear. (*B*) Fix the fluid line in a loop with second strip of adhesive tape. (*C*) Fix the fluid line to the opposite ear with a third strip of adhesive tape. (*D*) Administration of 5 L isotonic saline spiked with 250 mL 8.4% sodium bicarbonate by ear vein catheterization under field conditions.

8. Spray the catheterization site again (or scrub with iodine solution and swab with alcohol) to achieve easier sliding of catheter.
9. Identify a suitable ear vein after allowing some time for the vessels to distend. A straight and 2-cm long vein is suitable (see **Fig. 3**A).
10. If the vein does not properly distend in severely dehydrated or hypothermic calves, apply a sponge or gauze soaked with warm water to increase blood flow to the ear.
11. Prepare the catheter by gently moving the needle of the catheter back and forth to allow easy retraction of the needle after being inserted. Hold ear straight with one hand and bend the ear a little.
12. Advance the tip of the catheter into the distended vein at least 0.5 in (1 cm) in one movement. Expect some head and/or ear shaking and be prepared to move with the calf.
13. Confirm that the catheter is in the vein by watching for blood flow into the hub of the catheter before slightly withdrawing the needle (**Fig. 3**B).
14. Advance the catheter completely into the vein and then remove the needle. Do not reinsert the needle into the catheter after withdrawing it because this may shear the catheter and potentially result in damage to the blood vessel.
15. Fix catheter with first tape strip to the ear and press tape firmly (**Fig. 4**A).
16. Remove tourniquet (rubber band) with razor or scissors.
17. Check for correct catheter placement by examining for blood flow out of the catheter hub or by flushing the catheter.
18. Hang the fluids, connect the fluid line (include an extension set if necessary), connect the fluid line, and open the fluids completely (again checking for correct catheter placement).
19. Tape the catheter with a loop of the fluid line (extension set) to the ear with a second strip of tape (**Fig. 4**B). If necessary, place a gauze roll of adequate size inside the ear to allow better and more forceful taping. Do not tape in front of the catheter tip.
20. Tape the fluid line to the base of the opposite ear with third strip of tape (**Fig. 4**C).
21. Avoid stress and manipulation in severely compromised calves. Usually calves with severe dehydration and acidosis are depressed or comatose. These cases require almost no assistance from another person to place an ear catheter. If calves are more active, however, it is the authors' preference to use the least amount of restraint possible and attempt placement of the catheter without assistance. If necessary, light sedation can be used.

Catheter-Related Complications

Over-the-needle catheters slide out easily when the animal moves or during manipulation of the catheter before securing it with tape.[97] For secure fixation, the catheter can be sutured to the ear using an injection needle and monofilament suture material.[73] Suturing the catheter to the ear is usually not necessary because most calves that require IV fluids are depressed or comatose and do not move vigorously. Attaching the catheter to the pinna with cyanoacrylate (tissue glue),[92] using a gauze roll placed inside the ear, and taping the catheter with bandage material have been recommended for better catheter fixation.[91] The risk of damaging catheters in ear veins attached with two strips of tape is minimal if the calf is confined. If the calf is able to move its head in and out of a gate or a hole in the hutch, however, the ear catheter may dislodge or the fluid line may become disconnected from the catheter. To avoid this complication, calves can be tethered during IV fluid therapy. The fluid line is not easily accessible for chewing or biting if the fluid bag is hanging above the calf.

Puncturing a vein damages the wall of the blood vessel and traumatizes the surrounding tissue. Bacterial contamination of the vessel often follows. Complications of IV catheterization include phlebitis and extravasation of fluids or blood with infiltration of surrounding tissue forming subcutaneous edema or hematoma.[95,97] The perivascular administration of fluids normally does not result in serious complications in calves if isotonic or mildly hypertonic solutions are administered. If the catheter is not correctly placed or is not advanced far enough into the vein, movement of the animal may cause displacement of the catheter. The signs of perivascular infusion include a slower infusion rate and swelling around the injection site. If the tip of the catheter is located close to the base of the ear, flow rates may be negatively affected.

Reports on catheter-related complications in cattle have focused primarily on problems associated with jugular vein catheterization. Thrombosis is the most frequent complication and results in thrombophlebitis, periphlebitis, and systemic infection.[95,97–99] Severe thrombophlebitis of the jugular veins in cattle is characterized by a painful and warm swelling around the jugular vein, increased rectal temperature, reduced feed intake, and abnormal behavior.[99] Auricular vein catheterization is believed to result in fewer complications compared with jugular vein catheterization.[91,95] Severe infections have not been observed by the author after using the ear vein catheterization technique in hundreds of calves. Arterial puncture is a common complication of jugular catheterization, resulting in the formation of large hematomas. Puncture of the artery is also a serious complication of ear vein catheterization, although it can be avoided by identifying this vessel. If an ear artery is catheterized accidentally, the brighter color of the blood or a slow infusion rate is usually obvious. An ear vein catheter can be left in place for several days without significant complications. In the authors' experience, calves with ear catheters left in place for up to 7 days had only minor swelling with no evidence of thrombophlebitis. Most catheters can be removed by the producer after 2 days if the calf is able to suckle and maintain a normal hydration status. Changing ear catheters is not needed as often as compared with jugular catheters.[91] Although it tends to be a common criticism of ear vein catheters, slow fluid flow rates are almost never a problem; however, ear catheters do tend to occlude more than jugular catheters.[91]

ADMINISTRATION OF INTRAVENOUS FLUIDS

Many studies have presented various protocols for IV fluid therapy in calves; however, clinical research comparing the effectiveness of different protocols in dehydrated calves with diarrhea has not been done.[80] In practice, fluid therapy has to be simple and cost effective and must be based on clinical signs that are easily assessed. **Fig. 2** shows a simple flow chart with guidelines for resuscitation of dehydrated calves. The focus of this algorithm is on restoration of the suckle reflex to allow for further rehydration and maintenance fluid therapy to be given orally. European teaching hospitals and practitioners have recommended larger quantities (5–20 L) of volume-expanding and maintenance IV fluids for periods of 24 hours or longer.[35,78] To determine daily fluid requirements, estimated amounts for replacement, maintenance, and ongoing losses (for diarrhea) must be calculated. The quantity of replacement fluid in liters is calculated by multiplying the estimated dehydration in percentage with body weight in kilograms according to the following formula:

Replacement fluid [L] = dehydration[%] × bodyweight [kg]

A maximum rate of 80 mL/kg/h for IV fluid administration has been used without inducing significant overhydration and hypertension.[64] This rate is equivalent to a maximum fluid volume of 2.8 L/h for a 35-kg (77-lb) calf or 1 gallon (3.8 L) per hour for a 47-kg (104-lb) severely dehydrated calf. Higher flow rates are not recommended. Slower infusion rates of 30 to 50 mL/kg/h are often used to avoid overhydration and pulmonary edema. A recent study gave the first liter within 30 minutes and the subsequent dose of 3 L over the following 2.5 hours,[100] which is in agreement with the slower rate of 30 to 40 mL/kg/h reported by Roussel.[101] With a rate of 30 to 40 mL/kg/h, a 40-kg calf with 10% dehydration can be rehydrated within 3 to 4 hours. Daily maintenance fluid volumes of 80 to 100 mL/kg and ongoing losses of up to 7 L/d should be added to calculate the daily fluid requirements. If a calf can suckle after initial resuscitation, however, these fluid requirements can be given orally to reduce costs.

Measurements of buffer needs are based on formulas for extracellular base excess (from blood gas analysis) or plasma total carbon dioxide concentration. Values calculated from blood gas analysis multiply base deficit with body weight and with a factor that considers the volume of distribution for bicarbonate ions in the body (0.5–0.6) according to the following formula:[51,101]

$$\text{Bicarbonate requirement [mEq]} = \text{body weight [kg]}$$
$$\times \text{ base deficit [mEq/L]}$$
$$\times 0.5 - 0.6 \text{ [L/kg]}$$

Values above 1.0 for calculating bicarbonate requirements have been reported—a finding that was attributed to ongoing fecal and renal losses of bicarbonate, along with ongoing production of organic acids in the gastrointestinal tract.[50] Another study recommended a distribution factor of 1.0 to consider the ongoing losses that accompany diarrhea.[93] Values of 1.0 or more seem much too high to be used to correct existing deficits as supported by a report from Japan, which found a much lower distribution factor of bicarbonate (0.367) in dehydrated calves with diarrhea.[84] More recent research showed that calves with acidemia from D-lactic acidosis need more sodium bicarbonate to buffer the metabolic acidosis and to decrease D-lactate concentration below 3 mmol/L.[43]

Practitioners must rely on clinical signs and the guidelines developed by Naylor based on standing ability, suckling force, and age of calves with diarrhea to predict if alkalinizing therapy is indicated and how much isotonic sodium bicarbonate should be administered. Because determining the severity of acidosis on the farm is difficult and costly, buffer administration is commonly done without any laboratory data. The clinical response of the calf to IV fluid therapy must be monitored. Urination within 30 to 60 minutes, improvement of mental and hydration status, and, most importantly, restoration of the suckle reflex are monitored as responses to treatment.[78,102] Recumbent calves should stand within a few hours of IV fluid therapy. If the suckle reflex does not return after IV buffer therapy, other diseases, such as septicemia, omphalitis, or pneumonia, should be ruled out.[103]

An easy but successful guideline for the treatment of severely dehydrated calves with diarrhea and acidosis is administration of isotonic sodium bicarbonate solution at approximately 10% body weight over a period of several hours.[94] This protocol had a success rate of 91% without calculating buffer requirements, fluid rates, or maintenance requirements. Ninety calves with a mean base deficit of −19.0 ± 3.8 mEq/L (pH 7.06 ± 0.22) received approximately 10% of their body weight as isotonic sodium bicarbonate solution (1.26% = 12.6 g/L instead of the more widely used 1.3%). The first half was given rapidly over 2 to 3 hours, which equals an administration rate of approximately 20 mL/kg/h. After 3 hours, when approximately 5% body weight of isotonic sodium bicarbonate had been infused, 77% of the calves were able to suckle water again. Milk replacer was continuously fed in that study; however, oral electrolytes were not given. Additional replacement therapy with 2 to 4 L of Ringer's or isotonic sodium chloride was given to 16 calves.[94] Another practical technique for a 40- to 50-kg, severely dehydrated and comatose calf is to give 2 L of isotonic sodium bicarbonate rapidly and then switch fluid to an isotonic mixture of sodium chloride and sodium bicarbonate.[104]

A Simplified Protocol for Farm Intravenous Fluid Therapy

A simplified protocol for IV fluid therapy by ear vein catheterization in calves used in the authors' practice is presented in this section. Calves are examined for dehydration by evaluating the eyeball position within the orbit, for weakness and ability to stand by careful manipulation (not performed in comatose calves), for duration of anorexia by obtaining history and determining suckle reflex, and for hypothermia by palpating extremities and oral cavity and obtaining rectal temperature.

The standard treatment protocol for IV fluid therapy consists of a 5-L bag of isotonic saline (0.9% NaCl) to which 250 mL of 8.4% hypertonic sodium bicarbonate (total of 250 mEq HCO_3^-) is added (**Fig. 5**). This mixture creates a slightly hypertonic solution and is recommended for use in calves younger than 1 week. All solutions are commercially available, and isotonic saline solution is supplied in plastic bags that are easily attachable in the calf's environment (see **Fig. 4D**). Calves that present with relapses after administration of this standard protocol receive another treatment when they are able to suckle. Calves that fail to significantly improve in attitude, have a weak or absent suckle reflex, or show consistent weakness after one or two administrations of the standard (5-L) IV fluid solution are generally suspected of having a more severe acidosis. These calves receive fluids that contain a higher amount of sodium bicarbonate, especially when they are older than 1 week of age. Up to 750 mL of 8.4% sodium bicarbonate (750 mEq HCO_3^-) can be added to the 5-L bag of isotonic saline. Calves with ongoing relapses of dehydration or depression after repeated administrations of

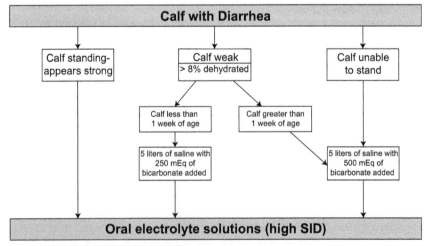

Fig. 5. Simplified algorithm for fluid therapy of dehydrated calves. This approach requires that the practitioner carry only 5-L bags of 0.9% saline and 250-mL or 500-mL bottles of hypertonic sodium bicarbonate in practice. 8.4% sodium bicarbonate contains 1 mEq of bicarbonate per milliliter (so a 250-mL bottle equals 250 mEq of bicarbonate). 5% sodium bicarbonate contains 0.6 mEq of bicarbonate per milliliter (so a 500-mL bottle contains 298 mEq of bicarbonate).

this standard IV protocol, with or without a higher dose of sodium bicarbonate, receive a transfusion of whole blood (800–1000 mL) through the same fluid line. All IV fluid therapy is performed by ear vein catheterization using a 22-gauge IV catheter placed under aseptic conditions. In calves with dehydration or severe depression, a maximum flow rate is preferred, which allows administration of 1 to 2 L/h. In normally hydrated calves, slower flow rates are used (0.5–0.75 L/h). Milk may be withheld for one feeding if D-lactic acidosis is suspected; however, milk feeding normally is continued.

COMPLICATIONS OF INTRAVENOUS FLUID THERAPY
Technical Problems

Complications associated with IV catheterization were previously described. Problems in maintaining a continuous fluid line on farm for extended periods of time are primarily caused by lack of observation. Fluids may run out, which is usually followed by clotting of the catheter. Twisting or kinking of the fluid line is frequently observed if the lines are in place for several days and if the calf begins to recover and starts moving around in the stall or hutch. It is difficult to perform long-term (maintenance) IV fluid therapy without fluid line problems in an unobserved calf. When the calf begins moving freely in its stall, the infusion line can be coiled and is often occluded after bending. Complications with maintaining a permanent fluid line can be reduced by using coiled infusion sets, self-retractable dog leashes, or elastic bands[92] to which the infusion line is taped. Because of the difficulty associated maintaining a fluid line for long-term fluid therapy, maintenance fluid therapy in calves is best performed orally.

Hypothermia

Hypothermia is often a significant pre-existing problem in newborn calves without a suckle reflex during the first 24 hours of life and in calves with diarrhea and dehydration.[37] Particularly during periods of cold weather, administration of larger fluid volumes can exacerbate the hypothermia. IV therapy during cold weather conditions with large fluid volumes is almost impossible without creating or exacerbating hypothermia. Calves that receive IV fluids should be moved inside a building where external heating can be provided efficiently by heat lamps or some other type of heat source. The fluid line may be wrapped or looped around a heat lamp or passed through the metal cage of the heat lamp. In freezing weather conditions, however, it is almost impossible to avoid creating some degree of hypothermia in sick calves with or without dehydration that receive large volumes of IV fluids.

Overhydration

Overhydration may occur when fluids are administered too rapidly or with administration rates that increase intravascular pressure to an extent that pulmonary edema develops.[105] Clinical signs of overhydration and pulmonary edema include nasal discharge, tachypnea, tachycardia, coughing, and wet lung sounds (crackles).[95] If the central venous pressure exceeds 12 cm of water (measured at the level of the scapulohumeral joint in calves), the vascular pressure is too high and the infusion rate should be reduced or stopped temporarily.[64] In a study that used a high flow rate (80 mL/kg/h), central venous pressure increased in almost one third of dehydrated calves but signs of pulmonary edema were not detected.[64] In practice, it is not possible to determine an accurate body weight. An infusion rate slower than 80 mL/kg/h is preferred to avoid overhydration and development of pulmonary, interstitial, or cerebral edema. Anemia and hypoproteinemia also may follow overhydration, leading to hypoxia if the packed cell volume falls below 15%. Formation of interstitial edema occurs if total protein concentrations drop below 4 mg/dL.[95] To the authors' knowledge, these complications have not been reported in the literature of calves and may be overlooked because of lack of observation on the farm. It seems unlikely that severe overhydration of calves would occur with flow rates that can be accomplished through a small (22-gauge) ear vein catheter, however.

Other Potential Adverse Effects of Intravenous Fluid Administration

The ideal composition of IV fluids for the treatment of calves with diarrhea and dehydration is unknown, and no studies have compared the effectiveness of different IV fluid therapy protocols on long-term survival of calves with diarrhea. Potential adverse effects of IV fluid administration on serum concentration of electrolytes, enzymatic activities, and voluntary intake of milk or oral electrolytes have not been investigated extensively. One study reported that the administration of isotonic sodium bicarbonate in calves with diarrhea was followed by a decrease in concentrations of potassium, magnesium, total calcium, and ionized calcium.[22] The clinical significance of these findings is unknown, and the authors did not recommend any treatments other than the administration of sodium bicarbonate or calcium.[22] In newborn calves with a mixed respiratory and metabolic acidosis (birth asphyxia), the administration of a hypertonic 5% sodium bicarbonate solution was followed by a decrease in total calcium concentration; however, concentrations of potassium, magnesium, and inorganic phosphorus were not affected 120 minutes after treatment.[57] A study on the long-term effects of neonatal diarrhea and its treatment with IV sodium bicarbonate, glucose, and electrolyte solutions followed by oral electrolytes found significantly lower serum concentrations of sodium, magnesium, and total calcium up to 10 days after the last treatment was administered compared with healthy control calves.[30] Base excess values of treated calves were significantly lower than those found in healthy control calves, and potassium concentrations were lower, although not statistically significant.

REFERENCES

1. United States Department of Agriculture. Part II: changes in the United States dairy industry, 1991–2002. #N388.0603. Fort Collins (CO): National Animal Health Monitoring System; 2002.
2. Svensson C, Linder A, Olsson SO. Mortality in Swedish dairy calves and replacement heifers. J Dairy Sci 2006;89:4769–77.
3. Haschek B, Klein D, Benetka V, et al. Detection of bovine torovirus in neonatal calf diarrhoea in lower Austria and Styria (Austria). J Vet Med B Infect Dis Vet Public Health 2006;53:160–5.
4. Constable PD. Antimicrobial use in the treatment of calf diarrhea. J Vet Intern Med 2004;18:8–17.
5. Naylor JM, Zello GA, Abeysekara S. Advances in oral and intravenous fluid therapy of calves with gastrointestinal disease. In: Proceedings of the 24th World Buiatrics Congress. Nice, France; 2006. p. 139–50.
6. Ewaschuk JB, Naylor JM, Zello GA. Anion gap correlates with serum D- and DL-lactate concentration in diarrheic neonatal calves. J Vet Intern Med 2003;17:940–2.
7. Ewaschuk JB, Naylor JM, Palmer R, et al. D-Lactate production and excretion in diarrheic calves. J Vet Intern Med 2004;18:744–7.
8. Ewaschuk JB, Naylor JM, Zello GA. D-Lactate in human and ruminant metabolism. J Nutr 2005;135:1619–25.

9. Lorenz I. Investigations on the influence of serum D-lactate levels on clinical signs in calves with metabolic acidosis. Vet J 2004;168:323–7.

10. Lorenz I. Influence of D-lactate on metabolic acidosis and on prognosis in neonatal calves with diarrhoea. J Vet Med A Physiol Pathol Clin Med 2004;51:425–8.

11. Lorenz I. D-Lactic acidosis in calves. Vet J, in press; corrected proof available online doi:10.1016/j.tvjl.2007.08.028.

12. Navetat H, Biron P, Contrepois M, et al. Paralysing gastroenteritis: disease or syndrome? Bull Acad Vét Fr 1997;70:327–36.

13. Omole OO, Nappert G, Naylor JM, et al. Both L- and D-lactate contribute to metabolic acidosis in diarrheic calves. J Nutr 2001;131:2128–31.

14. Schelcher F, Marcillaud S, Braun JP, et al. Metabolic acidosis without dehydration and no or minimal diarrhoea in suckler calves is caused by hyper-D-lactatemia. In: Proceedings of the 20th World Buiatrics Congress. Sydney, Australia; 1998. p. 371–4.

15. Gentile A, Sconza S, Lorenz I, et al. D-Lactic acidosis in calves as a consequence of experimentally induced ruminal acidosis. J Vet Med A Physiol Pathol Clin Med 2004;51:64–70.

16. Bleul U, Schwantag S, Stocker H, et al. Floppy kid syndrome caused by D-lactic acidosis in goat kids. J Vet Intern Med 2006;20:1003–8.

17. Lorenz I, Gentile A, Klee W. Investigations of D-lactate metabolism and the clinical signs of D-lactataemia in calves. Vet Rec 2005;156:412–5.

18. Abeysekara S, Naylor JM, Wassef AWA, et al. D-Lactic acid-induced neurotoxicity in a calf model. Am J Physiol 2007;293:E558–65.

19. Hartmann H, Finsterbusch L, Lesche R. Fluid balance of calves. II. Fluid volume in relation to age and the influence of diarrhoea. Arch Exp Vet Med 1984;38:913–22.

20. Doll K, Weirather P, Küchle HM. Calf diarrhoea as a herd problem: effects of husbandry and management and frequent errors in treatment. Prakt Tierarzt 1995;76:995–1004.

21. Hartmann H, Reder S. Effect of dehydration on functional indicators of fluid metabolism in calves and the efficacy of rehydration with crystalline or colloidal saline infusions. Tierärztl Prax 1995;23:342–50.

22. Grove-White D, Michell AR. Iatrogenic hypocalcemia during parenteral fluid therapy of diarrhoeic calves. Vet Rec 2001;149:203–7.

23. Doll K. Studies on the secretory process and osmotic mechanism in the pathogenesis of neonatal diarrhoea in calves. In: Proceedings of the 18th World Buiatrics Congress. Bologna, Italy; 1994. p. 411–4.

24. Grove-White DH, White DG. Diagnosis and treatment of metabolic acidosis in calves: a field study. Vet Rec 1993;133:499–501.

25. Berchtold J. Untersuchungen zur Diagnose und Behandlung systemischer Azidosen bei Kälbern [thesis]. [Investigations on the diagnosis and treatment of systemic acidosis in calves]. Berlin: Free University of Berlin; 1998 [in German].

26. Abutarbush SM, Petrie L. Treatment of hypernatremia in neonatal calves with diarrhea. Can Vet J 2007;48:184–7.

27. Maach L, Gründer HD, Boujija A. Clinical and haematological investigations in newborn Holstein-Friesian calves with diarrhoea in Morocco. Dtsch Tierärztl Wochenschr 1992;99:133–40.

28. Constable PD, Walker PG, Morin DE, et al. Clinical and laboratory assessment of hydration status of neonatal calves with diarrhea. J Am Vet Med Assoc 1998;212:991–6.

29. Constable PD, Stämpfli HR, Navetat H, et al. Use of a quantitative strong ion approach to determine the mechanism for acid-base abnormalities in sick calves with or without diarrhea. J Vet Intern Med 2005;19:581–9.

30. Bostedt H, Hermühlheim H, Bleul U, et al. Studies on the convalescent phase of calves after neonatal diarrhoea. Prakt Tierarzt 2000;81:301–12.

31. Fayet JC. Plasma and fecal osmolality, water kinetics, and body fluid compartments in neonatal calves with diarrhoea. Br Vet J 1971;127:37–44.

32. Phillips RW, Lewis LD, Knox KL. Alterations in body water turnover and distribution in neonatal calves with acute diarrhea. Ann N Y Acad Sci 1971;176:321–43.

33. Phillips RW, Lewis LD. Viral induced changes in intestinal transport and resultant body fluid alterations in neonatal calves. Ann Rech Vet 1973;4:87–98.

34. Hartmann H, Meyer H, Steinbach G, et al. Influence of diarrhoea on electrolyte content and osmolarity of the blood of calves. Monatsh Veterinarmed 1983;38:292–6.

35. Rademacher G, Lorenz I, Klee W. Feeding and treatment of calves with neonatal diarrhoea. Tierärztl Umsch 2002;57:177–89.

36. Naylor JM. A retrospective study of the relationship between clinical signs and severity of acidosis in diarrheic calves. Can Vet J 1989;30:577–80.

37. Cambier C, Clerbaux T, Detry B, et al. Effects of intravenous infusions of sodium bicarbonate on blood oxygen binding in calves with diarrhoea. Vet Rec 2005; 156:706–10.

38. Gökce G, Gökce HI, Erdogan HM, et al. Investigation of the coagulation profile in calves with neonatal diarrhea. Turk J Vet Anim Sci 2006;30:223–7.

39. Berchtold J, Prechtl J. Orale und parenterale Flüssigkeitstherapie – Das Kalb als Intensivpatient in der Praxis. Nutztierpraxis Aktuell 2002;2:12–5.

40. Berchtold J, Prechtl J. Technik der Ohrvenen-Infusion beim Kalb. Fachpraxis – Zeitschrift für die Tierarztpraxis 2003;(27):5–8.

41. Prechtl J, Berchtold J, Brunner B. Simplified intravenous (IV) fluid therapy of calves in practice [abstract 538]. In: Proceedings of the 22nd World Buiatrics Congress. Hannover, Germany; 2002. p. 171–2.

42. Dunlop RH, Hammond PB. D-lactic acidosis of ruminants. Ann N Y Acad Sci 1965;119:1109–32.

43. Lorenz I, Vogt S. Investigations on the association of D-lactate blood concentration with the outcome of therapy of acidosis, and with posture and demeanor in young calves with diarrhoea. J Vet Med A 2006;53:490–4.

44. Grude T. Laktat in Blut, Harn und Pansensaft von Kälbern, insbesondere bei "Pansentrinkern" [Lactate levels in blood, urine, and rumen liquor in calves, with special reference to "ruminal drinkers"] [thesis]. Munich: University of Munich; 1999 [in German].

45. Ewaschuk JB, Zello GA, Naylor JM, et al. Metabolic acidosis: separation methods and biological relevance of organic acids and lactic acid enantiomers. J Chromatogr B Analyt Technol Biomed Life Sci 2002;781:39–56.

46. Tennant B, Harrold D, Reina-Guerra M. Physiologic and metabolic factors in the pathogenesis of neonatal infections in calves. J Am Vet Med Assoc 1972;161: 993–1007.

47. Groutides C, Michell AR. Changes in plasma composition in calves surviving or dying from diarrhea. Br Vet J 1990;146:205–10.

48. Hartmann H, Berchtold J, Hofmann W. Pathophysiological aspects of acidosis in diarrhoeic calves. Tierärztl Umsch 1997;52:568–74.

49. Stocker H, Lutz H, Kaufmann C, et al. Acid-base disorders in milk-fed calves with chronic indigestion. Vet Rec 1999;145:340–6.

50. Grove-White DH. Pathophysiology and treatment of metabolic acidosis in the diarrhoeic calf. Bovine Practitioner 1997;31:56–60.
51. Naylor JM. Severity and nature of acidosis in diarrheic calves over and under one week of age. Can Vet J 1987;28:168–73.
52. Kasari TR, Naylor JM. Further studies on the clinical features and clinicopathological findings of a syndrome of metabolic acidosis with minimal or no dehydration in neonatal calves. Can J Vet Res 1986;50:502–8.
53. Walker PG, Constable PD, Morin DE, et al. A reliable, practical, and economical protocol for inducing diarrhea and severe dehydration in the neonatal calf. Can J Vet Res 1998;62:205–13.
54. Zello GA, Janzen A, Abeysekara S, et al. Urinary excretion of both D- and L-lactate using a calf-infusion model. FASEB J 2008;22(1205):5 [abstract].
55. Berchtold JF, Constable PD, Smith GW, et al. Effects of intravenous hyperosmotic sodium bicarbonate on arterial and cerebrospinal fluid acid-base status and cardiovascular function in calves with experimentally induced respiratory and strong ion acidosis. J Vet Intern Med 2005;19:240–51.
56. Bleul U, Bachofner C, Stocker H, et al. Comparison of sodium bicarbonate and carbicarb for the treatment of metabolic acidosis in newborn calves. Vet Rec 2005;156:202–6.
57. Bleul UT, Schwantag SC, Kähn WK. Effects of hypertonic sodium bicarbonate solution on electrolyte concentrations and enzyme activities in newborn calves with respiratory and metabolic acidosis. Am J Vet Res 2007;68:850–7.
58. Fecteau G, Paré J, Van Metre DC, et al. Use of a clinical sepsis score for predicting bacteremia in neonatal dairy calves on a calf rearing farm. Can Vet J 1997; 38:101–4.
59. Lofstedt J, Dohoo IR, Duizer G. Model to predict septicemia in diarrheic calves. J Vet Intern Med 1999;13:81–8.
60. Constable PD, Walker PG, Morin DE, et al. Use of peripheral temperature and core-temperature difference to predict cardiac output in dehydrated calves housed in a thermoneutral environment. Am J Vet Res 1998;59:874–80.
61. Nappert G, Naylor JM. A comparison of pH determination methods in food animal practice. Can Vet J 2001;42:364–7.
62. Rollin F. Tools for a prompt cowside diagnosis: what can be implemented by the bovine practitioner? In: Proceedings of the 24th World Buiatrics Congress. Nice, France; 2006. p. 89–99.
63. Lorenz I, Hartmann I, Gentile A. Determination of D-lactate in calf serum samples: an automated assay. Comp Clin Path 2003;12:169–71.
64. Kasari TR, Naylor JM. Clinical evaluation of sodium bicarbonate, sodium L-lactate, and sodium acetate for the treatment of acidosis in diarrheic calves. J Am Vet Med Assoc 1985;187:392–7.
65. Geishauser T, Thünker B. Metabolic acidosis in diarrhoeic neonatal calves: estimation using suckling reflex and standing ability. Prakt Tierarzt 1997;78:600–5.
66. Grove-White D, Michell AR. Comparison of the measurement of total carbon dioxide and strong ion difference for the evaluation of metabolic acidosis in diarrhoeic calves. Vet Rec 2001;148:365–70.
67. Koch A, Kaske M. Clinical efficacy of intravenous hypertonic saline solution or hypertonic bicarbonate solution in the treatment of inappetent calves with neonatal diarrhea. J Vet Intern Med 2008;22:202–11.
68. Naylor JM. Neonatal ruminant diarrhea. In: Smith BP, editor. Large animal internal medicine. 4th edition. St. Louis: Elsevier; 2008. p. 356.

69. Geishauser T, Thünker B. Metabolic acidosis in diarrhoeic calves: treatment using isomolar sodium bicarbonate. Prakt Tierarzt 1997;78:595–600.
70. Kasari TR, Naylor JM. Metabolic acidosis without clinical signs of dehydration in young calves. Can Vet J 1984;25:394–9.
71. Gentile A, Lorenz I, Sconza S, et al. Experimentally induced systemic hyperchloremic acidosis in calves. J Vet Intern Med 2008;22:190–5.
72. Wendel H, Sobotka R, Rademacher G. Studies on the correlation between blood acidosis and clinical signs in calves with neonatal diarrhoea. Tierärztl Umsch 2001;56:351–6.
73. Berchtold J. Intravenous fluid therapy of calves. Vet Clin North Am Food Anim Pract 1999;15:505–31.
74. Constable PD, Gohar HM, Morin DE, et al. Use of hypertonic saline-dextran solution to resuscitate hypovolemic calves with diarrhea. Am J Vet Res 1996; 57:97–104.
75. Ewaschuk JB, Zello GA, Naylor JM. Lactobacillus GG does not affect D-lactic acidosis in diarrheic calves in a clinical setting. J Vet Intern Med 2006;20:614–9.
76. Gareis A. Die Bedeutung von Glukosezusatz zur Infusionslösung bei Kälbern mit Neugeborenendiarrhoe [Significance of glucose additions to infusions in calves with neonatal diarrhea] [thesis]. Munich: University of Munich; 2003 [in German].
77. Grünberg W, Morin DE, Drackley JK, et al. Effect of continuous intravenous administration of a 50% dextrose solution on phosphorus homeostasis in dairy cows. J Am Vet Med Assoc 2006;229:413–20.
78. Grove-White D. Practical intravenous fluid therapy in the diarrhoeic calf. In Pract 2007;29:404–8.
79. Corke MJ. Economical preparation of fluids for intravenous use in cattle practice. Vet Rec 1988;122:305–7.
80. Constable PD. Fluid and electrolyte therapy in ruminants. Vet Clin North Am Food Anim Pract 2003;19:557–97.
81. Groutides C, Michell AR. Intravenous solutions for fluid therapy in calf diarrhoea. Res Vet Sci 1990;49:292–7.
82. Roussel AR, Cohen ND, Holland PS, et al. Alterations in acid-base balance and serum electrolyte concentrations in cattle: 632 cases (1984–1994). J Am Vet Med Assoc 1998;212:1769–75.
83. Iwabuchi S, Suzuki K, Abe I, et al. Comparison of the effects of isotonic and hypertonic sodium bicarbonate solutions on acidemic calves experimentally induced by ammonium chloride administration. J Vet Med Sci 2003;65: 1369–71.
84. Suzuki K, Abe I, Iwabuchi S, et al. Evaluation of isotonic sodium bicarbonate solution for alkalizing effects in conscious calves. J Vet Med Sci 2002;64:699–703.
85. Suzuki K, Kato T, Tsunoda G, et al. Effect of intravenous infusion of isotonic sodium bicarbonate solution on acidemic calves with diarrhea. J Vet Med Sci 2002; 64:1173–5.
86. Zello GA, Abeysekara S, Lohmann KL, et al. Bicarbonate treatment of acidosis produces paradoxical acidosis in the brain. FASEB J 2007;21:838.4 [abstract].
87. Naylor JM, Forsyth GW. The alkalinizing effects of metabolizable bases in the healthy calf. Can J Vet Res 1986;50:509–16.
88. Walker PG, Constable PD, Morin DE, et al. Comparison of hypertonic saline-dextran solution and lactated Ringer's solution for resuscitating severely dehydrated calves with diarrhea. J Am Vet Med Assoc 1998;213:113–21.
89. Schmid G, Rüsse M. Technique for the continuous infusion into an ear vein of the newborn calf. Berl Münch Tierärztl Wochenschr 1983;96:189–91.

90. Glawischnig E, Gerber N, Schlerka G. Continuous drip infusion for calves with severe acidosis. Tierärztl Umsch 1990;45:562–9.
91. Roussel AJ, Taliofera L, Navarre CB, et al. Catheterization of the auricular vein in cattle: 68 cases (1991–1994). J Am Vet Med Assoc 1996;208:905–7.
92. Garcia JP. A practitioner's views on fluid therapy in calves. Vet Clin North Am Food Anim Pract 1999;15:533–43.
93. Geishauser T. Intravenöse Dauertropfinfusion zur Durchfallbehandlung beim Kalb. Prakt Tierarzt 1992;78:595–600.
94. Kümper H. Kälberdurchfall mit schwerer Allgemeinstörung: Therapiemöglichkeiten unter Praxisbedingungen. In: Proceedings (Large Animal) BpT-Kongress. Münster, Germany; 1997. p. 27–9.
95. Hartmann H. Technik, Überwachung und Komplikationen der Infusionstherapie. In: Hartmann H, Staufenbiel R, editors. Flüssigkeitstherapie bei Tieren. Jena–Stuttgart (Germany): Gustav Fischer Verlag; 1995. p. 112–59.
96. van Leengoed LA, de Vrey P, Verheijden JHM, et al. Intravenous catheterization in pigs: an evaluation of two methods. Zentralbl Veterinarmed A 1987;34:549–56.
97. Hansen BD. Technical aspects of fluid therapy. In: DiBartola SP, editor. Fluid, electrolyte, and acid-base disorders in small animal practice. 3rd edition. St. Louis (MO): Saunders Elsevier; 2006. p. 344–76.
98. Pusterla N, Braun U. Prophylaxis of intravenous catheter-related thrombophlebitis in cattle. Vet Rec 1996;139:287–9.
99. Pusterla N, Braun U. Ultrasonographic evaluation of the jugular vein of cows with catheter-related thrombophlebitis. Vet Rec 1995;137:431–4.
100. Bouda J, Medina CM, Nunez OL, et al. Microbiology and clinicopathological findings in calves with acute diarrhea and suggested intravenous fluid therapy. In: Proceedings of the 20th World Buiatrics Congress. Sydney, Australia; 1998. p. 375–9.
101. Roussel AJ. Principles and mechanics of fluid therapy in calves. Compend Cont Educ Pract Vet 1983;5:S332–6.
102. Roussel AJ, Kasari TR. Using fluid and electrolyte replacement therapy to help diarrheic calves. Vet Med 1990;85:303–4.
103. Rebhun WC. Infectious diseases of the gastrointestinal tract. In: Rebhun WC, editor. Diseases of dairy cattle. Philadelphia: Lippincott Williams & Wilkins; 1995. p. 161–2.
104. Radostits OM. Treatment and control of neonatal diarrhea in calves. J Dairy Sci 1975;58:464–70.
105. Rollin F. Practical parenteral fluid therapy in the bovine species. Ann Méd Vét 1997;141:89–111.

Treatment of Calf Diarrhea: Antimicrobial and Ancillary Treatments

Peter D. Constable, BVSc (Hons), MS, PhD, MRCVS

KEYWORDS

- Fluoroquinolones • Cephalosporins • Halofuginone
- Azithromycin • Acetate • Propionate

There are six major causes of diarrhea in calves less than 21 days of age: enterotoxigenic *Escherichia coli* (ETEC), rotavirus, coronavirus, *Cryptosporidium parvum* (*C parvum*) type II, *Salmonella enterica* (*S enterica*) subsp. *enterica* serovars, and nutritional. Regardless of the etiology, calves with diarrhea often have increased coliform bacterial numbers in the small intestine; small intestinal bacterial overgrowth is associated with altered small intestinal function, morphologic damage, and increased susceptibility to bacteremia and endotoxemia.[1–3] The importance of bacterial overgrowth in calf diarrhea has garnered renewed attention with the realization that D-lactic acid plays an important role in the development of acidemia in calves with diarrhea. Production of D-lactic acid results from bacterial fermentation in the gastrointestinal tract and is a common finding in neonatal calves with and without diarrhea.[4–8] D-lactic acid is a major component of acidemia in diarrheic calves[6,8,9] and is accompanied by systemic signs of weakness and ataxia.[10]

This review focuses on adjunct therapy of diarrhea in the first 3 weeks of life and therefore does not address the efficacy of adjunct treatment for calf diarrhea due to *Eimeria bovis*, *Eimeria zurneii*, or *Giardia duodenalis*. The main principles of ancillary treatment in neonatal calves with diarrhea and systemic illness are: (1) treat or prevent Gram-negative septicemia and bacteremia; (2) decrease the numbers of coliform bacteria in the proximal small intestine and abomasum; (3) increase nonspecific resistance; (4) provide nutrients that facilitate repair of damaged intestine and prevent negative energy balance; and (5) provide analgesia and reduce stress to the calf. Treatment goals for all calves with diarrhea are accomplished by the parenteral

Dr. Constable has received funding support related to the treatment of calf diarrhea from Boehringher-Ingelheim Inc, CEVA-Animal Health, and Vetoquinol.

Department of Veterinary Clinical Sciences, School of Veterinary Medicine, Purdue University, 625 Harrison Street, West Lafayette, IN 47907-2026, USA

E-mail address: constabl@purdue.edu

administration of antimicrobials with a predominantly Gram-negative spectrum of activity, short-term administration of nonsteroidal anti-inflammatory agents such as flunixin meglumine or meloxicam, and continued milk feeding. For calves with diarrhea caused by *C parvum*, the oral administration of halofuginone or azithromycin appears to be effective in decreasing the duration and severity of diarrhea, as well as in decreasing fecal oocyst concentration and environmental contamination. Theoretically efficacious treatments include the administration of oral rehydration therapy solutions that contain acetate and propionate, and the administration of parenteral B vitamins and fat-soluble vitamins in calves that have chronic diarrhea. There is no evidence to support the efficacy of corticosteroids, motility modifiers, immunostimulants, intestinal "protectants" or "absorbants," or probiotic substances in the treatment of calf diarrhea, and the administration of any of these items is not currently recommended.

RECOMMENDED TREATMENTS
Antimicrobials

Although some consider the use of antimicrobials to treat calf diarrhea to be controversial and not indicated,[11,12] a systematic review of the literature provided strong and unequivocal evidence that specific antimicrobials are efficacious in the treatment of calf diarrhea.[1] The initial concern about antimicrobial use in calf diarrhea was derived from the results of studies that indicated oral administration of penicillin, chloramphenicol, and neomycin increased the incidence of diarrhea in healthy calves, produced malabsorption, or reduced growth rate.[1] More recent concerns about antimicrobial use in calf diarrhea have focused on whether antimicrobial administration promotes antimicrobial resistance of enteric pathogens and facilitates the emergence of multiple resistant strains of *Salmonella enterica* subsp. *enterica serovars* typhimurium and newport. Important considerations when administering antimicrobials as part of the treatment of calves with diarrhea are: (1) administering as directed on the label or by a veterinarian whenever possible; (2) selecting an antimicrobial agent with an appropriate spectrum of activity; (3) using a dosage protocol that attains and maintains an effective therapeutic concentration at the site of infection; (4) treating for an appropriate duration; (5) avoiding adverse local or systemic effects and violative residues; and (6) minimizing the potential for transfer of antimicrobial resistance genes.[13] The overarching philosophy is that veterinarians should use and prescribe antimicrobials conservatively to minimize potential adverse effects on animal or human health.[14]

Calves with diarrhea have small intestinal overgrowth with *E coli* bacteria, regardless of the inciting cause for the diarrhea (**Fig. 1**),[1] and 20%–30% of systemically ill calves with diarrhea have bacteremia, predominantly due to *E coli*.[15–17] The frequency of bacteremia is high enough that treatment of calves with diarrhea that are systemically ill (as indicated by decreased appetite and activity or the presence of fever) should include routine treatment against potential bacteremia, with emphasis on treating potential *E coli* bacteremia. Bacteremia should also be suspected to be present in 100% of calves with clinical signs of *Salmonella* diarrhea, although the prevalence of bacteremia in calves with salmonellosis does not appear to have been determined.[18] A clinical sepsis score to predict bacteremia[19] does not appear to be sufficiently accurate to guide antimicrobial treatment decisions.

Antimicrobial treatment of diarrheic calves with systemic illness should be focused against *E coli* in the blood (due to bacteremia) and small intestine (due to bacterial overgrowth), as these constitute the two sites of bacterial infection. Fecal bacterial culture and antimicrobial susceptibility testing is not recommended in calves with

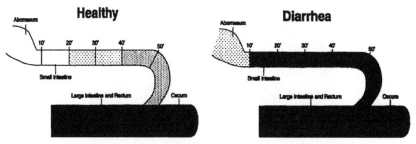

Fig. 1. Schematic of the distribution and concentration of *Escherichia coli* bacteria in the intestinal tract of a calf with undifferentiated diarrhea and a similarly aged calf without diarrhea. (*Adapted from* Reisinger RC. Pathogenesis and prevention of infectious diarrhea (scours) of newborn calves. J Am Vet Med Assoc 1965;147:1377–86.) The figure indicates that the number of *E coli* in the large intestine of diarrheic and healthy calves is similar but that diarrheic calves have increased *E coli* numbers in their small intestine, particularly in the distal jejunum and ileum. (*Reprinted from* Constable PD. Antimicrobial use in the treatment of calf diarrhea. J Vet Intern Med 2004a;18:8–17; with permission.)

diarrhea because fecal bacterial populations do not accurately reflect small intestinal or blood bacterial populations, and because the breakpoints for susceptibility test results have not been validated for calves with diarrhea.[1] Antimicrobial efficacy is therefore best evaluated by the clinical response to treatment. Antimicrobial treatment may also be effective in eliminating D-lactate–producing bacteria from the gastro-intestinal tract of calves with diarrhea[3,7] and thereby hasten the time course of clinical improvement, although this supposition needs to be verified.

Oxytetracycline and sulfachloropyridiazine administered parenterally and amoxicillin, chlortetracycline, neomycin, oxytetracycline, streptomycin, sulfachloropyridazine, sulfamethazine, and tetracycline administered orally have been labeled by the US Food and Drug Administration (FDA) for the treatment of bacterial enteritis (scours, colibacillosis) caused by *E coli* bacteria susceptible to the antimicrobial.[1] Studies supporting the efficacy of parenteral oxytetracycline and sulfachloropyridiazine, and of oral amoxicillin, chlortetracycline, neomycin, oxytetracycline, streptomycin, sulfachloropyridiazine, sulfamethazine, and tetracycline at labeled doses in treating calves with naturally acquired diarrhea do not appear to have been published in peer-reviewed journals.[1] Oral amoxicillin was effective in the treatment of experimentally induced diarrhea[20,21] but was not efficacious in the treatment of naturally acquired diarrhea in beef calves.[22] In view of the apparent lack of published studies documenting clinical efficacy of antimicrobials with a label claim for the treatment of naturally occurring calf diarrhea, and because the health of the animal is threatened (suffering or death may result from failure to treat systemically ill calves), extralabel antimicrobial use (excluding prohibited antimicrobials) is justified for the treatment of calf diarrhea.[1]

Antimicrobials should be administered to all calves with diarrhea that exhibit systemic signs of illness (as indicated by inappetance, dehydration, lethargy, or pyrexia) (**Fig. 2**); or have blood or mucosal shreds in their stool (**Fig. 3**); the latter indicates breakdown of the blood-gut barrier and a presumed increased risk of bacteremia. Parenteral administration of antimicrobials is preferred to oral administration, with the ideal parenteral antimicrobial being bactericidal and predominantly Gram-negative in spectrum.[1] The ideal parenteral antimicrobial should also be excreted in an active form in bile that results in a local antimicrobial effect in the small intestine.[1] Current evidence suggests that antimicrobials should not be administered

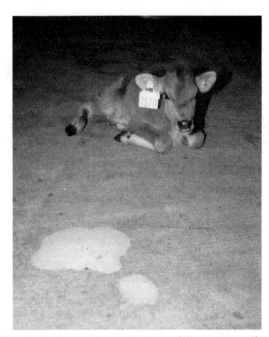

Fig. 2. A Jersey calf with diarrhea and systemic signs of illness. The calf is reluctant to stand and has a weak suckle reflex. Current knowledge indicates that this calf will benefit from parenteral antimicrobial administration, such as amoxicillin, ampicillin, or a third or fourth generation cephalosporin in countries where there use is permitted. Parenteral fluoroquinolone administration is not indicated because the calf does not need intravenous fluid therapy.

to diarrheic calves that have a normal appetite, activity level, rectal temperature, and hydration status and the absence of concurrent infections such as pneumonia or omphalophlebitis (**Fig. 4**).[23] Instead, these calves should be separated from other calves and their health status monitored frequently.

The success of antimicrobial therapy varies with the route of administration and whether the antimicrobial is dissolved in milk, oral electrolyte solutions, or water. Oral antimicrobials administered as bolus, tablet, or in a gelatin capsule maybe swallowed into the rumen and exhibit a different serum concentration-time profile to antimicrobials dissolved in milk replacer that are suckled by the calf.[13] Antimicrobials that bypass the rumen are not thought to alter rumen microflora, potentially permitting bacterial recolonization of the small intestine from the rumen. Individual antimicrobial treatment of sick calves increases the level of resistance in fecal *E coli* isolates, but the change in antimicrobial susceptibility is only transient.[24]

First choice antimicrobials for the treatment of diarrhea in systemically ill calves include parenteral amoxicillin or ampicillin (10 mg/kg, intramuscularly [IM] every 12 hours), parenteral potentiated sulfonamides (25 mg/kg, IV or IM every 24 hours), and oral amoxicillin trihydrate (10 mg/kg every 12 hours) alone or combined with the inhibitor clavulanate potassium (12.5 mg combined drug/kg every 12 hours).[1,13,25] Second choice antimicrobials in those countries where cephalosporin administration is permitted are third and fourth generation cephalosporins, such as ceftiofur and cefquinome.[1,13] Parenteral ceftiofur has evidence of efficacy in experimentally-induced *S*

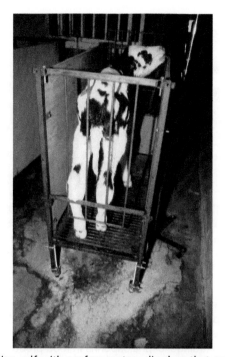

Fig. 3. A Holstein-Friesian calf with profuse watery diarrhea that contains blood. The calf was admitted in lateral recumbency, and was pyrexic, markedly depressed, and inappetant. The calf was treated intravenously with 2 L of 1.4% sodium bicarbonate solution containing glucose and was able to stand within 2 hours of treatment. Current knowledge indicates that this calf should be treated with parenteral antimicrobials and a nonsteroidal anti-inflammatory agent such as meloxicam or flunixin meglumine. Parenteral fluoroquinolone or third or fourth generation cephalosporin administration may be indicated in countries where such administration is permitted because the calf needed intravenous fluid therapy. The extralabel administration of fluoroquinolones in food producing animals in the United States is prohibited by law because of concerns regarding facilitating the emergence of bacteria with multiple antimicrobial resistance, particularly pathogenic enteric bacteria in humans.

enterica subsp enterica serovar dublin infection.[18] Last choice antimicrobials are fluoroquinolones in those countries where fluoroquinolone administration is permitted to treat calves with E coli diarrhea and salmonellosis. However, parenteral fluoroquinolones should be administered only to critically ill calves, such as those calves requiring intravenous fluid administration.[13] Aminoglycosides should also not be administered orally because they are very poorly absorbed from the gastrointestinal tract. Aminoglycosides should not be administered parenterally because of prolonged withdrawal times for slaughter, potential for nephrotoxicity in dehydrated calves, and minimal excretion in bile.[1] The results of a 2002 survey of Italian cattle veterinarians indicated that fluoroquinolones and aminoglycosides were the first choice antimicrobials for treating calf diarrhea by 54% and 14% of respondents, respectively.[26]

Even though oral and parenteral fluoroquinolones have documented efficacy in treating calves with diarrhea and systemic illness,[1] the extralabel administration of fluoroquinolones in food-producing animals in the United States is prohibited by law because of concerns regarding facilitating the emergence of bacteria with multiple

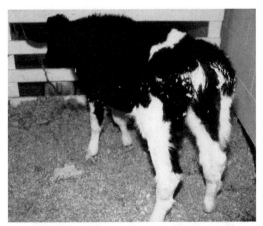

Fig. 4. A Holstein-Friesian calf with diarrhea but no systemic signs of illness. The calf is eager to stand and has a good suckle reflex. Current knowledge indicates that this calf does not need parenteral or oral antimicrobial administration.

antimicrobial resistance, particularly pathogenic enteric bacteria in humans. Another important issue is the potential ban on extralabel use of cephalosporins in the United States. At the time this article was written, the US FDA had proposed a final rule prohibiting any use of extralabel cephalosporins in food producing animals. Because there are no third or fourth generation cephalosporins specifically approved for the treatment of diarrhea in calves, their use would not be permitted if this rule is not amended.

Analgesic and Anti-Inflammatory Agents

Diarrhea can be accompanied by intestinal cramping and abdominal pain. The administration of an effective analgesic may therefore be beneficial as part of the treatment of calf diarrhea, provided that the side effects of such treatment are not deleterious. Meloxicam is an analgesic and anti-inflammatory agent that is labeled in Europe for the treatment of calf diarrhea when used in conjunction with oral rehydration therapy. In a randomized multilocation trial of 191 calves in Europe, a single IV injection of meloxicam (0.5 mg/kg bodyweight) in conjunction with a standard treatment (oral electrolyte rehydration solution therapy and parenteral gentamicin) increased feed intake, hydration score, and fecal consistency, and decreased the signs of visceral pain, relative to standard treatment alone.[27] In a recent randomized study of 56 calves in Ontario Canada, the subcutaneous administration of meloxicam (0.5 mg/kg, once) resulted in treated calves consuming starter rations earlier than placebo-treated calves. Treated calves also had improved starter ration intakes, a higher body weight gain, and increased activity level than placebo-treated calves.[28] Taken together, these results suggest that meloxicam should be considered as part of the initial treatment of calves with diarrhea and systemic illness in those countries where meloxicam is labeled for use in calves.

Two broad categories of anti-inflammatory agents could potentially be used as part of the treatment for calf diarrhea: corticosteroids and nonsteroidal anti-inflammatory agents (NSAIDs). The major therapeutic goals of anti-inflammatory administration are to decrease inflammation in the gastrointestinal tract and to ameliorate the effects of endotoxemia and septicemia secondary to translocation of enteric bacteria across damaged intestinal epithelium. Although studies evaluating the prevalence of endotoxemia in calves with diarrhea do not appear to have been done, the results of a recent study in neonatal lambs with diarrhea indicated that affected lambs were frequently endotoxemic, as assessed by the Limulus amoebocyte lysate assay.[2]

The routine administration of corticosteroids to diarrheic calves is not recommended. This is because calves with diarrhea have higher plasma corticosteroid concentrations, relative to healthy calves,[29,30] and because corticosteroids suppress the immune system.

The routine administration of NSAIDs, such as meloxicam or flunixin meglumine, is recommended as part of the initial treatment in calves with diarrhea that are systemically ill. An empiric guideline for the treatment of diarrhea is to administer meloxicam once at a dose of 0.5 mg/kg bodyweight (0.22 mg/lb) or flunixin meglumine once at a dose 2.2 mg/kg (1.0 mg/lb), and not to exceed 3 doses of either meloxicam or flunixin meglumine. This recommendation is based on the need to avoid damaging the abomasal mucosa, particularly in intensive calf-rearing facilities with a history of calf deaths due to perforated abomasal ulcers.[3] The beneficial effects of meloxicam and flunixin meglumine could be caused by their analgesic, anti-inflammatory, antipyretic, or antisecretory properties, or due to underdetermined effects on intestinal motility. It is currently not clear which of these potential effects is the most important.

The administration of one dose of flunixin meglumine (2.2 mg/kg [1.0 mg/lb] intramuscularly) as an adjunct treatment for naturally occurring diarrhea resulted in fewer morbid-days and antimicrobial treatments, but only when calves had fresh blood visible in their feces.[31] In calves administered STa toxin as a model for experimentally induced ETEC infection, intramuscular administration of flunixin meglumine (2.2 mg/kg [1.0 mg/lb] every 8 hours) reduced fecal output, possibly by acting as an antisecretory agent.[32] Blockade of both cyclo-oxygenase isoforms (COX-1 and COX-2) is required to facilitate the uptake of sodium from the intestinal ileum of calves with diarrhea due to *C parvum*.[33] The clinical relevance of this finding remains unclear because the ileum is not a quantitatively important site of fluid flux in calves with diarrhea[34,35] and because doses needed for effective in vitro COX-1 and COX-2 blockade[33] have not been related to those obtained in vivo using standard dosage protocols for meloxicam or flunixin meglumine. An important effect of flunixin meglumine administration is the clinical impression that calves show improved suckle behavior and general well being after treatment.[3,36]

Calves administered a high dose of ketoprofen (6 mg/kg bodyweight, IV, twice 4 hours apart) tended ($P = .059$) to have reduced fecal output, relative to untreated controls,[37] whereas a lower dose of ketoprofen (3 mg/kg bodyweight, IV, twice 4 hours apart) had no effect. Orally administered aspirin (acetylsalicylic acid, 100 mg/kg bodyweight, once) was not effective in decreasing STa-induced intestinal secretion in calves, whereas intravenously administered sodium salicylate was effective when administered at a dose calculated to maintain a therapeutic serum salicylate concentration of 30 μg/mL.[38] Subsalicylate, a component in bismuth subsalicylate ("Peptobismol" in the United States) is believed to exert a similar effect to aspirin. Bismuth subsalicylate may therefore decrease intestinal epithelial secretion mediated by cAMP or cGMP in calves with diarrhea, although this has not been verified. There does not appear to be a persuasive reason to prefer bismuth subsalicylate, aspirin, or ketoprofen over meloxicam or flunixin meglumine as an ancillary treatment for calf diarrhea. Until such data is available, bismuth subsalicylate, aspirin, and ketoprofen are not recommended as ancillary treatments for calf diarrhea.

Halofuginone and Azithromycin for Cryptosporidiosis

Specific therapy of presumed Cryptosporidial infection in calves remains an active area of research. The results of studies indicate that halofuginone, azithromycin, and possibly lasalocid can be effective in the treatment of cryptosporidial diarrhea in calves. It is currently believed that fresh cow's milk should be fed in small quantities several times daily to optimize digestion and to minimize loss of body weight. Feeding of cow's milk may also be beneficial as a source of dietary lipid, which has been shown to be a potent inhibitor of cryptosporidium-host cell adhesion in vitro.[39]

Halofuginone, a quinazoline of unknown mode of action, is licensed in a number of countries in Europe for the prevention and treatment of cryptosporidiosis in newborn calves. Halofuginone (0.06 to 0.12 mg/kg bodyweight by mouth daily) improved the clinical status and decreased fecal oocyst excretion and mortality in a dose-dependent manner in calves with experimentally induced cryptosporidial infection.[40] A toxicity study indicated that 0.5 mg/kg daily by mouth was close to the toxic dose.[41] Halofuginone (5 mg orally daily from approximately day 7 to day 14 of life, equivalent to 0.1 mg/kg bodyweight daily), was efficacious in decreasing oocyst excretion, but had no effect on the prevalence of diarrhea, fecal water percentage, or the severity of dehydration in naturally infected calves in Quebec, compared with untreated controls.[42] In contrast, the results of a large 2007 study in the Czech Republic indicated that halofuginone (0.1 mg/kg bodyweight daily for 7 days, orally) decreased the intensity of diarrhea and the fecal oocyst count, when started on day 1 or day 8 of life.[43] The preponderance of evidence indicates that halofuginone (0.1 mg/kg bodyweight daily orally) is an effective treatment for cryptosporidial diarrhea in calves.

Azithromycin (1–2 g/calf orally once daily for 7 days, equivalent to 30–40 mg/kg daily) decreased the mortality rate and fecal oocyst shedding, and increased the clinical health and weight gain, of 10-day-old calves with naturally acquired C parvum infection in Turkey.[44] Azithromycin is a macrolide antibiotic that is well absorbed from the small intestine and is likely to have some prokinetic and antimicrobial effects, based on its structural similarity to erythromycin.[45–47] The results of the above study suggest that azithromycin is an effective treatment for cryptosporidial diarrhea in calves. However, because this macrolide is widely used in the treatment of respiratory disease in humans and is expensive, the administration of azithromycin should be restricted to sick calves with documented Cryptosporidial diarrhea that have not responded to treatment with oral halofuginone.

Decoquinate, a hydroxyquinolone that inhibits cytochrome-mediated electron transport in mitochondria, has been used to prevent and treat cryptosporidia in calves. However, decoquinate (125 mg orally daily from approximately day 7 to day 14 of life in a solid premix, equivalent to 2.5 mg/kg bodyweight daily) had no effect on oocyst excretion, the prevalence of diarrhea, fecal water percentage, or the severity of dehydration in calves, compared with untreated controls.[42] Decoquinate (2 mg/kg bodyweight orally daily from approximately day 1 onwards of life in a soluble formulation in milk replacer) had no effect on oocyst excretion, the total number of days of diarrhea, or mortality rate in calves, compared with untreated controls.[48] These studies suggest that decoquinate is not an effective treatment for cryptosporidial diarrhea in calves.

Paromomycin sulfate solution (100–200 mg paromomycin/kg bodyweight by mouth daily for 2 to 3 days) was effective in decreasing oocyst excretion and the prevalence of diarrhea in lambs with naturally acquired C parvum diarrhea.[49] Paromomycin is an aminoglycoside antibiotic that is poorly absorbed from the gastrointestinal tract but is efficacious in treating immunocompromised humans with cryptosporidosis. The mechanism of paromomycin's effect remains unknown.

Lasalocid, an ionophore, is an effective treatment for naturally acquired and experimentally-induced cryptosporidial diarrhea in calves,[50] with a daily oral dose rate of 15 mg/kg bodyweight. In an uncontrolled trial of calves in Turkey with naturally acquired *C parvum* diarrhea, the oral administration of Lasolocid (8 mg/kg bodyweight, daily) in milk was associated with a decrease in fecal oocyst count,[51] although such a decrease was likely to occur in untreated calves because of age-related changes in fecal oocyst shedding.

Continued Feeding of Cow's Milk

It has become increasingly evident over the past 20 years that a damaged intestine needs metabolic fuel to optimize repair, and that fresh cow's milk provides an excellent, inexpensive, and readily available source of nutrition and growth factors to facilitate repair. Milk is also more energy dense than oral rehydration therapy (ORT) solutions and continued milk feeding minimizes the weight loss associated with chronic diarrhea in calves.[52] Concurrent feeding of milk and ORT solutions results in improved intestinal morphology, compared with that from ORT solutions alone.

Glutamine supplementation has been investigated as an ancillary treatment of calf diarrhea, but the results of two studies indicate the addition of glutamine had deleterious effects on small intestinal villus height and villus surface area, and glutamine-treated calves had a lower mitotic rate in the small intestine than control calves.[53,54] It is currently believed that glutamine offers no advantage in improving gut morphology in diarrheic calves.[55]

TREATMENTS THAT MAY BE EFFECTIVE
B Vitamins and Fat Soluble Vitamins

Parenteral administration of B-vitamins and fat-soluble vitamins may have beneficial effects in calves with chronic diarrhea.[3] However, there is a lack of data supporting the beneficial effects of vitamins in the treatment of calf diarrhea.

Oligosaccharides

Oligosaccharides are sugar polymers present in cow milk that contain a small number of (usually up to ten) component sugars that are either *O*- or *N*-linked to compatible amino acids in proteins (called glycoproteins) or lipids. Because many Gram-negative bacteria attach to the intestinal epithelium via receptors that have a similar structure to oligosaccharides, milk oligosaccharides may provide competitive binding sites for the K99 (F5) fimbrae from enterotoxigenic *E coli*.[56] Bacteria bound to oligosaccharides move along the intestine with intestinal peristalsis and are eliminated in the feces because oligosaccharides are not enzymatically digested in the small intestine.[57]

The administration of exogenous oligosaccharides in water to neonatal calves decreased intestinal *E coli* counts in the small intestine of calves inoculated with ETEC.[56] Prophylactic addition of exogenous oligosaccharides to milk replacer resulted in fecal scores (scours) in calves which were similar to those observed when calves were fed milk replacer containing antibiotics.[57-59] It must be noted that data on morbidity and mortality were either low or remained undetermined in these studies,[58] and that scours may well have had nutritional rather than an infectious origin.[57]

Oligosaccharides show promise as a non–antimicrobial method for preventing ETEC or treating ETEC diarrhea in calves. However, the experimental studies performed to date do not support the routine administration of oligosaccharides to sick calves with diarrhea.

Increasing Nonspecific Resistance

Nonspecific resistance is conferred by factors such as low abomasal pH, short chain fatty acids (acetate, propionate), lactoferrin and leukocytes in colostrum, oligosaccharides in colostrum and fresh milk,[60] and the lactoperoxidase system, lysozyme, and medium chain fatty acids (particularly n-decanoic and n-octanic acid) in fresh milk.[61,62]

Abomasal pH of the calf is 4.4 at birth[63] and after colostrum ingestion ranges from 5.9 to 7.2 over the first 20 hours of life.[64] The mean preprandial pH is constant between 1.4 and 1.7 after day 5 of life.[65,66] The relatively high pH during the first day of life ensures ingested colostral immunoglobulins are minimally degraded before arriving in the small intestine, which is the site of immunoglobulin absorption. Unfortunately, the high abomasal pH also allows ingested E coli and Salmonella spp. to escape the "abomasal sterilizer" and large numbers of viable pathogenic bacteria can therefore arrive in the small intestine if colostrum is heavily contaminated.

As outlined in the following section, the administration of acidified ORT solutions, or the availability of acidified water or milk replacer that acidify the small intestinal lumen, is likely to be beneficial in the treatment of diarrhea due to E coli and Salmonella. Indeed, acidified water has gained widespread acceptance as a simple and effective method for decreasing the incidence and severity of diarrhea in weaned pigs.

Acidifying the small intestinal lumen

E coli cause two common diseases of neonatal calves: ETEC, in which the bacteria are localized to the lumen and mucosal surface of the small intestine, and colisepticemia, in which the bacteria invade the systemic circulation.[67] The main features of the pathogenesis of ETEC diarrhea are: (1) ingestion of ETEC; (2) passage through the low pH environment of the abomasum; (3) attachment by K99 (F5) fimbrae to epithelial cells in the ileum with colonization; (4) progressive anterior movement of colonization to involve the entire small intestine; (5) production of a heat stable enterotoxin (STa); and (6) binding of STa to intestinal epithelial cells and stimulation of secretion. This chain of events leads to acute profuse watery diarrhea and death in severe cases.[67] The main features of the pathogenesis of colisepticemia are: (1) ingestion of serum resistant strains of E coli; (2) passage through the low pH environment of the abomasum; (3) multiplication in the small intestinal lumen; and (4) translocation across intestinal epithelium to produce bacteremia and septicemia.

Mixed enteric infections are commonly diagnosed in diarrheic calves.[68,69] Primary viral damage facilitates small intestinal overgrowth with E coli that, in turn, exacerbates the morphologic damage and predisposes the calf to colisepticemia[70] and E coli bacteremia.[15–17] E coli bacterial numbers are increased 5 to 10,000 fold in the lumen of the duodenum, jejunum, and ileum of calves with naturally acquired diarrhea,[68,69,71–74] even when the diarrhea is not due to ETEC (**Fig. 1**). In calves with naturally acquired diarrhea, increased small intestinal colonization with E coli has been associated with impaired glucose, xylose, and fat absorption.[74] Calves with ETEC and non-ETEC diarrhea therefore have increased numbers of E coli bacteria in the small intestine, and this increase is deleterious to the calf's health.

The growth rate and viability of E coli varies markedly with pH. In gastric juice aspirated from human infants, a pH < 2.5 for 60 minutes was bactericidal for Gram-negative bacteria; an increase in pH from 2.5 to 5.0 was associated with an increased growth rate of Gram-negative bacteria; and the fastest growth rate occurred when pH > 5.0.[75] In an unpublished study using a small number of bovine ETEC and colisepticemic strains cultured in abomasal contents and other fluids, E coli was killed when pH $\leq$ 3.0 but multiplied when pH $\geq$ 5.0.[76] In a related unpublished in vivo study, abomasal luminal pH influenced the numbers of E coli recovered from the abomasum and small intestine of calves infected with a mixture of ETEC and colisepticemic strains. At abomasal pH of 3.0 to 3.7, < 10% of the inoculum dose was recovered, with ETEC strains being more resistant to pH-mediated killing than colisepticemic strains. At abomasal luminal pH of 5.0, both ETEC and colisepticemic strains proliferated.[76] Taken together, these studies suggest that E coli is killed when pH ≤ 3.0 and multiplies when pH ≥ 5.0.

The abomasum and anterior small intestine of the suckling calf are much more acidic than caudal aspects of the intestinal tract (**Fig. 5**).[77,78] Preliminary data of the magnitude of the relative acidity of the proximal small intestine has been obtained from 13 healthy calves aged 2–14 days[73] and four calves aged <30 days.[78,79] Alimentary tract pH was measured 2 hours after ingestion of milk, with the following median values: abomasum, 4.9; small intestine (divided into 7 equal parts, from orad to aborad), 5.9, 6.1, 6.3, 6.5, 6.8, 7.2, 8.1; large intestine, 6.6; rectum, 6.0.[73] In another study, the median small intestinal pH in fasted suckling calves was 6.0 at 30% of the distance from the abomasum, 6.5 (at 50%), 8.1 (at 70%), and 8.0 (ileum).[79] Mean duodenal pH for 12 hours after feeding also decreases with age, being: 3.7 at 7 days, 3.5 at 24 days, and 3.0 at 63 days.[80] Because bovine ETEC strains do not express K99 pili when pH < 6.5,[81] the relative acidity of the proximal small intestine explains why ETEC bacteria first colonize the distal small intestine, followed by anterior progression of bacterial adhesion.[82] Maintaining a luminal pH < 6.5 should therefore increase nonspecific resistance to ETEC diarrhea.

Decreasing proximal intestinal pH also decreases STa production by attached ETEC, because production of STa enterotoxin is greatly decreased when pH < 7.2[83]

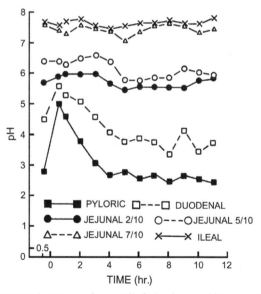

Fig. 5. The pH of intestinal contents from milk fed calves suckling cow's milk at time = 0 hours. Note that the pH fluctuates with milk feeding in the abomasum and anterior small intestine but is more stable in the distal half of the small intestine. Note also that luminal pH becomes increasingly alkaline moving aborad from duodenum toward the ileum. (*Reprinted from* Mylrea PJ. Gastro-intestinal disorders and the functioning of the digestive tract of young calves. Res Vet Sci 1968;9:14–28; with permission.)

and because STa toxin is a much more potent secretagogue in the proximal small intestine. Although STa receptor affinity and density are greatest in the ileum and distal jejunum of the neonatal calf,[84] in studies using ligated intestinal segments of Jersey calves aged 3 to 7 days and Holstein calves aged 1 day inoculated with ETEC, a much larger secretory volume was obtained from segments in the proximal small intestine, with the terminal jejunum and ileum producing very little volume following inoculation.[34,35] The mean volumes secreted in the small intestine following ETEC inoculation were as follows (with the intestine divided into six equal parts, from orad to aborad): 36, 24, 30, 13, 10, 0 mL.[34] Colonization of the proximal intestine is therefore the critical determinant of the severity of dehydration following infection with ETEC because colonization of the ileum and distal jejunum with ETEC has minimal effect on hydration status as STa is an ineffective secretagogue in this section of the intestinal tract. In summary, decreasing luminal pH in the proximal small intestine will increase nonspecific resistance to ETEC by preventing adherence to epithelial cells by K99 pili and preventing secretion of STa enterotoxin. This observation suggests that feeding ORT solution or water of acidic pH will be beneficial in treating and preventing calf diarrhea. Moreover, alkalinization induced by bicarbonate-containing ORT solutions potentially facilitates growth of ETEC bacteria, expression of K99 pili, and production of STa enterotoxin in the small intestine.

Neonatal calves are particularly susceptible to infection by *Salmonella enterica* subsp. *enterica* because of their immature immune system and suspected high abomasal pH during the first 24 hours of life.[85–87] Calves on endemically infected farms are exposed to *Salmonella* immediately after birth through ingestion of feces and colostrum of their dams;[88] in the first week of life from the environment and via contaminated colostrum, milk, feeding utensils, and farm personnel;[86] and after weaning by drinking water from a continuously replenished water tank with a pH >8.[89] Cows that are chronically infected may shed up to 10^5 salmonella/mL of milk, with 10^2 to 10^3 being the most frequent.[90] *Salmonella* readily multiply in pooled unrefrigerated waste milk, and outbreaks of salmonellosis in calves have been associated with feeding of unrefrigerated waste milk[86] or colostrum from another cow.[91] One study found that 58% (43/74) of dairy calves on a California dairy shed *Salmonella* in their stool within 24 hours of birth, and 85% shed *Salmonella* within 7 days of birth.[92]

Calves develop an age-dependent resistance to *Salmonella* that appears to be associated with development of a functional rumen, presence of a diverse small intestinal bacterial population, and low abomasal pH.[93,94] The optimum pH for *Salmonella* growth is generally accepted to fall between 6.5 and 7.5,[95] and *Salmonella* are sensitive to destruction by exposure to low pH.[96–98] Abomasal acidity therefore provides a natural barrier to ingested salmonellae.[94] *Salmonella* isolated from a small number of cattle were killed when pH ≤ 3.4 and multiplied when pH ≥ 5.5.[97] Maintaining a low abomasal pH will therefore decrease the number of viable *Salmonella* bacteria reaching the small intestine, thereby increasing nonspecific resistance to intestinal colonization and decreasing the incidence of infection and clinical disease.

Acetate and propionate inhibit the growth of Salmonella

The presence of bacteria can inhibit the growth of *Salmonella*, and this inhibition appears to be mediated by bacterial metabolic waste products, such as short chain fatty acids.[95,96,99] Acetate, propionate, and butyrate inhibit the growth of *Salmonella*, even in concentrations as low as 20 mmol/L[95,96] that are frequently found in ORT solutions administered to diarrheic calves.[100] This finding suggests that the addition of acetate or propionate may have beneficial effects separate from those obtained by sodium coupled intestinal absorption, systemic alkalinization, preventing excessive intestinal alkalinization, and being a source of nutrition.[100]

TREATMENTS THAT ARE NOT CURRENTLY RECOMMENDED
Probiotics

Probiotics are lyophilized or live bacterial cultures that are added to animal feeds or administered individually to animals in an attempt to improve performance or increase resistance to enteric pathogens. Probiotics may be more correctly termed as direct-fed microbials. There has recently been an emphasis on differentiating probiotics from prebiotics; the latter are foods that nourish beneficial bacteria that already reside in the digestive tract, such as *Bifidobacteria* and *Lactobacillus* species.

Administration of probiotics to diarrheic calves is done in some dairy herds, but the practice cannot currently be recommended. Daily administration of lyophilized lactic-acid producing bacteria in milk for the first 10 days of life had no effect on *C parvum* infection in dairy calves in California.[101] In calves with spontaneous diarrhea, the administration of *Lactobacillus rhamnosus* GG, an extensively studied probiotic isolated from the human gastrointestinal tract, for therapy of diarrhea did not change the mortality rate of the incidence of diarrhea.[7] Of real concern are the results of a recent study in neonatal foals that indicated administration of a different *Lactobacillus* strain for the prevention of diarrhea was associated with the development of diarrhea and clinical abnormalities requiring veterinary intervention.[102] This foal study contradicts widely held beliefs that "probiotics can't hurt."

The results of a recent study under field conditions in Germany indicated that the prophylactic administration of the probiotic bacteria *E coli* strain Nissle 1917 for the first 10 or 12 days of life to calves with unknown status of passive transfer was associated with a significant decrease in the number of calves developing diarrhea.[103] Based on these reports, administration of *E coli* strain Nissle 1917 may be helpful in preventing or treating diarrhea in calves, but additional studies are needed. This product is sold in Germany under the trade name Ponsocol for the prevention of neonatal diarrhea.

Intestinal "Protectants" and "Absorbants"

Administration of intestinal "protectants," such as kaolin (natural hydrated aluminum silicate), activated attapulgite (hydrated magnesium aluminum trisilicate), and pectin (natural polygalacturonic acids) or "absorbants," such as activated charcoal, kaolin, and attapulgite, are not recommended. Protectants are believed to protect damaged intestinal mucosa and absorbants purportedly neutralize luminal toxins by preventing binding to epithelial cell receptors. No data on treatment efficacy is available in calves.[3] More importantly, the results of a recent prospective randomized study indicated that non-antibiotic treatments for calf diarrhea, including bismuth, kaolin-pectin, activated attapulgite, and activated charcoal, resulted in a longer duration of treatment and increased risk for morbidity and mortality, compared with oral antibiotics in milk replacer (neomycin sulfate and chlortetracycline hydrochloride) and parenteral administration of ceftiofur hydrochloride (2.2 mg/kg, 3 to 5 days).[36]

Gastrointestinal Motility Modifiers

Intestinal motility is altered in diarrhea, but this change does not mean that abnormal motility is deleterious and that therapeutic manipulation of intestinal motility in calves with diarrhea will be beneficial. Drugs that inhibit intestinal motility are not indicated as part of the routine treatment of calf diarrhea, even though induction of complete intestinal paralysis may be viewed as a successful treatment of calf diarrhea if success were measured on the basis of fecal production.[104] Indeed, if the daily volume of feces is an important criterion of treatment success, then mere starvation of the calf would be viewed as an excellent therapy! Reduction of intestinal motility means that toxins and bacteria present in the intestinal lumen are not flushed away, increasing their local concentration and the possibility of a pathogenic effect.

Administration of agents that decrease intestinal motility, such as hyoscine N-butyl-bromide or atropine, are not recommended, despite their widespread use. No data on their treatment efficacy in calves with naturally acquired diarrhea is available.[3] One study in calves with nutritional diarrhea caused by sucrose administration found that hyoscine/dipyrone caused a modest reduction in fecal water losses.[105] Combined administration of the centrally acting muscarinic antagonist dexetimide (Benzetimide; 15 µg/kg bodyweight IM) and antibiotics caused a faster resolution of diarrhea in calves than did administration of antibiotics alone.[106] Dexetimide has been widely used to treat neuroleptic-induced Parkinsonism in humans, and its role, if any, in the treatment of calf diarrhea remains unclear.

Parenteral Administration of Mycobacterial Cell Wall Extracts

A product that was derived from mycobacterial cell wall extracts was developed in the 1990s in the United States. Parenteral administration of the product (Immunoboost, Bioniche Animal Health USA, Inc) during the first 24 hours of life purportedly decreased the prevalence of diarrhea,[107] suggesting that the product may have some efficacy as an ancillary treatment for calf diarrhea. However, peer-reviewed publications documenting treatment efficacy do not appear to be available.

Homeopathic Treatments, Such As Podophyllum or Oregano

Veterinary homeopathy is increasing in popularity, particularly in Europe, where priority is often given to veterinary homeopathic treatment rather than allopathic veterinary medicine on organic farms.[11] The homeopathic agent podophyllum is derived from *Podophyllum peltatum* (mayapple), and it has been used as a medicine by Native American Indians as a laxative or a treatment for intestinal parasites. The results of a double-blind placebo-controlled clinical trial of podophyllum (dose not stated) in 44 calves with diarrhea in Sweden indicated that podophyllum had no effect on the duration of diarrhea or the presence of depression, inappetance, and fever.[11]

Allicin, a sulfur-containing component of garlic that prevents the growth of some bacteria, fungi, viruses, and protozoa, had no effect on weight gain or duration of diarrhea due to *C parvum* in calves.[108] Anecdotal reports of the use of nutmeg as a treatment for calf diarrhea exist,[109] but treatment efficacy has not been formally evaluated.

Oregano contains oils (carvacrol and thymol) that have antimicrobial activity. The effects of oral administration of oregano essential oils (10 mg/kg bodyweight by mouth daily) was compared with that of a purported positive control (oral neomycin, 10 mg/kg bodyweight by mouth daily) in calves with naturally acquired diarrhea in Greece.[110] No difference in duration of diarrhea or severity of diarrhea was observed between the two treatments. Because a study documenting the efficacy of oral neomycin at labeled doses in treating calves with naturally acquired diarrhea does not appear to have been published in a peer-reviewed journal,[1] oregano cannot be recommended as an adjunct treatment for calf diarrhea.

SUMMARY

Adjunct treatment of calves with diarrhea should be routinely undertaken in all calves with systemic signs of illness, manifest as fever, inappetance, or lethargy. Ancillary treatments with documented efficacy in undifferentiated calf diarrhea include: parenteral administration of antimicrobials with a predominantly Gram-negative spectrum of activity; parenteral administration of the NSAID agents meloxicam and flunixin meglumine; and continued feeding of cow's milk. This recommended adjunct treatment protocol is similar to that used by a leading dairy veterinarian in Europe.[111] Finally, because halofuginone and azithromycin have documented efficacy in calves with diarrhea caused by *C parvum*, their administration may be considered in calves documented or suspected to have cryptosporidiosis.

REFERENCES

1. Constable PD. Antimicrobial use in the treatment of calf diarrhea. J Vet Intern Med 2004a;18:8–17.
2. Jiminez A, Sanchez J, Andres S, et al. Evaluation of endotoxemia in the prognosis and treatment of scouring merino lambs. J Vet Med A Physiol Pathol Clin Med 2007;54:103–6.
3. Berchtold J, Constable PD. Antibiotic treatment of diarrhea in preweaned calves. In: Anderson DE, Rings DM, editors. Current veterinary therapy—food animal practice. 5th edition. St. Louis (MO): Saunders Elsevier; 2008. p. 520–5.
4. Navetat H, Biron P, Contrepois M, et al. Les gastroentérites paralysantes: maladie ou syndrome? Bull Acad Vet Fr 1997;70:327–36.
5. Schelcher F, Marcillaud S, Braun JP, et al. Metabolic acidosis without dehydration and no or minimal diarrhoea in suckler calves is caused by hyper D-lactatemia. Proc World Buiatrics Congress 1998;XX:371.
6. Ewaschuk JB, Naylor JM, Zello GA, et al. Anion gap correlates with serum D- and DL-lactate concentration in diarrheic neonatal calves. J Vet Intern Med 2003;17:940–2.
7. Ewaschuk JB, Zello GM, Naylor JM, et al. Lactobacillus GG does not affect D-lactic acidosis in diarrheic calves in a clinical setting. J Vet Intern Med 2006;20:614–9.
8. Lorenz I. Influence of D-lactate on metabolic acidosis and on prognosis in neonatal calves with diarrhoea. J Vet Med A 2004a;51:425–8.
9. Constable PD, Staempfli HR, Navetat H, et al. Use of a quantitative strong ion approach to determine the mechanism for acid-base abnormalities in sick calves with or without diarrhea. J Vet Intern Med 2005;19:581–9.
10. Lorenz I. Investigations on the influence of serum D-lactate levels on clinical signs in calves with metabolic acidosis. Vet J 2004b;168:323–7.
11. de Verdier K, Ohagen P, Alenius S, et al. No effect of a homeopathic preparation on neonatal calf diarrhoea in a randomised double-blind, placebo-conrolled clinical trial. Acta Vet Scand 2003;44:97–101.
12. Grove-White DH. A rational approach to treatment of calf diarrhoea. Irish Vet J 2004;57:722–8.
13. Constable PD, Pyörälä S, Smith GW, et al. Antimicrobial use in cattle. In: Guardabassi L, Jensen LB, Kruse H, editors. Principles of prudent and rational use of antimicrobials in animals. Oxford (UK): Blackwell Publishing; 2008. p. 143–60.
14. Morley PS, Apley MD, Besser TE, et al. Antimicrobial drug use in veterinary medicine. J Vet Intern Med 2005;19:617–29.

15. Fecteau G, Van Metre DC, Pare J, et al. Bacteriological culture of blood from critically ill neonatal calves. Can Vet J 1997a;38:95–100.
16. Lofstedt J, Dohoo IR, Duizer G. Model to predict septicemia in diarrheic calves. J Vet Intern Med 1999;13:81–8.
17. Thomas E, Roy O, Skowronski V, et al. Comparative field efficacy study between cefquinome and gentamicin in neonatal calves with clinical signs of septicaemia. Revue Méd Vét 2004;155:489–93.
18. Fecteau ME, House JK, Kotarski SF, et al. Efficacy of ceftiofur for treatment of experimental salmonellosis in neonatal calves. Am J Vet Res 2003;64:918–25.
19. Fecteau G, Paré J, Van Metre DC, et al. Use of a clinical sepsis score for predicting bacteremia in neonatal dairy calves on a calf rearing farm. Can Vet J 1997b;38:101–4.
20. Bywater J. Evaluation of an oral glucose-glycine-electrolyte formulation and amoxicillin for treatment of diarrhea in calves. Am J Vet Res 1977;38:1983–6.
21. Palmer GH, Bywater RJ, Stanton A, et al. Absorption in calves of amoxicillin, ampicillin, and oxytetracycline in milk replacer, water, or an oral rehydration formulation. Am J Vet Res 1983;44:68–71.
22. Radostits OM, Rhodes CS, Mitchell ME, et al. A clinical evaluation of antimicrobial agents and temporary starvation in the treatment of acute undifferentiated diarrhea in newborn calves. Can Vet J 1975;16:219–27.
23. Ortman K, Svensson C. Use of antimicrobial drugs in Swedish dairy calves and replacement heifers. Vet Rec 2004;154:136–40.
24. Berge ACB, Moore DA, Sischo WM, et al. Field trial evaluating the influence of prophylactic and therapeutic antimicrobial administration on antimicrobial resistance of fecal Escherichia coli in dairy calves. Appl Environ Microbiol 2006a;72:3872–8.
25. White G, Piercy DWT, Gibbs HA, et al. Use of a calf salmonellosis model to evaluate the therapeutic properties of trimethoprim and sulphadiazine and their mutual potentiation in vivo. Res Vet Sci 1981;31:27–31.
26. Busani L, Graziani C, Franco A, et al. Survey of the knowledge, attitudes and practice of Italian beef and dairy cattle veterinarians concerning the use of antibiotics. Vet Rec 2004;155:733–8.
27. Phillip H, Schmidt H, During F, et al. Efficacy of meloxicam (Metacam®) as adjunct to a basic therapy for the treatment of diarrhea in calves. Acta Vet Scand Suppl 2003;98:273.
28. Todd CG, McKnight DR, Millman ST, et al. An evaluation of meloxicam (Metacam®) as an adjunctive therapy for calves with neonatal diarrhea complex. J Anim Sci 2007;85(Suppl 1):369.
29. Lopez GA, Phillips RW, Lewis LD, et al. Plasma corticoid changes during diarrhea in neonatal calves. Am J Vet Res 1975;36:1245–7.
30. Hudson S, Mullord M, Whittlestone WG, et al. Plasma corticoid levels in healthy and diarrheic calves from birth to twenty days of age. Br Vet J 1976;132:551–6.
31. Barnett SC, Sischo WM, Moore DA, et al. Evaluation of flunixin meglumine as an adjunct treatment for diarrhea in dairy calves. J Am Vet Med Assoc 2003;223:1329–33.
32. Roussel AJ, Sriranganathan N, Brown SA, et al. Effect of flunixin meglumine on Escherichia coli heat-stable enterotoxin-induced diarrhea in calves. Am J Vet Res 1988;49:1431–3.
33. Cole J, Blikslager A, Hunt E, et al. Cyclo-oxygenase blockade and exogenous glutamine enhance sodium absorption in infected bovine ileum. Am J Phys 2003;284:G516–24.

34. Smith HW, Halls S. Observations by the ligated intestinal segment and oral inoculation methods on *Escherichia coli* infections in pigs, calves, lambs, and rabbits. J Pathol Bacteriol 1967;93:499–529.
35. Tennant B, Harrold D, Reina-Guerra M, et al. Physiologic and metabolic factors in the pathogenesis of neonatal enteric infections in calves. J Am Vet Med Assoc 1972;161:993–1007.
36. Berge ACB, Lindeque P, Moore DA, et al. A clinical trial evaluating prophylactic and therapeutic antibiotic use on health and performance of preweaned calves. J Dairy Sci 2005;88:2166–77.
37. Roussel AJ, Dodson SL, Brumbaugh GW, et al. Effect of ketoprofen on *Escherichia coli* heat-stable enterotoxin-induced diarrhea of calves. Am J Vet Res 1993;54:2088–90.
38. Wise CM, Knight AP, Lucas MJ, et al. Effect of salicylates on intestinal secretion in calves given (intestinal loops) *Escherichia coli* heat-stable enterotoxin. Am J Vet Res 1983;44:2221–5.
39. Johnson JK, Schmidt J, Gelberg HB, et al. Microbial adhesion of *Cryptosporidium parvum* sporozoites: purification of an inhibitory lipid from bovine mucosa. J Parasitol 2004;90:980–90.
40. Naciri M, Mancassola R, Yvore P, et al. The effect of halofuginone lactate on experimental *Cryptosporidium parvum* infections in calves. Vet Parasitol 1993; 45:199–207.
41. Villacorta I, Peeters JE, Vanopdenbosch E, et al. Efficacy of halofuginone lactate against *Cryptosporidium parvum* in calves. Antimicrobial Agents Chemother 1991;35:283–7.
42. Lallemond M, Villeneuve A, Belda J, et al. Field study of the efficacy of halofuginone and decoquinate in the treatment of cryptosporidiosis in veal calves. Vet Rec 2006;159:672–7.
43. Klein P. Preventive and therapeutic efficacy of halofuginone-lactate against *Cryptosporidium parvum* in spontaneously infected calves: a centralized, randomized, double-blind, placebo-controlled study. Vet J 2008;177: 429–31.
44. Elitok B, Elitok OM, Pulat H, et al. Efficacy of azithromycin dihydrate in treatment of cryptosporidosis in naturally infected dairy calves. J Vet Intern Med 2005;19: 590–3.
45. Nouri M, Hajkolaee MR, Constable PD, et al. Effect of erythromycin and gentamicin on abomasal emptying rate in suckling calves. J Vet Intern Med 2008;22:196–201.
46. Nouri M, Constable PD. Effect of parenteral administration of erythromycin, tilmicosin, and tylosin on abomasal emptying rate in suckling calves. Am J Vet Res 2007;68:1392–8.
47. Ashfari G, Banihassan E, Dwzfuli MRM, et al. The effect of parenteral administration of ivermectin and erythromycin on abomasal emptying rate in suckling calves. Am J Vet Res, in press.
48. Moore DA, Atwill ER, Kirk JH, et al. Prophylactic use of decoquinate for infections with *Cryptosporidium parvum* in experimentally challenged neonatal calves. J Am Vet Med Assoc 2003;223:839–45.
49. Viu M, Quilez J, Sanchez-Acedo C, et al. Field trial on the therapeutic efficacy of paromyomycin on natural *Cryptosporidium parvum* infections in lambs. Vet Parasitol 2000;90:163–70.
50. Gobel F. Diagnosis and treatment of acute cryptosporidiosis in the calf. Tierartz Umschau 1987;42:863–9.

51. Sahal M, Karaer Z, Yas Duru S, et al. Cryptosporidiosis in newborn calves in Ankara region: clinical, haematological findings and treatment with Lasalocid-Na. Dtsch Tierarztl Wschenschr 2005;112:203–10.

52. Heath SE, Naylor JM, Guedo BL, et al. The effects of feeding milk to diarrheic calves supplemented with oral electrolytes. Can J Vet Res 1989;53:477–85.

53. Brooks HW, Hall GA, Wagstaff AJ, et al. Detrimental effects on villus form during conventional oral rehydration therapy for diarrhea in calves: Alleviation by a nutrient oral rehydration solution containing glutamine. Vet J 1998;155:263–74.

54. Naylor JM, Leibel T, Middleton DM, et al. Effect of glutamine or glycine containing oral electrolyte solutions on mucosal morphology, clinical and biochemical findings, in calves with viral induced diarrhea. Can J Vet Res 1997;61:43–8.

55. Naylor JM. Oral electrolyte therapy in Roussel AJ, Constable PD. Vet Clin Food Anim 1999;15(3):487–504.

56. Mouricout M, Petit JM, Carias JR, et al. Glycoprotein glycans that inhibit adhesion of Escherichia coli mediated by K99 fimbrae: Treatment of experimental colibacillosis. Infect Immun 1990;58:98–106.

57. Heinrichs AJ, Jones CM, Heinrichs BS, et al. Effects of mannan oligosaccharide or antibiotics in neonatal diets on health and growth of dairy calves. J Dairy Sci 2003;86:4064–9.

58. Quigley JD III, Drewry JJ, Murray LM, et al. Body weight gain, feed efficiency, and fecal scores of dairy calves in response to galactosyl-lactose or antibiotics in milk replacers. J Dairy Sci 1997;80:1751–4.

59. Donovan DC, Franklin ST, Chase CCL, et al. Growth and health of Holstein calves fed milk replacers supplemented with antibiotics or Enteroguard. J Dairy Sci 2002;85:947–50.

60. Brody EP. Biological activities of bovine glycomacropeptide. Br J Nutr 2000; 84(Suppl 1):S39–46.

61. Reiter B. Review of nonspecific antimicrobial factors in colostrum. Ann Rech Vet 1978;9:205–24.

62. Ward GE, Nelson DI. Effects of dietary milk fat (whole milk) and propionic acid on intestinal coliforms and lactobacilli in calves. Am J Vet Res 1982;43:1165–7.

63. Parrish DB, Fountaine FC. Contents of the alimentary tract of calves at birth. J Dairy Sci 1953;36:839–45.

64. Fey H. Immunology of the newborn calf: It's relationship to colisepticemia. Annal NY Acad Sci 1971;176:49–66.

65. Ahmed AF, Constable PD, Misk NA, et al. Effect of an orally administered antacid agent containing aluminum hydroxide and magnesium hydroxide on abomasal luminal pH in clinically normal milk-fed calves. J Am Vet Med Assoc 2002a;220:74–9.

66. Ahmed AF, Constable PD, Misk NA, et al. Effect of feeding frequency and route of administration on abomasal luminal pH in dairy calves fed milk replacer. J Dairy Sci 2002b;85:1502–8.

67. Acres SD. Enterotoxigenic Escherichia coli infections in newborn calves: a review. J Dairy Sci 1985;68:229–56.

68. Morin M, Lariviere S, Lallier R, et al. Pathological and microbiological observations made on spontaneous cases of acute neonatal calf diarrhea. Can J Comp Med 1976;40:228–40.

69. Isaacson RE, Moon HW, Schneider RA, et al. Distribution and virulence of Escherichia coli in the small intestines of calves with and without diarrhea. Am J Vet Res 1978;39:1750–5.

70. Mebus CA, Stair EL, Underdahl NR, et al. Pathology of neonatal calf diarrhea induced by a Reo-like virus. Vet Pathol 1971;8:490–505.
71. Carpenter CM, Woods G. The distribution of the colon-aerogenes group of bacteria in the alimentary tract of calves. Cornell Vet 1924;14:218–25.
72. Smith T, Orcutt ML. The bacteriology of the intestinal tract of young calves with special reference to early diarrhea. J Exp Med 1925;41:89–106.
73. Smith HW. Observations on the etiology of neonatal diarrhoea (scours) in calves. J Pathol Bacteriol 1962;84:147–68.
74. Youanes YD, Herdt TH. Changes in small intestinal morphology and flora associated with decreased energy digestibility in calves with naturally occurring diarrhea. Am J Vet Res 1987;48:719–25.
75. Maffei HVL, Nobrega FJ. Gastric pH and microflora of normal and diarrhoeic infants. Gut 1975;16:719–26.
76. Haddad JJ. Factors in the establishment of enteropathogenic escherichia coli in the small intestine of calves. PhD thesis. University of Guelph, 1981.
77. Reisinger RC. Pathogenesis and prevention of infectious diarrhea (scours) of newborn calves. J Am Vet Med Assoc 1965;147:1377–86.
78. Mylrea PJ. Digestion in young calves fed whole milk ad lib and its relationship to calf scours. Res Vet Sci 1966;7:407–16.
79. Mylrea PJ. Gastro-intestinal disorders and the functioning of the digestive tract of young calves. Res Vet Sci 1968;9:14–28.
80. Ternouth JH, Roy HB. The effect of diet and feeding technique on digestive function in the calf. Ann Rech Vet 1973;4:19–30.
81. Francis DH, Allen SD, White RD, et al. Influence of bovine intestinal fluid on the expression of K99 pili by *Escherichia coli*. Am J Vet Res 1989;50:822–6.
82. Pearson GR, Logan EF. The pathogenesis of enteric colibacillosis in neonatal suckled calves. Vet Rec 1979;105:159–64.
83. Mitchell IG, Tame MJ, Kenworthy R, et al. Conditions for the production of *Escherichia coli* enterotoxin in a defined medium. J Med Microbiol 1974;7: 395–400.
84. Al-Majali AM, Asem EK, Lamar CH, et al. Studies on the mechanism of diarrhea induced by *Escherichia coli* heat-stable enterotoxin (STa) in newborn calves. Vet Res Commun 2000;24:327–38.
85. Roden LD, Smith BP, Spier SJ, et al. Effect of calf age and Salmonella bacterin type on the ability to produce immunoglobulins directed against Salmonella whole cells or lipopolysaccharide. Am J Vet Res 1992;53:1895–9.
86. House JK, Smith BP. Current strategies for managing salmonella infections in cattle. Vet Med 1998;756–64.
87. Anderson M, Blanchard P. The clinical syndromes caused by Salmonella infection. Vet Med 1989;816–9.
88. Osborne AD, Pearson H, Linton AH, et al. Epidemiology of salmonella infection in calves: The source of calfhood infection by *Salmonella Dublin*. Vet Rec 1977; 101:513–6.
89. Kirk J, Atwill E, Holmberg C, et al. Prevalence of and risk factors for salmonella in water offered to weaned dairy calves in California, USA. Prev Vet Med 2002;54: 169–78.
90. Smith BP, Oliver DG, Singh P, et al. Detection of *Salmonella dublin* mammary gland infection in carrier cows, using an enzyme-linked immunosorbent assay for antibody in milk or serum. Am J Vet Res 1989;50:1352–60.

91. Veling J, Wilpshaar H, Frankena K, et al. Risk factors for clinical *Salmonella enterica* subsp. *enterica* serovar Typhimurium infection on Dutch dairy farms. Prev Vet Med 2002;54:157–68.
92. House JK, Ontiveros MM, Blackmer NM, et al. Evaluation of an autogenous Salmonella bacterin and a modified live salmonella serotype choleraesuis vaccine on a commercial dairy farm. Am J Vet Res 2001;62:1897–902.
93. Robinson RA, Loken KI. Age susceptibility and excretion of salmonella typhimurium in calves. J Hyg 1968;66:207–16.
94. Segall T, Lindberg AA. Experimental oral Salmonella dublin infection in calves. A bacteriological and pathological study. Zentralbl Veterinarmed B 1991;38: 169–85.
95. Chung KC, Goepfert JM. Growth of Salmonella at low pH. J Food Sci 1970;35: 326–8.
96. Bohnhoff M, Miller CP, Martin WR, et al. Resistance of the mouse's intestinal tract to experimental salmonella infection. J Exp Med 1964;120:805–16.
97. Wray C, Callow RJ. Studies on the survival of *Salmonella Dublin, S typhimurium*, and *E coli* in stored bovine colostrum. Vet Rec 1974;94:407–12.
98. Collins FM. Salmonellosis in orally infected specific pathogen-free C57B1 mice. Infect Immun 1972;5:191–8.
99. Chambers PG, Lysons RJ. The inhibitory effect of bovine rumen fluid on *Salmonella typhimurium*. Res Vet Sci 1979;26:273–6.
100. Constable PD, Thomas E, Boisrame B, et al. Comparison of two oral electrolyte solutions for the treatment of dehydrated calves with experimentally-induced diarrhoea. Vet J 2001;162:129–40.
101. Harp JA, Jardon P, Atwill ER, et al. Field testing of prophylactic measures against *Cryptosporidum parvum* infection in calves in a California dairy herd. Am J Vet Res 1996;57:1586–8.
102. Weese JS, Rousseau J. Evaluation of *Lactobacillus pentosus* WE7 for prevention of diarrhea in neonatal foals. J Am Vet Med Assoc 2005;226:2031–4.
103. von Buenau R, Jaekel L, Schubotz E, et al. *Escherichia coli* strain Nissle 1917: Significant reduction of neonatal calf diarrhea. J Dairy Sci 2005;88:317–23.
104. Roussel AJ, Brumbaugh GW. Treatment of diarrhea of neonatal calves. Vet Clin Food Anim 1991;7(3):713–28.
105. Fallon RJ, Quirke JF, Limper J, et al. The effects of buscopan compositum on calf nutritional diarrhoea. Vet Res Commun 1991;15:475–82.
106. Symoens J, Geerts H, Van Gestel J, et al. Benzetimide in the treatment of diarrhea in newborn calves and adult cattle. Vet Rec 1974;94:180–3.
107. Muscato TV, Tedeschi LO, Russell JB, et al. The effect of ruminal fluid preparations on the growth and health of newborn, milk-fed dairy calves. J Dairy Sci 2002;85:648–56.
108. Olson EJ, Epperson WB, Zeman DH, et al. Effects of an allicin-based product on cryptosporidiosis in neonatal calves. J Am Vet Med Assoc 1998;212:987–90.
109. Stamford IF, Bennett A. Treatment of diarrhoea in cattle and pigs. Vet Rec 1978; 103:14–5.
110. Bampidis VA, Christodoulou V, Florou-Paneri P, et al. Effect of dried oregano leaves versus neomycin in treating newborn calves with colibacillosis. J Vet Med A 2006;53:154–6.
111. Garcia JP. A practitioner's view on fluid therapy in calves. Vet Clin Food Anim 1999;15(3):533–43.

Respiratory Disease of the Bovine Neonate

Keith P. Poulsen, DVM[a,b,]*, Sheila M. McGuirk, DVM, PhD[a]

KEYWORDS

- Bovine • Calf • Neonate • Hypoxia
- Persistent pulmonary hypertension • Pneumonia
- Pneumothorax

Respiratory disease is a constant challenge for dairy replacement heifer rearing systems, and is responsible for 21.3% of mortality in preweaned calves and 50.4% of deaths in weaned heifers.[1] There are many negative long-term consequences for survivors of subclinical, clinical, and chronic calf pneumonia including poor growth, reproductive performance, milk production, and longevity.[2–4] These calves also become sources of infection for other calves, and can cause outbreaks after weaning in group pens.[5] Contamination of the environment with bacterial and viral pathogens is the obvious source of respiratory disease in calves. When reviewing the literature and examining cases seen both in the authors' hospital and during herd investigations, however, it was realized that treatment and prevention of calf pneumonia has evolved beyond recommendations for antibiotic therapy and vaccination protocols. The high cost of replacement heifers and the development of reproductive technologies have increased the need to detect and treat high-risk neonates suffering from respiratory disease. Many times those calves serve as sentinels for infectious disease that direct calf management decisions on the farm. This article discusses the normal physiologic changes from the uterine environment through parturition and methods to monitor the high-risk or abnormal neonate. Covered are causes of respiratory disease and different strategies for diagnosis and treatment that can be applied to herd investigations or individual animals. All herd investigation tools and forms can be found at the following Web site: http://www.vetmed.wisc.edu/dms/fapm/fapmtools/calves.htm.

THE POSTNATAL PERIOD, HYPOXIA, AND HYPERCAPNIA

Many physiologic changes occur rapidly in the transition from fetal life to the neonatal period. At parturition the neonate needs to assume responsibility for oxygenating its

[a] Department of Medical Sciences, University of Wisconsin-Madison School of Veterinary Medicine, 2015 Linden Drive, Madison, WI 53706, USA
[b] Department of Pathobiological Sciences, University of Wisconsin-Madison School of Veterinary Medicine, Madison, WI 53706, USA
* Corresponding author. Department of Medical Sciences, University of Wisconsin-Madison School of Veterinary Medicine, 2015 Linden Drive, Madison, WI 53706.
E-mail address: poulsenk@svm.vetmed.wisc.edu (K.P. Poulsen).

Vet Clin Food Anim 25 (2009) 121–137
doi:10.1016/j.cvfa.2008.10.007
0749-0720/08/$ – see front matter © 2009 Elsevier Inc. All rights reserved.

own blood from atmospheric air, and maintaining a normal blood pH and body temperature.[6] In utero, the numerous placentomes that are distributed on the endometrial surface provide oxygen and nutrient-rich blood to the fetal placenta. Distribution of the oxygen and nutrients is accomplished by the fetal circulation shunting blood away from the pulmonary circulation by way of the ductus arteriosus and foramen ovale, which is facilitated by hypoxia-induced pulmonary arterial constriction.[7] The fetus is quite hypoxic (80% O_2 saturation, Pao_2 of 38 mm Hg) relative to the dam (98%–100% O_2 saturation, Pao_2 of 100 mm Hg), but adapts well to this environment because of efficient O_2 extraction from maternal placental blood with fetal hemoglobin's high affinity for O_2[7–9] and by increasing blood flow from nonessential organs to the brain, heart, and adrenal glands.[10]

At birth massive changes in lung function and arterial blood gases occur as the fetal lung fluid is removed with uterine contractions and absorbed by the pulmonary circulation and lymphatics as the calf begins to breathe.[11] Before stage 2 labor, the fetus should not be hypoxic as long as the umbilical cord remains attached,[8] but during fetal expulsion, rupture of the fetal membranes and separation of the umbilical vessels lead to hypoxia and respiratory and metabolic acidosis.[12,13] Respiratory acidosis (hypercapnia), detected by the chemosensitive area in the medulla, is the most important stimulus for respiration. This is aided by tactile stimulation from the dam (ie, licking) and a decrease in environmental temperature relative to in utero conditions.[14,15] Hypoxia, detected by peripheral chemoreceptors in the carotid and aortic bodies, does not have a significant direct effect on the respiratory center in the brain.[14] Dystocia can result in a severe respiratory and metabolic acidosis that may require treatment or can result in long-term detrimental effects on the neonate, such as hypoxic-ischemic encephalopathy.[16] The degree of respiratory acidosis is dependent on the time between loss of maternal blood supply to the fetus and successful respiration.[8] Metabolic acidosis is caused by lactic acid accumulation during hypoxia.[17,18] Healthy calves have a surprising ability, however, to self-correct hypercapnia and hypoxia within the first hours of life.[19–21] As respiration continues to increase pulmonary blood flow and improve oxygenation, the foramen ovale and ductus arteriosus close to end fetal circulation.[8]

Several methods have been described to monitor acid-base status and pulmonary function, and predict morbidity and mortality caused by respiratory disease in the neonate. Sternal recumbency should be attained within 2 to 3 minutes and the normal calf should attempt to stand within 15 to 30 minutes after birth. Hypoxic neonates, likely to be affected by respiratory acidosis, have a weak to absent suckle reflex, have difficulty maintaining sternal recumbency, and require more time to stand.[22] The Apgar scoring index can be used to assess neonatal viability and predict early signs of peripartum asphyxia.[23] Perhaps more practical on the dairy, Schuijt and Taverne[24] described the time to attain sternal recumbency as a measure of neonatal viability. They reported a negative correlation between neonatal vitality and increased time for the calf to achieve sternal recumbency after birth. Calves that took greater than 15 minutes to achieve sternal recumbency had an 84% predictive value for nonvitality. Other critical elements of the physical examination when assessing for the presence of respiratory disease include mucous membrane color (vulvar mucous membranes); character and frequency of the respiratory effort; and thoracic auscultation.

If available, pulse oximetry and blood gas analysis can be valuable to assess pulmonary function and acid-base status. Pulse oximetry was validated in the calf as a relatively accurate, noninvasive, immediate, and portable method to monitor oxygen saturation (Sao_2).[25] Bleul and Kähl[26] describe using pulse oximetry during stage 2 labor to assess pulmonary function in valuable calves during delivery, because fetal reflexes are poorly correlated with fetal vitality in cattle.[27] Despite the challenge of using the oximeter during parturition, calves with low Sao_2 (<30%) for at least 2 minutes in stage 2 labor had a high predictive value for acidosis (blood pH <7.2).[26] In a hospital setting, blood gas analysis is a direct measure of Po_2, Pco_2, concentration of bicarbonate (Hco_3^-), base excess, Sao_2, and pH. Reference values for acidotic calves (pH <7.2) and normal calves (pH ≥ 7.2) were recently reported (**Table 1**).[28] Evaluating pH and base excess values from venous blood are established methods;[12–15,29] however Po_2 and Pco_2 need to be measured from arterial blood because of the CO_2 and O_2 exchange in peripheral tissues.[30,31] There is no significant difference between using arterial blood from peripheral versus central arteries[32] and the brachial, lateral metatarsal, or the branches of the caudal auricular artery are suitable collection sites.[28,33] Plastic has replaced glass syringes in many settings because of cost, convenience, and resistance to breakage. It is important to note, however, that blood in plastic syringes needs to be analyzed immediately to ensure accuracy of the Po_2 measurement.[34,35]

Treatment of hypoxia and hypercapnia can be a challenge. Calves with significant hypoxia can be started on humidified oxygen by nasal administration at a rate of 2 to 10 L/min. Hypercapnia may persist despite oxygen therapy. The ventilatory drive caused by hypercapnia and associated respiratory acidosis is significantly stronger than the drive caused by hypoxemia. These calves might require treatment with respiratory stimulants, such as the methylxanthines (caffeine and aminophylline) or doxapram hydrochloride. Both of these drugs decrease the need for mechanical ventilation.[36] Methylxanthines directly stimulate the respiratory center, improve diaphragmatic contractility, and antagonize adenosine, which slows respiration.[36,37] Caffeine (NoDoz, 200 mg/tab) is readily available as an over-the-counter product but its oral bioavailability has been recently questioned in foals.[38] Extrapolated from equine doses, caffeine can be administered orally or per rectum with a 10 mg/kg loading dose followed by a 2.5 to 3 mg/kg every 24 hour maintenance dose.[39] When using aminophylline in the authors' hospital the doses reported for horses are used (4–10 mg/kg every 8–12 hours)[40] as a constant rate infusion (10–30 mg/kg/d). Doxapram hydrochloride stimulates the medullary respiratory centers by way of the aortic and carotid body chemoreceptors and can be given at a dose of 0.5 mg/kg IV or 5 to 10 mg/kg injected at the base of the tongue for emergency resuscitation and anoxia.[40–42] Doxapram has a history of poor availability to practitioners and has been reported to increase cerebral oxygen consumption and decrease cerebral blood flow, which has negative long-term consequences for the neonate.[43] A study in foals using an experimentally induced hypercapnia model, however, reported that doxapram restored ventilation without neurologic side effects in a dose-dependent manner.[38] Acupressure is an alternative therapy for anoxia that has occasionally been used in small and large animal neonatology. In calves, the authors use a 20-gauge, 1-in hypodermic needle placed in the nasal planum immediately after parturition if the calf is anoxic. The mechanism behind this technique is stimulation of the Renzhong acupoint, which increases phrenic nerve activity.[44] Ideally, serial blood gas analysis should be done to monitor the calf's response to whichever therapies are implemented. Calves with persistent hypercapnia despite therapeutic intervention are candidates for mechanical ventilation if available.

PERSISTENT PULMONARY HYPERTENSION

Persistent pulmonary hypertension is a syndrome characterized by significant cellular proliferation and extracellular matrix protein production in pulmonary endothelial cells.

Table 1
Mean (SD) values of arterial and venous blood gas and acid-base analyses in 57 newborn calves from birth to 24 hours

Variable	Blood	Time of Sampling					P^a	P^b
		At Birth	30 Minutes	4 hours	12 Hours	24 Hours		
pH	Arterial	7.30 (0.06)	7.36 (0.04)	7.38 (0.03)	7.42 (0.03)	7.43 (0.04)	<0.001	>0.05
	Venous	7.24 (0.09)	7.30 (0.04)	7.33 (0.03)	7.38 (0.04)	7.40 (0.06)	<0.001	
Pco_2 (mm Hg)	Arterial	57.31 (4.98)	52.58 (5.00)	48.70 (3.73)	43.71 (4.75)	44.22 (4.32)	<0.001	<0.001
	Venous	67.34 (10.39)	58.23 (6.45)	54.38 (6.10)	47.03 (5.75)	46.67 (6.24)	<0.001	
Po_2 (mm Hg)	Arterial	45.31 (16.02)	58.08 (13.12)	67.66 (14.55)	71.89 (8.32)	66.77 (14.21)	<0.001	<0.05
	Venous	20.94 (5.30)	27.95 (5.42)	29.15 (4.41)	29.33 (5.52)	27.62 (3.04)	<0.001	
Hco_3^- (mmol/l)	Arterial	26.76 (3.39)	28.01 (2.44)	27.40 (2.32)	26.96 (2.94)	28.31 (3.26)	>0.05	>0.05
	Venous	27.24 (3.70)	27.48 (3.81)	27.42 (3.18)	26.42 (2.82)	27.87 (3.35)	>0.05	
Base excess (mmol/L)	Arterial	0.86 (4.12)	2.9 (2.88)	2.52 (2.64)	2.78 (3.23)	4.42 (3.59)	>0.05	>0.05
	Venous	1.01 (3.49)	1.53 (4.37)	1.89 (3.48)	1.59 (3.08)	3.40 (3.92)	>0.05	
So_2 (%)	Arterial	64.16 (20.82)	82.08 (9.98)	89.23 (6.84)	92.84 (2.32)	89.75 (8.31)	<0.001	>0.05
	Venous	22.64 (10.00)	39.26 (10.98)	44.19 (9.39)	47.41 (12.06)	47.81 (15.41)	<0.001	

Abbreviations: Hco_3^-, bicarbonate; Pco_2, partial pressure of carbon dioxide; Po_2, partial pressure of oxygen; So_2, oxygen saturation.
[a] Analysis of variance for repeated measures within groups.
[b] Analysis of variance for repeated measures between groups.
Data from Bleul U, Lejeune B, Schwantag S, et al. Blood gas and acid-base analysis of arterial blood in 57 newborn calves. Vet Record 2007;161:688–91.

It occurs in response to persistent hypoxemia and vasoconstriction, which causes reversion to fetal pulmonary circulatory patterns with right-to-left shunting. Pulmonary hypertension can also be secondary to failure of the neonate's cardiopulmonary circulation to transition from the fetal state.[45–48] The disorder has been recognized in human and equine neonates, and the calf is used as a model to study pulmonary hypertension.[49–53] Pulmonary hypertension can be secondary to many different factors, such as persistent hypoxia caused by pneumonia, high altitude, or meconium aspiration, but the primary disorder is often idiopathic. Recently, persistent pulmonary hypertension has been increasingly recognized in calves derived from somatic cell clone technology.[54–58]

Calves with persistent pulmonary hypertension are hypoxic (Pao_2 <80 mm Hg) and tend to be hypercapnic. Diagnosis can be based on repeated arterial blood gas measurements when all other causes of hypoxemia are ruled out.[59] Other diagnostic tests for persistent pulmonary hypertension include radiographs or CT, cardiac catheterization, and echocardiography. Radiographs and CT show atelectasis and diminished vascular patterns from pulmonary hypoperfusion. Cardiac catheterization shows elevated pressure in the pulmonary artery, right ventricle, and right atrium.[60,61]

Treatment of persistent pulmonary hypertension centers on oxygen supplementation and mechanical ventilation if hypoxemia and hypercapnia persist. If acidosis is severe, bicarbonate therapy may be indicated. Nitric oxide is frequently used in human and equine neonates as a vasodilator.[62,63] Vasodilation with a phosphodiesterase-5 inhibitor, sildenafil (Viagra) given orally or as a suppository, has been used to treat persistent pulmonary hypertension in human infants[64,65] and foals[61] with varying success.

ASPIRATION PNEUMONIA

Aspiration pneumonia occurs when solid materials, typically a liquid or meconium, are inhaled. The most common cause of neonatal aspiration pneumonia seen in the authors' practice is from misuse of oral esophageal feeders. The use of oral esophageal feeders to "tube-feed" a calf has increased on farms to ensure timely feeding of an appropriate volume of clean, good-quality colostrum. Feeding calves with bottles can be time consuming and calves left to suckle the dam have high rates of failure of passive transfer.[66] Even though the esophageal groove does not close when using esophageal feeders, there is no significant difference in calf serum IgG concentrations or morbidity when compared with calves that suckle colostrum from a bottle.[67] Proper training of on-farm personnel is important to ensure placement of the feeder in the esophagus. Important points to review with personnel responsible for calf feeding are to use lubrication, to use an oral esophageal feeder that has a mechanism to control flow rates in case problems occur, and to maintain the calf's neutral head position during feeding while the calf is standing or in sternal recumbency.

Another cause of aspiration pneumonia, meconium aspiration, is associated with fetal distress syndrome and frequently results in increased mortality.[68] Gross and histopathologic lesions are similar to those described in human infants with meconium aspiration syndrome and consist of acute and long-term sequelae.[68] In the acute phase of the syndrome, complete and partial airway obstruction leads to hyperinflated pulmonary tissue, ventilation-perfusion mismatch, pulmonary hypertension, and increased risk for pneumothorax.[69–71] Chronic effects of meconium aspiration include chemical pneumonitis and disruption of surfactant function, which has been proposed to be a significant contributor to meconium aspiration syndrome.[72–82]

With large quantities of aspirated foreign material the calf may die acutely. Generally, the aspiration causes a gangrenous bronchopneumonia and animals display the typical clinical signs of depression, respiratory distress, fever, and malodorous breath. Auscultation of the lung fields bilaterally may reveal crackles, wheezes, and pleural friction rubs.[83] The calf may be hypoxic and hypercapnic on arterial blood gas analysis. History and clinical signs aid in diagnosis; however, hematology, radiographs, and pleural ultrasound examination are required to define better the extent of disease. Treatment almost always involves long-term antimicrobial and anti-inflammatory therapy.

BACTERIAL PNEUMONIA

Bacterial pneumonia in the first few days of life can be from sepsis, aspiration pneumonia, or gross bacterial contamination of colostrum. Most septic calves with pulmonary disease present depressed and lethargic. The physical examination, specifically thoracic auscultation, is not always consistent with pulmonary disease. The authors have found that inducing a cough by firmly shaking the trachea at the level of the larynx is helpful in confirming the diagnosis of pulmonary disease. Definitive diagnosis requires radiographs, transtracheal wash, or bronchial alveolar lavage. The authors have implemented bronchial alveolar lavage in the clinic and on-farm as an efficient way to get diagnostic samples representative of lower airway fluid for culture (Sheila M. McGuirk, DVM, PhD, unpublished data, 2007).

The bronchial alveolar lavage procedure is described next. Calves are sedated with xylazine (0.1 mg/kg IM) and the head is restrained by pushing the poll down while elevating the nose to ease placement of a flexible 10- × 36-in French catheter with a 3-mL balloon cuff (Mila International, Medical Instrumentation for Animals, Florence, Kentucky) into the trachea by way of the nares (**Fig. 1**). Repeated coughing is observed with proper placement of the catheter. The catheter is passed until it is wedged in a terminal bronchus and the balloon is inflated to create a seal to allow alveolar

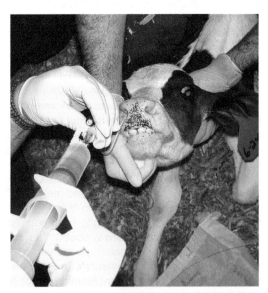

Fig. 1. This is an example of an on-farm bronchial alveolar lavage procedure. A flexible 10F catheter has been inserted into the trachea by the nares and advanced until it is wedged in a terminal bronchus. See text for further details on the procedure.

lavage. A total of 240 mL of 0.9% NaCl is lavaged (two separate 120-mL samples). Following administration, as much saline as possible is then aspirated back through the catheter. An appropriate sample volume is 10 to 40 mL of clear to mildly turbid, foamy fluid. The samples from both lavages are mixed and should be refrigerated or analyzed fresh within 2 hours. Five milliliters of sample should be submitted for aerobic and *Mycoplasma* cultures. The remaining fluid should be submitted for cytologic interpretation from cytospin and direct smear. Bronchial alveolar lavage fluid that yields homogenous ($>10^6$ CFU/mL) bacterial or positive *Mycoplasma bovis* culture is considered abnormal. A disproportionate decrease in the percentage of macrophages (<75%) or an elevation in neutrophils (>25%) provides evidence of an inflammatory response with or without a positive culture. Using this technique it is possible to sample six to eight calves in a 2-hour period. Identifying which calves are good candidates for bronchial alveolar lavage during an on-farm herd investigation can be challenging. The authors have developed a respiratory disease screening tool (**Fig. 2**) to identify these calves for diagnostic testing and treatment that can be used by veterinarians and farm personnel.[5,84,85] This tool can be found at http://www.vetmed.wisc.edu/dms/fapm/fapmtools/calves.htm.

Because the topic of interest is the calf, it is important to note that sepsis and bacteremia can cause interstitial pneumonia. Blood culture is important for diagnosis in these cases and fecal coliforms, most notably *Escherichia coli*, are the most commonly isolated bacteria from bacteremic calves.[86,87] Recently, *Salmonella dublin* has become increasingly more prevalent in septic calves admitted to the authors' hospital. *S dublin* is shed in colostrum and milk, and is associated with severe interstitial pneumonia along with fever, depression, and gastrointestinal disease.[88–90] Antemortem diagnostics submitted in the authors' hospital when *S dublin* is suspected include blood culture, fecal culture, and bronchial alveolar lavage. It is important to send *Salmonella* isolates for speciation. Postmortem samples should also include culture of liver, lung, and spleen.

Treatment is often initiated at the farm with one or more broad-spectrum antibiotics. Antibiotic therapy can be tailored to culture and sensitivity results, and in the authors' opinion should be continued for a minimum of 6 days (**Table 2**). For herd investigations, nasal swabs can be used to screen for *Mycoplasma* sp and to guide antibiotic therapy. To accomplish this, six untreated calves are sampled with two deep nasal swabs with flexible culturettes that contain transport media for aerobic and anaerobic bacteria (BBL Culture Swab Plus, Benton Dickenson, Sparks, Maryland). One swab is used for bacterial culture and the other is submitted for *Mycoplasma* sp culture.[5] Clinical response to therapy or complete blood cell analysis with fibrinogen can be used in the decision to extend antibiotic therapy. Depending on severity of clinical signs, supportive care with anti-inflammatory drugs, nutritional support, and nasal administration of oxygen may be indicated.

Prevention of bacterial sepsis and associated pneumonia centers on providing the calf with appropriate amounts of maternal antibodies for passive transfer by maternal colostrum.[81] Herds that have problems with gross bacterial contamination of colostrum or those that are trying to decrease the prevalence of pathogens present in maternal colostrum including *Mycobacterium paratuberculosis*, *S dublin*, and bovine leukosis virus should use a colostrum replacement product that provides the calf with a minimum of 175 g of immunoglobulin.[89,91–96] Prompt removal of the calf from the maternity pen is perhaps equally important in preventing exposure of the animal to a highly contaminated environment. The early environment poses a high risk for pathogen exposure to the calf trying to stand and frequently crashing head first into the maternity pen pack. In addition, calves attempting to nurse frequently suckle other

A

SCHOOL of
VETERINARY MEDICINE
University of Wisconsin-Madison

Calf Respiratory Scoring Chart

Farm Name: _____

Date: _____

Calf Scores	(Total respiratory score: 4 – watch, 5 or more – treat.)					
Animal ID	Age	Temp-erature	Nasal discharge	Cough – spontaneous or induced	Eye or ear	Total respiratory score

B

Calf Health Scoring Criteria			
0	**1**	**2**	**3**
Rectal temperature			
100-100.9	101-101.9	102-102.9	≥103
Cough			
None	Induce single cough	Induced repeated coughs or occasional spontaneous cough	Repeated spontaneous coughs
Nasal discharge			
Normal serous discharge	Small amount of unilateral cloudy discharge	Bilateral, cloudy or excessive mucus discharge	Copious bilateral mucopurulent discharge
Eye scores			
Normal	Small amount of ocular discharge	Moderate amount of bilateral discharge	Heavy ocular discharge
Ear scores			
Normal	Ear flick or head shake	Slight unilateral droop	Head tilt or bilateral droop

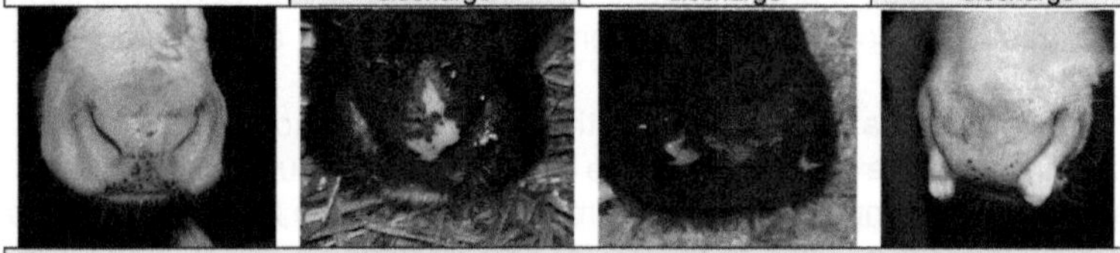

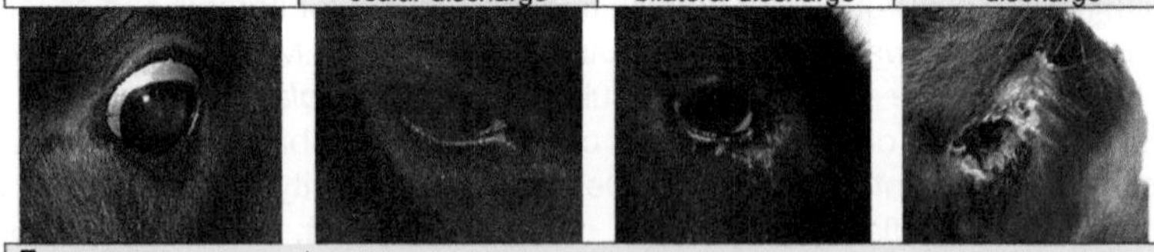

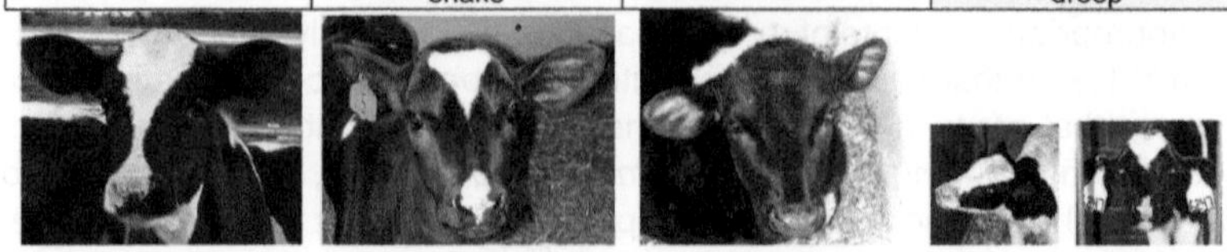

Fig. 2. (*A*) Calf respiratory scoring chart developed to identify calves for diagnostic treatment and treatment. Calves are assessed based on four categories: rectal temperature, nasal discharge, cough, and eye or ear. Scores from each category are combined to come up with a total respiratory score. (*B*) Calf health scoring criteria for the scoring chart pictured in (*A*).

Table 2
Antibiotics commonly used to treat respiratory disease in dairy replacement heifers

Drug	Antibiotic Class	Trade Name	Dosage	Dose for 45-kg (100-lb) Calf	Route	Frequency	Label for Mycoplasma?
Trimethoprim-sulfa	Sulfonamides	Tribrissen	20 mg/kg, 40 mg/kg loading dose	(960 mg tablet) 1 tablet, 2 tablet loading dose	Oral	1. Calves <2 wk: BID for 6 d 2. Calves 2–3 wk: TID for 6 d	No
Ceftiofur	β-lactams	Naxcel	2.2 mg/kg	2 mL	IM, SQ, or IV	SID	No
		Excenel	2.2 mg/kg	2 mL	IM or SQ	SID	No
		Exceed	6 mg/kg	1.5 mL	SQ at the base of the ear	Once	No
Florfenicol	Florfenicols	Nuflor	20 mg/kg 40 mg/kg	3 mL 6 mL	IM in the neck SQ in the neck	Q 48 h, 3 doses Once	No No
Tilmicosin	Macrolides	Micotil	10 mg/kg	1.5 mL	SQ in the neck	Q 48 h, 3 doses	No
Tulathromycin	Macrolides	Draxxin	2.5 mg/kg	1.1 mL	SQ in the neck	Once	Yes
Enrofloxacin	Fluoroquinolones	Baytril 100	7.5–12.5 mg/kg 2.5–5 mg/kg	3.5–5.5 mL 1.5–2 mL	SQ SQ	Once SID for 6 d	No[a] No[a]

[a] Labeled for treatment of bovine respiratory disease in dairy replacement heifers less than 20 months of age. Off-label use of fluoroquinolones is strictly prohibited. In mixed respiratory infections, Mycoplasma bovis has been shown to be susceptible to enrofloxacin.[124,125]

prepartum cows and make erratic nursing attempts on potentially heavily contaminated areas (tail, hock, brisket).[97–99] These normal behaviors in the maternity pen put calves at risk of massive oral contamination and possible colonization of the gastrointestinal tract. This along with an exposed umbilicus and high concentration of aerosolized bacteria are potential causes of sepsis.[87]

The calf's environment after the maternity pen is another source of bacterial pathogens that can cause respiratory disease. Calf raisers continue to build naturally ventilated barns to be more efficient and provide a more hospitable environment for labor despite the long-standing recommendations that individual hutches are the ideal environment to raise preweaned replacement heifers.[100–102] Lago and colleagues[84] reported that these naturally ventilated calf barns frequently have poor air quality and despite ventilation, calf stalls may continue to have high aerosolized bacterial counts. Their recommendations for calf stalls are that there should be a minimum area of 3 m^2 or more per calf, solid panels on two sides to provide a physical barrier between calves, mesh panels in the front and rear to allow air flow, and deep loose bedding in colder temperatures. A more thorough review of calf barn design can be found in a previous edition of this publication.[103]

VIRAL PNEUMONIA

The most commonly identified causes of viral pneumonia in calves during the first few weeks of life are bovine herpes virus type 1 or infectious bovine rhinotracheitis and bovine respiratory syncytial virus. Parainfluenza-3 and bovine viral diarrhea virus are also capable of infecting the respiratory tract and predisposing calves to bacterial pneumonia.[104–109] Prevention of viral pneumonia, as with bacterial pneumonia, centers on passive transfer of maternal antibodies and the innate immune response. As maternal antibody levels decline, active immunity and vaccination become mainstays of prevention for both viral and bacterial pneumonia. Vaccination recommendations for calves have been reviewed recently by Chase and colleagues,[110] and in the article by Cortese elsewhere in this issue. Treatment for viral pneumonia is primarily supportive and includes metaphylactic or prophylactic antibiotic therapy.

TRAUMATIC INJURY, PNEUMOTHORAX, AND ANAPHYLAXIS

Traumatic injury to the lung has declined over the years because fewer animals have horns. Fractures are possible in calves if they are stepped on in the maternity pen or may occur following dystocia.[111] Rib fractures are diagnosed during physical examination and confirmed with radiographs. Treatment is usually not required unless complications, such as myocardial injury, hemothorax, or pneumothorax, occur.[112]

Pneumothorax of clinical significance is rare in cattle and little information exists in the literature. Most reports are of adult cattle with rupture of emphysematous bullae associated with straining, coughing, or parturition.[113–116] Pneumothorax has been reported in a preweaned calf as a result of bovine respiratory syncytial virus and in neonates that have undergone mechanical ventilation, both of which may lead to bullae formation and rupture.[117] In a retrospective study of 30 animals, 2 of the cases were neonates. Traumatic injury was not identified in those cases but blunt thoracic trauma could not be definitively ruled out.[118] The authors suggested idiopathic pneumothorax secondary to rupture of subpleural blebs or cysts as possible causes.[119,120] Meconium aspiration leading to pneumothorax has been reported to be a significant risk in human infants.[121–124] Slack and colleagues[118] described pneumothorax and pneumomediastinum in a calf born by caesarian section with substantial meconium staining. The calf was resuscitated with mechanical ventilation, however, so both of these could have been contributory. Calves with pneumothorax frequently have dyspnea, tachypnea, and absent lung sounds in the dorsal lung field. Cattle have a complete mediastinum, and pneumothorax may be limited to one hemithorax depending on the inciting cause. Treatment of pneumothorax involves therapy for the primary disease together with evacuation of air from the pleural space. In the field, suction of air can be done with a teat cannula or an 18-gauge 3.5-in (51-mm) catheter, a three-way valve, and a syringe. This procedure may need to be repeated as dictated by the clinical signs of the calf. Severe, persistent pneumothorax may require hospitalization and continuous suction with a device as described by Peek and colleagues.[117]

Dyspnea and tachypnea from pulmonary edema or laryngeal edema can occur with anaphylactic reactions in calves induced by exogenous antigens. Anaphylactic reactions are type 1 hypersensitivity reactions mediated by IgE. Antibiotic therapy with penicillin G, sulfonamides, tetracyclines, epidural analgesia with lidocaine or Carbocaine, and vitamin E and selenium injection have been associated with anaphylactic reactions in cattle.[115] Plasma and other blood products have the potential for anaphylaxis and animals receiving transfusions need to be monitored closely. Treatment is dependent on severity of clinical signs and can include epinephrine (0.01 mg/kg); corticosteroids (dexamethasone, 0.1–0.2 mg/kg); antihistamines (tripelennamine hydrochloride, 1 mg/kg IM or SQ); furosemide (0.05–1 mg/kg IM or IV), nonsteroidal anti-inflammatory drugs (flunixin meglumine, 1.1 mg/kg IM or IV); and nasal administration of oxygen.[115,117]

REFERENCES

1. USDA. Part I: Reference of dairy health and management in the United States. Fort Collins (CO): USDA: APHIS: VS, CEAH, National Animal Health Monitoring System; 2002. #N377.1202.
2. Donavan GA, Dohoo IR, Montgomery DM, et al. Calf and disease factors affecting growth in female Holstein claves in Florida, USA. Prev Vet Med 1998;33:1–10.
3. Waltner-Toews D, Martin SW, Meek AH. The effect of early calfhood health status on survivorship and age at first calving. Can J Vet Res 1986;50:314–7.
4. Warnick LD, Erb HN, White ME. The relationship of calfhood morbidity with survival after calving in 25 New York Holstein herds. Prev Vet Med 1997;31:263–73.
5. McGuirk SM. Disease management of dairy calves and heifers. Vet Clin North Am Food Anim Pract 2008;24:139–53.
6. Kasari TR. Physiologic mechanisms of adaptation in the fetal calf at birth. Vet Clin Food Anim 1994;10:127–36.
7. Ardran GM, Dawes GS, Prichard MM, et al. The effect of ventilation of the fetal lungs upon the pulmonary circulation. J Physiol 1952;118:12–22.
8. Detweiler DK, Riedesel DH. Regional and fetal circulations. In: Swenson MJ, Reece WO, editors. Duke's physiology of domestic animals. 11th edition. Ithaca (NY): Cornell University Press; 1993. p. 227.
9. Harvey JW. Hemoglobin oxygen affinity. In: Kaneko JJ, editor. Clinical biochemistry of domestic animals: erythrocyte metabolism. 4th edition. San Diego (CA): Academic Press; 1989. p. 185.
10. Rurak DW, Richardson BS, Patrick JE, et al. Blood flow an oxygen delivery to fetal organs and tissues during sustained hypoxemia. Am J Phys 1990;258: R1116–22.
11. Harding R, Sigger JN, Wickham PJ. The regulation of flow of pulmonary fluid in fetal sheep. Respir Physiol 1984;57:47–59.

12. Eigenmann U. Der einfluss geburtshilflicher massnahmen auf die lebensfahigkeit neugeborener kalber [Effect of obstetric measures on the survival of newborn calves]. Prakt Tierarzt 1985;62:933–42.

13. Szenci O, Taverne MAM, Bakonyi S. Comparison between pre- and postnatal acid-base status of calves and their perinatal mortality. Vet Q 1988;10:140–4.

14. Guyton AC, Hall JE. Regulation of respiration. In: Guyton AC, Hall JE, editors. Medical physiology. 11th edition. Elsevier Saunders: Philadelphia; 2006. p. 516–23.

15. Maurer-Schweizer H, Wilhelm U, Walser K. Blutgase und säure-basen-haushalt bei lebensfrischen kälbern in der ersten 24 lebensstunden. Berl Münch Tierärztl Wochenschr 1977;90:192–6.

16. Gardiner RM. Cerebral blood flow and oxidative metabolism during hypoxia and asphyxia in the new-born calf and lamb. J Physiol 1980;305:357–76.

17. Edwards AV. Resistance to hypoglycaemia in the newborn calf. J Physiol 1964;171:46–9.

18. Comline RS, Silver M. Some aspects of foetal and uteroplacental metabolism in cows with indwelling umbilical and uterine vascular catheters. J Physiol 1976;260:571–7.

19. Varga J, Mester L, Börzsönyi L, et al. Improved pulmonary adaptation in newborn calves with postnatal acidosis. Vet J 2001;162:226–32.

20. Szenci O. Role of acid-base disturbances in perinatal mortality of calves. Acta Vet Hung. 1985;33:205–30.

21. Adams R, Garry FB, Holland MD. Clinicopathologic measurements in newborn beef calves experiencing mild to moderate degrees of dystocia. Agri-Practice 1995;16:5–11.

22. Dufty JH, Sloss V. Anoxia in the bovine foetus. Aust Vet J 1977;53:262–7.

23. Vaala WE, House JK. Routine postpartum care of the newborn foal. In: Smith BP, editor. Large animal internal medicine. 3rd edition. St. Louis: Mosby; 2002. p. 278.

24. Schuijt G, Taverne MA. The interval between birth and sternal recumbency as an objective measure of the vitality of newborn calves. Vet Rec 1994;135:111–5.

25. Uystepruyst CH, Coghe J, Bureau F, et al. Evaluation of accuracy of pulse oximetry in newborn calves. Vet J 2000;159:71–6.

26. Bleul U, Kähl W. Monitoring the bovine fetus during stage II of parturition using pulse oximetry. Theriogenology 2008;69:302–11.

27. Held T. Klinisch and blutgasanalytisch Unteruchungen bei kalbenden Rindern und deren Feten. Dr med vet Thesis. Klinik für Geburtshilfe und Gynäkologie des Rindes. Tierärztliche Hochschule. Hannover 1983.

28. Bleul U, Lejeune B, Schwantag S, et al. Blood gas and acid-base analysis of arterial blood in 57 newborn calves. Vet Rec 2007;161:688–91.

29. Held T, Eigenmann UJE, Grunert E. Findings obtained from blood-gas analysis of bovine fetuses in dilatation phase of parturition. Monatsh Veterinarmed 1985;40:405–9.

30. Waizenhöfer H, Mülling M. Behaviour of pHact, PO_2 and PCO_2 in venous, capillary and arterial blood of newborn calves. Berl Münch Tierärztl Wochenschr 1978;91:173–6.

31. Pickel M, Zaremba W, Grunert E. Comparison of arterial and venous blood gas and acid-base values in prematurely born healthy calves or calves with late asphyxia. Zentralbl Veterinarmed A 1989;36:653–63.

32. Nagy O, Kovac G, Seidel H, et al. The effect of arterial blood sampling sites on blood gases and acid-base balance parameters in calves. Acta Vet Hung 2001;49:331–40.

33. Adams R, Holland MD, Aldridge B, et al. Arterial blood sample collection from the newborn calf. Vet Res Commun 1991;15:387–94.
34. Picandet V, Jeanneret S, Lavoie JP. Effects of syringe type and storage temperature on results of blood gas analysis in arterial blood of horses. J Vet Intern Med 2007;21:476–81.
35. Knowles TP, Mullin RA, Hunter JA, et al. Effects of syringe material, sample storage time, and temperature on blood gases and oxygen saturation in arterialized human blood samples. Respir Care 2006;51:732–6.
36. Stark AR. Apnea. In: Cloherty JP, Eichenwald EC, Stark AR, editors. Manual of neonatal care. Philadelphia: Lippincott Williams & Wilkins; 2004. p. 388–93.
37. Comer AM, Perry CM, Figgitt DP. Caffeine citrate: a review of its use in apnoea of prematurity. Paediatr Drugs 2001;3:61–79.
38. Giguère S, Sanchez LC, Shih A, et al. Comparison of the effects of caffeine and doxapram on respiratory and cardiovascular function in foals with induced respiratory acidosis. Am J Vet Res 2007;68:1407–16.
39. Palmer JE. In: Divers TJ, Orsini JA, editors. Manual of equine emergencies. 3rd edition. Philadelphia: Saunders; 2008. p. 502.
40. Sullivan Hackett E, Orsini JA, Divers TJ. In: Divers TJ, Orsini JA, editors. Manual of equine emergencies. 3rd edition. Philadelphia: Saunders; 2008. p. 740–3.
41. Bhatt-Mehta V, Schumacher RE. Treatment of apnea of prematurity. Paediatr Drugs 2003;5:195–210.
42. Plumb DC. Doxapram hydrochloride. In: Veterinary drug handbook. 5th edition. Stockholm: PharmaVet; 2005. p. 403–5.
43. Dani C, Bertini G, Pezzati M, et al. Brain hemodynamic effects of doxapram in preterm infants. Biol Neonate 2006;89:69–74.
44. Zhang M, Zhang H, Liu L. The study of effect of pain in the change of respiration by stimulating renzhong acupoint. Zhen Ci Yan Jiu 1990;15:147–9.
45. McKenzie JC, Clancy J, Klein RM. Autoradiographic analysis of cell proliferation and protein synthesis in the pulmonary trunk of rats during the early development of hypoxia-induced pulmonary hypertension. Blood Vessels 1984;21:81–9.
46. Meyrick B, Reid L. Hypoxia and incorporation of ^{3}H-thymidine by cells of the rat pulmonary arteries and alveolar wall. Am J Pathol 1979;96:51–70.
47. Meyrick B, Reid L. Normal postnatal development of the media of the rat hilar pulmonary artery and its remodeling by chronic hypoxia. Lab Invest 1982;46:505–14.
48. Murphy JD, Rabinovitch M, Goldstein JD, et al. The structural basis of persistent pulmonary hypertension of the newborn infant. J Pediatr 1981;98:962–7.
49. Czarnecki SW, Rosenbaum HM, Wachtel HL. The occurrence of primary pulmonary hypertension in twin with a review of etiological considerations. Am Heart J 1968;75:240–6.
50. Drummond WH, Peckham GJ, Fox WW. The clinical profile of the newborn with persistent pulmonary hypertension: observations in 19 affected neonates. Clin Pediatr (Phila) 1977;16:335–41.
51. Drummond WH. Neonatal pulmonary hypertension. Equine Vet J 1987;19:169–71.
52. Cottrill CM, O'Connor WN, Cudd T, et al. Persistence of fetal circulatory pathways in a newborn foal. Equine Vet J 1987;19:252–5.
53. Stenmark KR, Fasules J, Hyde DM, et al. Severe pulmonary hypertension an arterial adventitial changes in newborn calves at 4,300 m. J Appl Phys 1987;62:821–30.
54. Chavatte-Palmer P, Heyman Y, Richard C, et al. Clinical, hormonal, and hematologic characteristics of bovine calves derived from nuclei from somatic cells. Biol Reprod 2002;66:1596–603.

55. Hill JR, Edwards JF, Sawyer N, et al. Placental anomalies in a viable cloned calf. Cloning 2001;3:83–8.

56. Heyman Y, Chavatte-Palmer P, LeBourhis D, et al. Frequency and occurrence of late-gestation losses from cattle cloned embryos. Biol Reprod 2002;66:6–13.

57. Tsunoda Y, Kato Y. Recent progress and problems in animal cloning. Differentiation 2002;69:158–61.

58. Hill JR, Roussel AJ, Cibelli JB, et al. Clinical and pathologic features of cloned transgenic calves and fetuses (13 case studies). Theriogenology 1999;51:1451–65.

59. Fecteau ME, Palmer JE, Wilkins PA. Neonatal care of high-risk cloned and transgenic calves. Vet Clin Food Anim 2005;21:637–53.

60. Reef VB, McGuirk SM. Diseases of the cardiovascular system. In: Smith BP, editor. Large animal internal medicine. 3rd edition. St. Louis: Mosby; 2002. p. 459.

61. Mazan MR. Noninfectious respiratory problems. In: Paradis MR, editor. Equine neonatal medicine: a case based approach. Philadelphia: Elsevier Saunders; 2006. p. 142.

62. Abman SH. Role of inhaled nitric oxide in treatment of neonatal pulmonary hypertension. Zhongguo Yao Li Xue Bao 1997;18(6):542–5.

63. Wilkins PA, Seahorn T. Acute respiratory distress syndrome. Vet Clin North Am Equine Pract 2004;20:253–73.

64. Shekerdemian LS, Ravn HB, Penny DJ. Intravenous sildenafil lowers pulmonary vascular resistance in a model of neonatal pulmonary hypertension. Am J Respir Crit Care Med 2002;165:1098–102.

65. Baquero H, Soliz A, Neira F, et al. Oral sildenafil in infants with persistent pulmonary hypertension of the newborn: a pilot randomized blinded study. Pediatrics 2006;117:1077–83.

66. Besser TE, Gay CC, Pritchett L. Comparison of three methods of feeding colostrum to dairy calves. J Am Vet Med Assoc 1991;198:419–22.

67. Adams GD, Bush LD, Horner JL, et al. Two methods for administering colostrum to newborn calves. J Dairy Sci 1985;68:773–5.

68. Lopez A, Bildfell R. Pulmonary inflammation associated with aspirated meconium and epithelial cells in calves. Vet Pathol 1992;29:104–11.

69. Rossi EM, Philipson EH, Williams TG, et al. Meconium aspiration syndrome: intrapartum and neonatal attributes. Am J Obstet Gynecol 1989;161:1106–10.

70. Patterson K, Kapur SP, Chandra RS. Persistent pulmonary hypertension of the newborn: pulmonary pathologic aspects. Perspect Pediatr Pathol 1988;15:389–413.

71. Spitzer AR, David J, Bernbaum J, et al. Pulmonary hypertension and persistent fetal circulation in the newborn. Clin Perinatol 1988;15:389–413.

72. Wu JM, Yeh TF, Wang JY, et al. The role of pulmonary inflammation in the development of pulmonary hypertension in newborn with meconium aspiration syndrome (MAS). Pediatr Pulmonol 1999;18:205–8.

73. Soukka H, Rautanen M, Halkola L, et al. Meconium aspiration induces ARDS-like pulmonary response in lungs of ten-week-old pigs. Pediatr Pulmonol 1997;23:205–11.

74. Cleary GM, Antunes MJ, Ciesielka DA, et al. Exudative lung injury is associated with decreased level of surfactant proteins in a rat model of meconium aspiration. Pediatrics 1997;100:998–1003.

75. Tyler DC, Murphy J, Cheney FW. Mechanical and chemical damage to lung tissue caused by meconium aspiration. Pediatrics 1978;62:454–9.

76. Davey AM, Becker JD, Davis JM. Meconium aspiration syndrome: physiological and inflammatory changes in a newborn piglet model. Pediatr Pulmonol 1993; 16:101–8.
77. Sun B, Curstedt T, Robertson B. Surfactant inhibition in experimental meconium aspiration. Acta Paediatr 1993;82:182–9.
78. Moses D, Holm BA, Spitaale P, et al. Inhibition of pulmonary surfactant function by meconium. Am J Obstet Gynecol 1991;164:477–81.
79. Paranka MS, Walsh WF, Stancombe BB. Surfactant lavage in a piglet model of meconium aspiration syndrome. Pediatr Res 1992;31:625–8.
80. Chen CT, Toung TJK, Rogers MC. Effect of intra-alveolar meconium on pulmonary surface tension properties. Crit Care Med 1985;13:233–6.
81. Clark DA, Niieman GF, Thompson JE, et al. Surfactant displacement by meconium free fatty acids: an alternative explanation for atelectasis in meconium aspiration syndrome. J Pediatr 1987;110:765–70.
82. Sun B, Curstedt T, Song G, et al. Surfactant improves lung function and morphology in newborn rabbits with meconium aspiration. Biol Neonate 1993;63:96–104.
83. Wikse SE. Diseases of the respiratory system: other pneumonias. In: Smith BP, editor. Large animal internal medicine. 3rd edition. St. Louis: Mosby; 2002. p. 584.
84. Lago A, McGuirk SM, Bennett TB, et al. Calf respiratory disease and pen microenvironments in naturally ventilated calf barns in winter. J Dairy Sci 2006;89: 4014–25.
85. McGuirk SM. Troubleshooting dairy calf pneumonia problems. In: Proceedings of the Twenty Fifth Annual ACVIM Forum. Seattle, Washington, June 6–9, 2007.
86. Aldridge BM, Garry FB, Adams R. Neonatal septicemia in calves: 25 cases (1985–1990). J Am Vet Med Assoc 1993;203:1324–9.
87. Fecteau G, Van Metre DC, Pare J, et al. Bacteriological culture of blood from critically ill neonatal calves. Can Vet J 1997;38:95–100.
88. Smith BP, Oliver DG, Singh P, et al. Detection of *Salmonella dublin* mammary gland infection in carrier cows, using an enzyme-linked immunosorbent assay for antibody in milk or serum. Am J Vet Res 1989;50:1352–60.
89. Spier SJ, Smith BP, Cullor JS, et al. Persistent experimental *Salmonella dublin* intramammary infection in dairy cows. J Vet Intern Med 1991;5:341–50.
90. Van Metre DC, Tennant BC, Whitlock RH. Infectious diseases of the gastrointestinal tract. In: Divers TJ, Peek SF, editors. Diseases of dairy cattle. 2nd edition. St. Louis: Saunders; 2008. p. 221.
91. James RE, Polan CE, Cummings KA. Influence of administered indigenous microorganisms on uptake of I125g-globulin in vivo by intestinal segments of neonatal calves. J Dairy Sci 1981;50:1352–60.
92. Poulsen KP, Hartmann FA, McGuirk SM. Bacteria in colostrum: impact on calf health. J Vet Intern Med 2002;16:339 [abstract].
93. Staley TE, Bush LJ. Receptor mechanisms of the neonatal intestine and their relationship to immunoglobulin absorption and disease. J Dairy Sci 1985;68:184–205.
94. Streeter RN, Hoffsis GF, Bech-Nielsen S, et al. Isolation of *Mycobacterium paratuberculosis* from colostrum and milk of subclinically infected cows. Am J Vet Res 1995;56:1322–4.
95. Sweeney RW, Whitlock RH, Rosenberger AE. *Mycobacterium paratuberculosis* cultured from milk and supramammary lymph nodes of infection asymptomatic cows. J Clin Microbiol 1992;30:166–71.
96. Poulsen KP, Foley AL, Collins MT, et al. Efficacy of a colostrum replacement product. J Vet Intern Med 2003;17:391 [abstract].

97. Roy JHB. The calf, 5th edition. In: Management of health, vol. 1. Toronto: Butter-worths; 1990. p. 38–58.
98. Curtis CR, Scarlett JM, Hollis EN, et al. Path model of individual-calf risk factors for calfhood morbidity and mortality in New York Holstein herds. Prev Vet Med 1988;6:43–62.
99. Hancock D. Epidemiologic diagnosis of neonatal diarrhea in dairy calves. Proc Annu Conv Am Assoc Bovine Pract 1983;15:15–22.
100. Brand A, Noordhuizen JPTM, Schukken YH. Herd health and production man-agement in dairy practice. Wageningen, The Netherlands: Wageningen Pers; 1996. p. 128.
101. McFarland D. Calves, heifers, and dairy profitability. Ithaca (NY): NRAES-74 NRAES; 1996. p. 82–94.
102. Holmes B. Dairy freestall housing and equipment, MWPS-7. Midwest plan ser-vice. 7th edition. Ames (IA): Iowa State University; 1996. p. 27–45.
103. Nordlund KV. Practical considerations for ventilating calf barns in winter. Vet Clin Food Anim 2008;24:41–54.
104. Martin SW, Bateman KG, Shewen PE, et al. The frequency, distribution and effects of antibodies, to seven putative respiratory pathogens, on respiratory disease and weight gain in feedlot calves in Ontario. Can J Vet Res 1989;53: 355–62.
105. Potgieter LN. Immunology of bovine viral diarrhea virus. Vet Clin Food Anim 1995;11:501–20.
106. Martin SW, Nagy E, Amrstrong D, et al. The associations of viral and mycoplas-mal antibody titers with respiratory disease and weight gain in feedlot calves. Can Vet J 1999;40:560–70.
107. Fulton RW, Purdy CW, Confer AW, et al. Bovine viral diarrhea viral infections in feeder calves with respiratory disease: interactions with *Pasteurella* spp., para-influenza-3 virus, and bovine respiratory syncytial virus. Can J Vet Res 2000;64: 151–9.
108. Fulton RW, Ridpath JF, Saliki JE, et al. Bovine viral diarrhea virus (BVDV) 1b: pre-dominant BVDV subtype in calves with respiratory disease. Can J Vet Res 2002; 66:181–90.
109. Todd JD. Immune response of cattle to intranasally or parenterally administered parainfluenza type 3 virus vaccines. Dev Biol Stand 1975;28:473–6.
110. Chase CL, Hurley DJ, Reber AJ. Neonatal immune development in the calf and its impact on vaccine response. Vet Clin Food Anim 2008;24:87–104.
111. Schuijt G. Iatrogenic fractures of ribs and vertebrae during delivery in perinatally dying calves: 235 cases (1978–1988). J Am Vet Med Assoc 1990;197:1196–202.
112. Wilkins PA. Lower respiratory problems of the neonate. Vet Clin North Am Equine Pract 2003;19:12–33.
113. Smith JA. Pneumothorax. In: Smith BP, editor. Large animal internal medicine. 3rd edition. St Louis: Mosby; 2002. p. 590.
114. Smith JA. Pneumothorax. In: Smith BP, editor. Large animal internal medicine. 3rd edition. St Louis: Mosby; 2002. p. 590.
115. Divers TJ. Pneumothorax. In: Peek SP, Divers TJ, editors. Respiratory diseases, diseases of dairy cattle. 2nd edition. Philadelphia: Saunders Elsevier; 2008. p. 121.
116. Gilroy B, CK Cebra. Pulmonary bullous emphysema with pneumothorax and subcutaneous emphysema: What's your diagnosis? J Am Vet Med Assoc 1999;215:475–6.
117. Peek SF, Slack JA, McGuirk SM. Management of pneumothorax in cattle by con-tinuous-flow evacuation. J Vet Intern Med 2003;17:119–22.

118. Slack JA, Thomas CB, Peek SF. Pneumothorax in dairy cattle: 30 cases (1990–2003). J Am Vet Med Assoc 2004;224:732–5.
119. Carey B. Neonatal air leaks: pneumothorax, pneumomediastinum, pulmonary interstitial emphysema, pneumopericardium. Neonatal Netw 1999;18:81–4.
120. Evrard V, Ceulemans J, Coosemans W, et al. Congenital malformations of the lung. World J Surg 1999;23:1123–32.
121. Cleary GM, Wiswell TE. Meconium-stained amniotic fluid and the meconium aspiration syndrome. An update. Pediatr Clin North Am 1998;45:511–29.
122. Wiswell TE, Bent RC. Meconium staining and the meconium aspiration syndrome: unresolved issues. Pediatr Clin North Am 1993;40:955–81.
123. Francoz D, Fortin M, Fecteau G, et al. Determination of mycoplasma bovis susceptibilities against six antimicrobial agents using the E test method. Vet Microbiol 2005;105:57–64.
124. Rosenbusch RF, Kinyon JM, Apley M, et al. In vitro antimicrobial inhibition profiles of *Mycoplasma bovis* isolates recovered from various regions of the United States from 2002 to 2003. J Vet Diagn Invest 2005;17:436–41.

Mycoplasma bovis Infections in Young Calves

Fiona P. Maunsell, BVSc, PhD[a],*, G. Arthur Donovan, DVM, MSc[b]

KEYWORDS

- *Mycoplasma bovis* • Calves • Respiratory disease
- Pneumonia • Otitis media

Mycoplasma bovis was first isolated from a case of severe mastitis in a US dairy cow in 1961, almost half a century ago.[1] It is now recognized as a worldwide pathogen of intensively farmed cattle and in recent years has emerged as an important cause of disease in young dairy and veal calves in North America and Europe. Pneumonia, otitis media, and arthritis are common manifestations of *M bovis* infection in young calves, and have been collectively termed *Mycoplasma bovis*–associated disease (*Mb*AD). *Mycoplasma bovis* also continues to be an important cause of mastitis in adult cows[2–5] and respiratory disease and arthritis in stocker and feeder cattle.[6–10] Readers are referred to recent reviews of mycoplasmal mastitis[5,11] and *Mb*AD in feedlot cattle[10,12] in North America; this article will focus on the clinical aspects of *M bovis* infections in young calves.

ETIOLOGY AND PATHOPHYSIOLOGY

Mycoplasma bovis belongs the class Mollicutes (from the Latin *mollis*, soft; *cutis*, skin), a group of bacteria so named because they lack cell walls and are instead enveloped by a complex plasma membrane. They are also characterized by their tiny physical size and correspondingly tiny genomes (0.58 to 2.2 megabases).[13] Perhaps as a direct consequence of the limited biosynthetic capacity of their small genome, mycoplasmas usually form an intimate association with host cells to obtain the growth and nutritional factors necessary for their survival.[14] Mycoplasmas typically inhabit mucosal surfaces, including those of the respiratory, urogenital, and gastrointestinal tracts; the eyes; and the mammary glands.[14] Their individual relationship with the host varies from primary or opportunistic pathogens to commensals.

[a] Department of Infectious Diseases and Pathology, College of Veterinary Medicine, University of Florida, P.O. Box 110880, Gainesville, FL 32611, USA
[b] Department of Large Animal Clinical Sciences, College of Veterinary Medicine, University of Florida, P.O. Box 100136, Gainesville, FL 32610, USA
* Corresponding author.
E-mail address: maunsellf@vetmed.ufl.edu (F.P. Maunsell).

Vet Clin Food Anim 25 (2009) 139–177
doi:10.1016/j.cvfa.2008.10.011
0749-0720/08/$ – see front matter © 2009 Elsevier Inc. All rights reserved.
vetfood.theclinics.com

Interactions between mycoplasmal pathogens and their hosts are much more complex than might be expected from their small genome and structural simplicity. Mycoplasmas can induce a broad range of immunomodulatory events by direct effects on macrophages, neutrophils, and lymphocytes, and by indirect effects through induction of cytokine secretion from these and other cells (eg, epithelial cells).[14] *Mycoplasma bovis* is no exception, and this pathogen is very effective at evading and modulating the host immune response, and the immune response contributes to the pathogenesis of *MbAD*.[15–19] The complicated relationship between mycoplasmas and their hosts means that many aspects of these interactions are poorly understood, even for the host-pathogen relationships for which there is a large body of research data. For *M bovis* infections, little is known about the factors that contribute to development of disease or to the production of an effective immune response.

Of those microbial factors that may contribute to *M bovis* pathogenesis, perhaps the best characterized is a large family of immunodominant variable surface lipoproteins (Vsps).[20–24] Surface lipoprotein variation in mycoplasmas is thought to be a means of adapting to varying environmental conditions, including the host response, and may be important in determining the chronic nature of many mycoplasmal infections.[25] The members of the Vsp family in *M bovis* undergo high-frequency phase and size variation, providing a vast capacity for antigenic variation.[21,22,24] Some *M bovis* Vsps have been shown to contain adhesive domains,[24] and others may play a role in biofilm formation;[26] however, the expression of particular Vsps has not been associated with disease severity, the site of infection, or with genotype.[27,28] It is important to recognize that Vsp expression is not a stable feature of any particular population of *M bovis* cells; instead, an *M bovis* population varies in Vsp expression over time.[29] Although variation in *M bovis* surface antigens likely contributes to immune evasion,[30] the precise roles that these highly immunogenic lipoproteins play in pathogenesis remain to be determined.

Typical of respiratory mycoplasmal pathogens, *M bovis* appears to be well adapted to colonize the upper respiratory tract (URT), where it may remain for long periods of time without causing clinical disease.[3,31] Disease occurs when host and/or pathogen factors result in replication and dissemination to other sites (eg, from the URT to the lower respiratory tract [LRT] or middle ear), and/or as a result of a detrimental host inflammatory response. Hematologic dissemination from sites of infection can occur, with the joints being a frequent site of secondary colonization.[32,33]

Dissemination of a bacterial infection to the middle ear can occur by several possible routes, including extension of external ear infections via the tympanic membrane, colonization of the oropharynx and extension into the tympanic bulla via the eustachian (auditory) tube, or by hematogenous spread.[34] In pigs, otitis media caused by *Mycoplasma hyorhinis* occurs by extension of URT infections to the middle ear via the eustachian tube.[35,36] In experimentally infected neonatal calves, *M bovis* colonization of the eustachian tubes occurred in almost all calves that had nasopharyngeal colonization, suggesting that ascending infection of the eustachian tube is the primary route by which *M bovis* enters the middle ear.[37]

As with other mycoplasmal respiratory infections,[38] innate responses and local humoral responses, especially phagocytosis and killing by alveolar macrophages facilitated by opsonization with specific antibody, are important in protection from *MbAD*. However, strong adaptive immune responses that develop after infection often fail to resolve the infection or prevent *MbAD*.[39] Modulation of the immune response by *M bovis*, including the widespread activation of macrophages and excessive recruitment of neutrophils and lymphocytes to sites of infection, appear to contribute to the development of *MbAD*.[39–41] The immune response in *M bovis*–associated respiratory disease has been recently reviewed,[12,15] and will not be covered in detail in this article.

THE IMPORTANCE OF *MYCOPLASMA*-ASSOCIATED CALF DISEASE
Evidence for Mycoplasmas as Etiologic Agents of Calf Disease

Mycoplasma bovis

It is now well established that *M bovis* plays a causal role in respiratory disease, otitis media, and arthritis in young calves. There are a number of reports of respiratory disease outbreaks where *M bovis* was the predominant bacteria isolated from lungs of affected calves.[42–47] In addition, although bovine pneumonia rarely involves a single infectious agent, experimental infection studies have shown that inoculation with *M bovis* alone can cause pneumonia in calves.[33,48,49] Seroconversion to *M bovis* is associated with increased respiratory disease rates[50] as well as decreased weight gain and increased number of antibiotic treatments in feedlot calves.[7,51] However, as with most bovine respiratory pathogens, colonization alone is not always sufficient to cause disease. *M bovis* can be isolated from the URT, trachea, and LRT of calves without clinical disease or gross lesions,[31,52–54] although its presence in the LRT may cause subclinical inflammation.[55] Despite these findings, isolation of *M bovis* as the predominant pathogen in numerous outbreaks of respiratory disease and experimental confirmation of its ability to cause pneumonia in calves verify its role as an important respiratory pathogen.

Field cases of respiratory disease caused by *M bovis* are sometimes accompanied by arthritis, and *M bovis* has been isolated in pure culture from affected joints, as well as from the lungs of calves with concurrent respiratory disease.[56–61] Consistent with the observations of natural disease, arthritis has been induced by inoculation of *M bovis* into joints or lungs, or intravenously.[33,48,56,62,63] Variation among clinical isolates of *M bovis* in their ability to cause arthritis in an experimental infection model has been reported.[58]

In addition to causing disease of the LRT and arthritis, *M bovis* is the predominant pathogen isolated from the middle ear of young calves with otitis media.[64–68] However, other bacteria, including *Mycoplasma bovirhinis*, *Mycoplasma alkalescens*, *Mycoplasma arginini*, *Pasteurella multocida*, *Mannheimia hemolytica*, *Histophilus somni*, and *Arcanobacterium pyogenes* are isolated sporadically, and some have been associated with outbreaks of otitis media, especially in feedlot cattle.[10,64,68–70] However, in the past 15 years, outbreaks of otitis media in groups of North American dairy calves have been largely attributable to *M bovis* infection.[64,65,68] In an experimental infection study, we inoculated immunocompetent calves at 7 to 10 days of age by feeding milk replacer containing a field strain of *M bovis*.[37] Inoculated calves were consistently colonized in the URT and the eustachian (auditory) tubes, and 37% of calves developed otitis media by 2 weeks postinoculation. No pathogens other than *M bovis* were isolated from the inoculated calves. Therefore, *M bovis* has been implicated as a primary pathogen of the middle ear in both natural and experimental infections.

Mycoplasmas other than Mycoplasma bovis

Disease in young calves is occasionally attributed to mycoplasmas other than *M bovis*, including *Mycoplasma dispar*, *Mycoplasma californicum*, *Mycoplasma canis*, *Mycoplasma alkalescens*, *Mycoplasma arginini*, *Mycoplasma bovirhinis*, *Mycoplasma bovigenitalium*, and *Mycoplasma bovoculi*, and a variety of other species have been isolated from the middle ear or LRT of diseased calves.[68,71–76] A number of these species are often found as part of the microbial flora of the URT in healthy calves and in most reports they have been isolated in mixed infections with other known pathogens.[77,78] Although specific episodes of disease are occasionally associated with one or more of these species, for the most part, their role in calfhood disease remains poorly defined. *M bovirhinis* is a particularly common inhabitant of the URT in intensively managed cattle and has been isolated from pneumonic lungs[71-73] and from the tympanic bulla of calves with otitis media;[68] however, it is believed to be an opportunistic invader and to play a minimal role in disease. In Australia, *Mycoplasma* species bovine group 7 has been isolated from cases of respiratory disease and arthritis in dairy calves, along with mastitis and abortion in cows.[79,80] Outbreaks of disease associated with this mycoplasma have been reported[80] but there are few data available to determine its overall importance to calf disease in that country.

M dispar is occasionally isolated from the respiratory tract of diseased cattle, typically in mixed infections with other pathogens such as *Mannheimia hemolytica*.[71-75] *M dispar* causes disruption of normal ciliary function in tracheal epithelium, suggesting that it could play a role in predisposing the LRT to infection with primary lung pathogens.[54,81,82] Experimental infection of calves with *M dispar* results in colonization of the LRT and occasionally causes pneumonia.[74,81] A rise in serologic titers to *M dispar* has been associated with increased risk of pneumonia[83] and with reduced weight gain[50] in feedlot cattle, supporting a role for *M dispar* in some cases of respiratory disease in feedlot cattle. There are few data on the importance of *M dispar* infections in young calves. In one case-control study, a rise in serologic titers to *M dispar* was associated with treatment for pneumonia during the first 3 months of life,[54] but there are few recent reports of its isolation from dairy calves in North America.

Prevalence

M bovis appears to be widespread within the North American dairy cattle population.[2,4,51,84,85] In the National Animal Health Monitoring System (NAHMS) Dairy 2002 study, 7.9% of 871 dairies tested positive for mycoplasmas upon culture of a single bulk tank milk sample; *M bovis* was identified in 86% of the positive herds. States in the Western region had a greater percentage of operations with positive *Mycoplasma* culture (9.4%) than states in the Midwest (2.2%), Northeast (2.8%), and Southeast (6.6%) regions. These values are likely an underestimate of true prevalence, as subclinically infected cows shed mycoplasmas intermittently in milk,[86,87] and milk from cows with clinical mastitis is usually withheld from the bulk tank. In a study of 463 dairy operations in the Northwestern United States (US), 20% (93) of herds had at least one *Mycoplasma*-positive bulk tank milk sample between 1998 and 2000.[4]

Because of the multifactorial nature of calfhood respiratory disease, it is very difficult to estimate the contribution of a single pathogen such as *M bovis*. This is further hampered by a lack of epidemiologic data on *M bovis* infections of calves in North America. In Europe it has been estimated that *M bovis* is responsible for 25% to 35% of calfhood respiratory disease.[88] Although specific data for *Mb*AD in dairy calves in North America have not been published, undifferentiated respiratory disease is the second most important cause of morbidity and mortality in US dairy heifers.[54,89-91] It is clear from the reports on outbreaks of *M bovis*–associated respiratory disease in North American dairy calves that *M bovis* can be a significant contributor to overall rates of disease and mortality in affected herds.[43,60,65,92] For example, in a 1996 prospective study of five New York dairies, 40 cases of pneumonia occurred in 78 calves that were prospectively followed for the first 3 months of life; and 22 (55%) of these cases were attributed to *M bovis* infection.[92]

Economic Losses

There are limited data available on the economic impact of *Mb*AD. Losses to the US beef industry as a result of reduced weight gain and carcass value because of *Mb*AD have been estimated at $32 million per year, and in the United Kingdom, it is estimated that *M bovis* contributes to at least a quarter of the economic loss due to bovine respiratory disease.[93] However, the cost of MbAD in dairy heifers has not been reported. In addition, there is scant recent information available on the cost of undifferentiated respiratory disease in dairy heifers in North America. In a 1990 study of Michigan dairy herds, the cost of respiratory disease in calves was estimated at $14.71 per calf year.[94] Esslemont and Kossaibati[95] estimated that the average cost of respiratory disease in dairy heifers in the UK was $61 per calf in the herd, based on 30% morbidity and 5% mortality rates. Economic costs associated with calf respiratory disease include treatment costs, labor costs, veterinary services, increased mortality, increased premature culling, reduced weight gain, reduced fertility, increased age at first calving, and possibly reduced milk production.[96–101] Without pathogen-specific data being available, it is reasonable to assume that MbAD incurs many of the same costs.

M bovis–associated disease tends to be debilitating and unresponsive to therapy.[42,44,47,102,103] Tschopp and colleagues[7] give an example of an outbreak of MbAD in which 54% of 415 calves introduced into an *M bovis*–endemic facility seroconverted to *M bovis*. Calves that seroconverted within 7 weeks of arrival experienced an 8% reduction in weight gain and required twice as many antibiotics as did seronegative calves. The proportion of clinical episodes of respiratory disease attributable to *M bovis* in these calves was 50.3%. In another reported outbreak of severe MbAD, 70% of the calves in one dairy herd required treatment for respiratory disease or otitis media before 3 months of age.[43] On the individual farm affected with *M bovis*–associated* calf disease, losses resulting from treatment costs, death, and culling can be substantial, and economically devastating outbreaks with very high morbidity rates and death losses of up to 30% have been observed.[7,42,44,45,57,60,64,65,104]

Animal Welfare

In addition to any economic consequences, *M bovis* must be considered important from a calf welfare perspective. MbAD is often chronic, responds poorly to antibiotic therapy, often affects a substantial proportion of calves in a herd, may cause permanent health issues for affected calves, and available vaccines appear to be, at best, of limited efficacy.[10,42,44,53,88,102,103] Taken together, these characteristics result in affected calves that may be subject to long periods of illness for which the producer or veterinarian can provide only limited relief.

EPIDEMIOLOGY OF *MYCOPLASMA* INFECTIONS IN CALVES
Colonization and Shedding

M bovis is a frequent colonizer of the URT of healthy or diseased calves. In diseased herds, nasal prevalences of up to 100% of calves have been reported.[31,37,43,52,105] Within-herd prevalence is generally higher in herds with a history of MbAD than in herds without such a history. For example, Bennett and Jasper[31] reported a nasal prevalence of 34% in dairy calves younger than 8 months of age in herds with MbAD, compared with 6% in nondiseased herds. Cattle can remain infected for long periods of time and may shed *M bovis* intermittently for many months and even years, acting as reservoirs of infection in the herd.[3,31] Chronic colonization of tonsils, with or without nasal shedding, has been described for mycoplasmal respiratory pathogens in other hosts,[106,107] and data from our experimental infection studies suggest that the tonsils are the primary site of URT colonization for *M bovis*.[37] In those studies, we infected calves by feeding milk replacer containing a field isolate of *M bovis*. All inoculated calves became heavily colonized at both palatine and pharyngeal tonsil sites by 2 weeks postinoculation, without significant nasal shedding of *M bovis* detected in most calves.

The significance of colonization of the URT with *M bovis* as a risk factor for the development of clinical disease in the individual animal is unknown. At the herd level, a high prevalence of nasal colonization is associated with increased rates of *Mb*AD and with isolation of *M bovis* from the LRT.[31,43,52,108] However, isolation of *M bovis* from nasal swabs in individual calves is generally poorly correlated with both clinical disease and the presence of *M bovis* in the LRT,[31,108,109] although a positive correlation between *M bovis* isolation from nasal swabs and clinical disease was reported in one study of backgrounding and stocker cattle.[110]

Little is known about the typical age of onset and duration of nasal shedding of *M bovis* in endemically infected herds. Bennett and Jasper[31] reported that in calves younger than 1 week of age, nasal prevalence was 38% in herds with *Mb*AD and 7.5% in nondiseased herds. Prevalence in the diseased herds peaked at 48% between 1 and 4 months of age. *M bovis* was still detected in nasal swabs from some calves at 8 months of age and from pre-partum heifers, although whether these represented new or chronic infections was not determined. Other investigators reported that almost 50% of calves in a herd with severe *M bovis* and *P multocida* pneumonia were shedding *M bovis* at 5 days of age and over 90% were shedding *M bovis* by 4 weeks. The onset of clinical disease in this herd peaked between 10 and 15 days of age.[45] Approximately 10% of the calves died as a result of severe pneumonia, and surviving calves had poor weight gain. In a Florida dairy experiencing an outbreak of *Mb*AD, *M bovis* was isolated before 14 days of age from nasal swabs of all of 50 calves sampled, and 70% of these calves required treatment for respiratory disease or otitis media.[43] In another study of 85 calves in a Florida dairy with a history of *Mb*AD, *M bovis* was isolated from weekly nasal swabs of every calf at least once before 90 days of age. Most calves were shedding *M bovis* by 3 weeks of age and remained shedders for several weeks.[37] It is apparent from these studies that calves in infected herds are often colonized when they are very young (even at less than 1 week of age), and that the highest rates of nasal shedding occur in the first 2 months of life. In addition, Bennett and Jasper[31] found that *M bovis* may be shed in nasal secretions of calves in herds with no history of *Mb*AD.

Although the URT is the most common site of infection, *M bovis* may similarly colonize and be shed from other body systems without causing clinical disease. In cows, subclinical *M bovis* mastitis is common, and infected cows may intermittently shed the bacteria in milk for months to years.[3,86] *M bovis* has also been isolated from the conjunctiva,[111] semen, and vaginal secretions[3] of cattle without clinical disease. Although both respiratory tract and mammary gland shedding have been implicated as reservoirs of infection within a herd,[3] colonization at other sites does not seem to play a major role in the epidemiology of *M bovis*. Long-term epidemiologic studies would be helpful to determine the impact of *M bovis* colonization or *Mb*AD in young calves on the risk of URT or mammary gland infection with *M bovis* as adults.

Transmission and Risk Factors

M bovis is thought to be introduced into *M bovis*–free herds by clinically healthy cattle that are carrying this microorganism.[5,7,86] Spread to uninfected animals may occur at the time of introduction into the herd or may be delayed until shedding occurs.[11] Little is published on the epidemiology of *M bovis* within young calf populations, but there are several potential routes of initial exposure. Calves could become infected from their dams or from other adult cows in the maternity area that are shedding *M bovis* in colostrum, vaginal, or respiratory secretions.[3] The isolation of *M bovis* from vaginal secretions of cows at calving[43] and congenital infection of calves[57,112] have been reported, although both events appear to occur infrequently and probably do not play a major role in transmission.

One of the major means of transmission to young calves is thought to be ingestion of milk from cows shedding *M bovis* from the mammary gland (**Fig. 1**).[43,60,65] Colonization of the URT by *M bovis* occurs more frequently in calves fed infected milk than in those fed uninfected milk,[31] and clinical disease has been documented following feeding of *M bovis*–contaminated waste milk or in calves nursing cows with *M bovis* mastitis.[43,56,60,65] Because milk in modern husbandry systems is typically batched for feeding to calves, a single cow shedding *M bovis* can potentially expose a large number of calves to infection, and calves may be repeatedly exposed over the milk-feeding period. In a field study to determine the method of transmission of *M bovis* in one Florida dairy herd, 100% of 50 calves exposed to *M bovis*–contaminated waste milk became colonized in the URT by 14 days of age.[43] Culture of nasal and vaginal swabs of cows at calving was only positive for *M bovis* in one instance each. This led the authors to conclude that the main method of spread of *M bovis* from dam to calf was through contaminated waste milk. This hypothesis has been supported by other investigators.[60,65] Additionally, in an experimental infection study using young calves, feeding of milk replacer containing a clinically relevant dose of *M bovis* consistently resulted in colonization of the URT and mild clinical disease by 14 days postinoculation.[37] However, feeding of unpasteurized waste milk is clearly not the only important factor in the epidemiology of *M bovis* in calves, because clinical disease can occur in herds that feed only milk replacer or in herds that effectively pasteurize milk before feeding.[68] The importance of colostrum as a source of *M bovis* infection in calves is unknown, although in one study, investigators did not isolate *M bovis* from 50 colostrum samples collected during an outbreak of *MbAD*.[43]

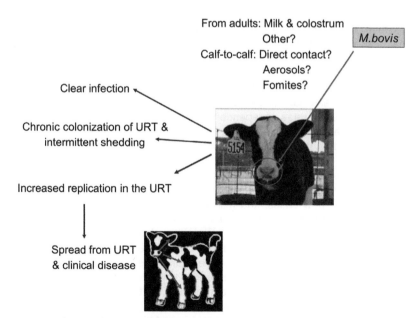

Fig. 1. Proposed transmission and infection dynamics of *M bovis* infections in young calves. URT, upper respiratory tract.

Whatever the mechanism (infected milk, colostrum, respiratory or vaginal secretions, or congenital infection) by which calves become infected, they may then shed *M bovis* in respiratory secretions (see **Fig. 1**). Once established on farms, *M bovis* becomes extremely difficult to eradicate, suggesting that continual transmission from older animals to incoming calves occurs.[31] Transmission is likely to be a result of direct or indirect contact of uninfected calves with calves that are shedding *M bovis* in respiratory secretions.[7,31,88]

In general, for bacterial pathogens involved in multifactorial diseases, the risk of infection and of developing clinical disease depends on a large number of pathogen, host, and environmental factors. With the exception of exposure to *M bovis*–contaminated milk (discussed previously), few specific risk factors for the transmission of *M bovis* or for outbreaks of clinical disease have been identified. Mixing of calves from different sources and the presence of at least one seropositive animal in new purchases increased the risk of MbAD on a ranch that raised dairy bull calves.[7] This result is in agreement with epidemiologic studies of *M bovis* mastitis, where one of the few consistently identified herd-level risk factors has been a history of purchasing cattle.[2] Herd size is the only other commonly identified risk factor for mycoplasmal mastitis.[4,113] Herd size was identified as a risk factor for an *M bovis*–positive bulk tank in the NAHMS Dairy 2002 study, with 21.7% of herds of 500 head or more having positive samples, compared with 3.9% and 2.1% of medium (100 to 400 head) and small (<100 head) herds, respectively.[84] Larger herd size was associated with increased rates of undifferentiated respiratory disease in calves in the 1991 to 1992 National Dairy Heifer Evaluation Project,[90] but the effect of herd size on MbAD in young calves has not been reported.

Despite the lack of published studies, other potential risk factors for *M bovis* infection in young calves can be identified from the limited research on *M bovis* epidemiology in calves, from studies of *M bovis* mastitis, and by extrapolating from what is known about risk factors for other respiratory pathogens in calves. For example, calves with MbAD shed huge numbers of bacteria[31] and are therefore likely to be the greatest contributors to the load of *Mycoplasma* within a calf-rearing facility, and the most important factor in calf-to-calf spread of disease. For undifferentiated respiratory disease, high bacterial counts in the air of calf pens are associated with increased disease prevalence.[114] Large numbers of *M bovis* can be isolated from the air in barns housing calves with MbAD.[115] Therefore, factors that influence airborne bacteria counts in calf pens, such as pen design, barn ventilation, and stocking density[114] may affect transmission rates. Independent of effects on bacterial load, poor air quality compromises respiratory defenses, which may increase the risk of respiratory disease.[99] However, this has not been specifically evaluated with respect to *M bovis* infections.

Mechanical transmission via fomites has been implicated in udder-to-udder spread of *M bovis* mastitis. Milking of uninfected and infected cows at the same time increases the risk for new cases, and milking equipment, teat dip, hands, sponges, washcloths, and poor hygiene during intramammary infusion of antibiotics have been implicated in the spread of *M bovis*.[5,115–117] It is plausible that similar mechanical means of transfer could occur in calf facilities. Despite being enveloped by only a thin cell membrane, some mycoplasmas survive well in the environment. *Mycoplasma bovis* was reported to survive at 4°C for nearly 2 months in sponges and milk, over 2 weeks on wood and in water, and 20 days in straw, although higher environmental temperatures dropped survival considerably.[3] In general, survival is best under cool, humid conditions.[3] In surveys of Florida dairy farms, *M bovis* was commonly isolated from cooling ponds and from dirt lots with recently calved cows on farms that had a history of *M bovis*–positive bulk tank milk culture.[118] These studies demonstrate that *M bovis* can survive well in the dairy environment, and that mechanical transmission via fomites could theoretically occur among calves. However, further studies are required to examine the role of fomites in the epidemiology of *M bovis* infection in calf-rearing facilities.

In a study of the effect of temperature and humidity on nasal shedding of mycoplasmas in calves, an abrupt change from warm (17°C) to cold (5°C) conditions was associated with increased rates of nasal shedding of *M bovis*. In addition, calves that were permanently housed at 5°C had higher rates of nasal shedding of *M bovis* than calves housed at 16°C.[119] Other investigators subjected healthy calves to extreme environmental temperatures (5°C or 35°C) for 4 hours; calves were housed at 18°C to 20°C before and after the exposure. Calves exposed to environmental extremes experienced significantly higher rates of respiratory disease over the following 3 weeks than did unexposed control calves. *Mycoplasma* spp were identified as the cause of respiratory disease in calves that were exposed to cold temperatures (5°C), whereas no mycoplasmas were isolated from the lungs of calves exposed to warmer temperatures (35°C) or in control calves.[120] Together, these findings suggest that mycoplasmal nasal shedding and, perhaps, clinical disease are favored by low environmental temperatures. However, epidemiologic studies to evaluate the association between temperature and MbAD have not been published.

Season may have some effect on *M bovis* infections in calves. Lamm and colleagues[68] reported that there was a seasonal distribution of cases of mycoplasmal otitis media in calves submitted for necropsy to a Californian diagnostic laboratory, with the highest proportion of cases submitted in the spring and the lowest in the summer months. Seasonal effects have been observed in some studies of mycoplasmal mastitis, with the incidence generally being higher in the cooler months of the year,[2,121] but not in others.[4,85] There are several possible explanations for increased rates of MbAD in winter or early spring compared with other times of year. Survival of mycoplasmas in the environment is best in cool, humid conditions[3] and the risk of indirect transmission between animals may be greatest when these conditions predominate. Second, a seasonal distribution could reflect an association of *M bovis* infection with exposure to cold environmental temperatures, as discussed above.[119,120] Last, air quality in enclosed cattle facilities may be worse in winter than at other times of the year, predisposing animals to increased rates of respiratory disease.[99,114] Further epidemiologic studies are required to definitively determine if there is a seasonal distribution of MbAD in calves.

The immune status of the calf is important in determining susceptibility to respiratory infections. Numerous investigators have found a strong association between failure of passive transfer of maternal immunoglobulins and increased risk and severity of respiratory disease in young calves.[51,91,122–124] However, whether maternal antibodies have any protective effects against *M bovis* infection is not clear. In one study, there was no significant association between *M bovis*–specific serum antibody titers in the first 2 weeks of life and occurrence of pneumonia in 325 colostrum-fed dairy calves.[51] Likewise, Brown and colleagues[43] did not find an association between *M bovis*–specific serum antibody concentrations at 7 days of age and occurrence of MbAD in 50 Holstein calves. Nonspecific respiratory defenses are important in protection from mycoplasmal respiratory infections in other hosts,[38] and it is logical that they would also be important in *M bovis* infections. The nonspecific respiratory defenses of calves can be compromised by a variety of factors including infection with viral pathogens, sudden changes in environmental temperature, heat or cold stress, overcrowding, transportation, poor air quality, and inadequate nutrition.[99,125] However, further studies are required to define the role of factors affecting the nonspecific respiratory defenses of calves as well as the role of passive immunity in *M bovis*–associated calf disease. Induction of specific immunity to *M bovis* will be discussed under vaccination later in this article.

Colonization of the URT of calves with *M bovis* often occurs within the first few weeks of life,[31,37,43] with the peak incidence of clinical disease at around a month of age. During this period, the immune system of the young calf is undergoing the rapid changes associated with maturation.[126,127] Therefore, age-specific features of the immune system are likely to be important in determining the susceptibility or resistance of the young dairy calf to *MbAD*. For example, the tendency toward an IgG_1-dominated humoral response in young calves may not be optimal for clearance of *M bovis*, given that IgG_2 is a superior opsonin for macrophage- and neutrophil-mediated killing of *M bovis*.[128] Additionally, the presence of age-specific immune responses means that vaccine strategies targeting young calves need to be tailored specifically to this age group. Readers are referred to the article in this issue on neonatal vaccination for more information on the challenges to successful vaccination of calves in this age group.

Genetic background is thought to play an important role in the susceptibility of cattle to infectious disease.[129,130] Genetic background is also important in determining susceptibility or resistance to mycoplasmal respiratory infections of nonbovine species. In many cases, genetic susceptibility to mycoplasmal respiratory disease appears to be a result of increased immunoreactivity of the host when compared with resistant animals.[131] Additionally, innate responses such as alveolar macrophage clearance of mycoplasmas from the lung early in the infection process are influenced by genetic background, at least in rodents.[132] Interestingly, male mice are more susceptible than females to mycoplasmal infection, suggesting that hormonal regulation may also be important in disease susceptibility.[133] Genetic susceptibility to mycoplasmal infections is not limited to rodents. In pigs that were bred for high or low cellular and humoral immune responses, high responders that were experimentally infected with *M hyorhinis* had more severe arthritis than did pigs bred for low immune response.[134] Given these findings coupled with the fact that immune responsiveness in cattle has a substantial genetic influence, it would not be surprising if genetic background is associated with susceptibility to *MbAD* in cattle. However, to date no studies have addressed the role of genetics in susceptibility of cattle to mycoplasmal infections.

Bovine respiratory disease frequently involves a number of viral and bacterial pathogens,[99,125] and *M bovis*–associated respiratory disease is no exception.[9,10,44,49,54,135–138] In fact, *M bovis* infection may predispose the respiratory tract to invasion by other bacterial pathogens.[10,49,54,139] Similarly, other pathogens may enhance *M bovis* infection. Viral infections can damage the respiratory mucosa, reduce ciliary activity, and impair secretory and cellular immune defenses in the respiratory tract.[99,140] Any or all of these changes could increase susceptibility to mycoplasmal infection. Studies in feedlot calves with chronic, antibiotic-resistant pneumonia suggest that there may be synergism between bovine viral diarrhea virus (BVDV) and *M bovis*.[141] Experimental infection studies have confirmed that *M bovis* plays a synergistic role with other respiratory pathogens,[33,142,143] especially *P multocida* and *M hemolytica*. In cases of *M bovis*–associated arthritis, mixed infections in affected joints are uncommon, although calves with arthritis often have concurrent respiratory disease from which multiple pathogens may be isolated.[6,60,68]

Mixed infections can occur in *M bovis*–associated otitis media, although their significance is unknown.[64,68] In other host species, viral infections of the URT are important risk factors for increased incidence, severity, and chronicity of bacterial otitis media. One mechanism by which viral infections can potentiate bacterial otitis media is by perturbing the ciliary clearance mechanisms of the eustachian tubes.[144,145] Specific viral etiologies have not been identified in the lungs of preweaned calves with *M bovis*–associated otitis media.[65,66,68,146] However, attempts to isolate viruses from lesions in the tympanic bullae have been reported only once,[66] and no attempts to isolate viruses from the nasopharynx or eustachian tubes of affected calves have been reported.

Susceptibility to *M bovis*–induced otitis media appears to be age related, with the peak incidence of clinical disease at 2 to 6 weeks of age.[64,65] *M bovis*–associated otitis media is uncommon in other age groups. In one recent study of feedlot cattle, *M bovis* was frequently isolated from the tympanic bullae of animals with no clinical or gross lesions of otitis media,[10] suggesting it is the expression of clinical disease rather than dissemination to the middle ear that is age related. Age-related susceptibility to otitis media is also observed in *M hyorhinis* infections of piglets, although age-specific factors contributing to susceptibility in this species have not been determined.[36,147] In other species, the age at which colonization of the nasopharynx or tonsils first occurs also affects the risk of developing otitis media. For example, infants who are first colonized in the nasopharynx with *Streptococcus pneumoniae, Haemophilus influenzae,* or *Moraxella catarrhalis* before 3 months of age have increased risk and severity of otitis media compared with infants who are first colonized after 3 months of age.[148] Colonization of the nasopharynx with bacterial pathogens within the first week of life is associated with extremely high rates of otitis media in infants. Interestingly, whereas complete eradication of *H influenzae* from the nasopharynx was highly effective at preventing otitis media, reduction of the bacterial load in the nasopharynx to below a critical threshold level appeared similarly effective.[149] These findings suggest that the ability to delay colonization by only a few weeks might have a dramatic impact on susceptibility to *M bovis*–associated otitis media in calves.

In summary, young calves can be infected at a very early age by ingestion of milk from cows infected with *M bovis*. They are also likely infected by direct or indirect transmission from other calves shedding *M bovis* in nasal secretions. However, other than the feeding of infected milk, few specific risk factors have been identified, and factors associated with dissemination from the URT to the LRT and clinical disease expression are poorly understood. Clearly, new epidemiologic studies would be helpful to establish risk factors and to provide guidance for calf producers to reduce *Mb*AD.

Molecular Epidemiology

M bovis is well equipped to generate genetically diverse populations, and has been observed to undergo DNA recombination and rearrangement events at high frequency.[21,24,28] The *M bovis* genome contains a large number of insertion sequences that are also likely to lead to heterogeneous populations.[150] There have been several molecular epidemiologic studies of *M bovis* using a variety of DNA fingerprinting techniques including randomly amplified polymorphic DNA analysis, amplified fragment length polymorphism analysis, restriction fragment length polymorphism analysis, pulsed-field gel electrophoresis (PFGE) analysis, and insertion sequence profile analysis.[27,150–154] Considerable genomic heterogeneity among field isolates of *M bovis* has been reported, especially when isolates were collected from diverse geographic regions and over a period of several years.[27,150,151] The significance of particular DNA fingerprint types in *M bovis* infections are currently unknown, and correlations between particular DNA fingerprint types and geographic location, year of isolation, and type or severity of pathology have not been reported.[27,150–152] However, the vast ability of *M bovis* to create genetically diverse populations as well as the frequent movement of cattle among herds in modern management systems may make it difficult to identify any such associations.

Comparison of PFGE patterns for isolates of *M bovis* or *Mycoplasma californicum* obtained at necropsy from multiple body sites in seven cows with mycoplasmal mastitis was reported.[154] Within each cow, the same PFGE pattern was found in 100% of isolates from sites in the mammary system (milk, mammary parenchyma, and supramammary lymph nodes). Forty-one percent of isolates obtained from the respiratory system and 90% of isolates obtained from other body systems had PFGE patterns identical to that of the mammary isolates. These findings indicate that the same strain of *M bovis* often colonizes multiple body sites, but also that multiple strains may be present within an animal. Isolates of *M bovis* from multiple sites of pathology within the same animal, or from multiple animals in the same disease outbreak, are typically closely related or identical by DNA typing methods, especially when the herd is closed.[152,153,155] In contrast, endemically infected open herds (including dairy calf ranches), harbor numerous genetically diverse strains of *M bovis*. This has been attributed to introduction of animals from multiple sources over time.[153] Further molecular epidemiologic studies will hopefully enhance the current understanding of the transmission dynamics of *M bovis*.

CLINICAL DISEASE IN CALVES

Clinical disease associated with *M bovis* infection of young calves typically presents as pneumonia, otitis media, or arthritis, or any combination of these.[43,45,56,60,65,67,68] *M bovis* has also been associated with a variety of other less common clinical manifestations in calves, including tenosynovitis, decubital abscesses, and meningitis.[57,59,104] The age of onset of clinical disease in affected calves is typically between 2 and 6 weeks,[43–45,65] but has been reported as early as 4 days of age.[57] Clinical disease caused by *M bovis* tends to be chronic, debilitating, and unresponsive to therapy.[10,42,44,53,102,103,141] Chronic endemic disease as well as epizootics can occur.[136]

M bovis–associated respiratory disease has a similar clinical presentation to other types of calf pneumonia. Fever, loss of appetite, nasal discharge, coughing, and both increased respiratory rate and effort are typically reported, and concurrent cases of otitis media and arthritis may occur.[43,45,59,65,67,68] As for undifferentiated calf pneumonia, auscultation reveals abnormal breath sounds including increased bronchial sounds, crackles, wheezes, and areas of cranioventral consolidation in severe cases.[99] Both acute and chronic disease can occur, and mixed infections are common.[9,42,44,49,54,81,137,138] Calves with chronic pneumonia often develop extreme dyspnea and emaciation.[99]

Otitis media has been an increasingly recognized form of MbAD in North American dairy calves over the past 15 years.[64,65,68] The clinical signs of otitis media observed include loss of appetite, fever, listlessness, ear pain evidenced by head shaking and scratching or rubbing ears, epiphora, ear droop, and signs of facial nerve paralysis (**Fig. 2A–C**).[43,65–67,146] One or both tympanic bullae can be affected. In some cases, purulent discharge from the ear canal is observed following rupture of the tympanic membrane.[65,67] In addition, calves with *M bovis*–induced otitis media often have concurrent pneumonia.[64–66,68]

Otitis interna is a common sequela to otitis media in calves, and affected animals exhibit varying degrees of vestibulocochlear dysfunction including head tilt, horizontal

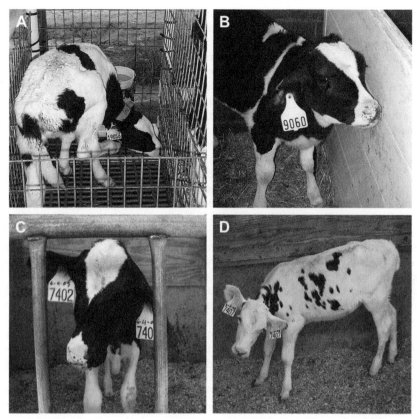

Fig. 2. Examples of the clinical manifestations of *Mycoplasma bovis*–associated otitis in calves. Ear scratching is frequently one of the earliest signs of otitis media (*A*), followed by unilateral or bilateral ear droop and epiphora (*B* and *C*). Head tilt is indicative of otitis interna and more advanced disease (*D*).

nystagmus, staggering, circling, falling, and/or lateral recumbency (**Fig 2**D).[64,66,68,146] Meningitis can occur as a complication of otitis interna.[57,67,68,146] Spontaneous regurgitation, loss of pharyngeal tone, and dysphagia have also been reported in calves with *M bovis*–associated otitis media-interna, indicative of glossopharyngeal nerve dysfunction with or without vagal nerve dysfunction.[146] Whether these nerves are affected by inflammation associated with meningitis or with inflammation at the sites where the nerves pass over the tympanic bullae is unknown. As is observed with *M bovis*–associated respiratory disease, calves with chronic otitis media-interna may become emaciated.[65,146]

Clinical cases of *M bovis*–induced arthritis in preweaned calves tend to be sporadic and are typically accompanied by respiratory disease within the herd and often within the same animal.[155,156] Clinical signs are typical of septic arthritis. Affected joints are painful and swollen, and calves exhibit varying degrees of lameness and may be febrile in the acute phase of disease.[57,61,157] Large rotator joints such as the shoulder, elbow, carpus, hip, stifle, and hock are most frequently involved.[10,57,59,157,158] One or multiple joints can be affected, and cattle with *M bovis* arthritis are frequently culled because of poor response to therapy.[59,61,159] Arthritis appears to be a less frequent clinical manifestation of *M bovis* infections in preweaned calves than in feedlot cattle. However, outbreaks of disease in young calves where arthritis was the predominant clinical presentation have been reported.[57,60]

M bovis also may cause a variety of less common clinical syndromes in calves, with or without concurrent respiratory disease. In addition to its occurrence as a sequela of otitis media,[66,67] meningitis has occurred as a consequence of mycoplasmemia in very young calves. For example, in one case report, 3- to 21-day-old calves developed polyarthritis and meningitis with high mortality rates. *M bovis* was the only pathogen isolated from joints and meninges of affected calves.[57] In very young calves, arthritis caused by *M bovis* must be distinguished from septic arthritis secondary to navel infections or other causes of bacterial sepsis.

M bovis infections can occur in or around tendons and synovial structures, and tenosynovitis and bursitis are commonly reported in feedlot calves with concurrent chronic *M bovis* arthritis.[59,157,158] In addition, intra-articular inoculation of *M bovis* in calves resulted in arthritis plus tenosynovitis.[56,63] In an unusual presentation of *M bovis* infection, an outbreak of subcutaneous decubital abscesses over carpal and stifle joints and over the brisket was reported in 50 calves fed unpasteurized waste milk on a California calf ranch.[104] *M bovis* was the only pathogen isolated from abscesses, which occurred at the sites of pressure sores. Whether the bacteria gained entry through skin abrasions or via hematogenous spread is unknown, but the authors hypothesized that *M bovis* in nasal secretions may have contaminated pressure sores when calves licked these areas. There was no evidence of joint involvement in affected calves, but at least one calf had concurrent *M bovis*–associated respiratory disease.

M bovis can be isolated from the conjunctiva of cattle in infected herds,[111] although *M bovis*–associated ocular disease is considered uncommon. However, there are several reports of outbreaks of keratoconjunctivitis involving *M bovis* alone, or in mixed infections with *Mycoplasma bovoculi*.[160–163] An outbreak of severe keratoconjunctivitis, from which *M bovis* was the only consistently isolated pathogen, was reported in a group of 20 calves. Clinical signs included mucopurulent ocular discharge, severe eyelid and conjunctival swelling, and corneal edema and ulceration. Most clinical signs resolved within 2 weeks but some animals had residual corneal scarring.[162] In a recent report, an outbreak of *M bovis*–associated keratoconjunctivitis in beef calves in Italy was followed by cases of pneumonia and arthritis.[160]

In summary, *M bovis* infections primarily result in pneumonia, otitis media, and, to a lesser extent, arthritis in young calves, but other more unusual clinical presentations affecting a wide variety of body systems can occur.

PATHOLOGY

The macroscopic and microscopic lesions of the respiratory tract in experimental *M bovis* infection vary considerably among studies, probably reflecting differences in the route of inoculation, the dose and strain of *M bovis*, the age and health status of the host, and the duration of infection. Gross lesions have consisted of cranioventral lung consolidation, sometimes accompanied by multiple necrotic foci.[33,48,136,143] Histologically, experimental lung infections with *M bovis* are characterized by peribronchiolar lymphoid hyperplasia or cuffing, often accompanied by acute or subacute suppurative bronchiolitis, thickening of alveolar septa as a result of cellular infiltration, atelectasis, and, in some cases, foci of coagulative necrosis.[33,48,125,136,143]

Lesions described for the lungs of cattle with natural *M bovis* infections are similar to those described for experimental disease, although typically of much greater severity. There are relatively few studies describing the naturally occurring pathology in young calves, so most information comes from feedlot cattle. The pathology associated with *M bovis* pneumonia in feedlot cattle has recently been reviewed.[10,12] Grossly, affected lung lobes are a deep red color and have varying degrees of consolidation, often accompanied in subacute to chronic cases by multifocal necrotizing lesions.[8,10,42,59,102,158,164] Similar lesions are observed in 6-month-old veal calves with *M bovis*–associated pneumonia.[165] Lesions usually have a cranioventral distribution, but can involve whole lung lobes and the cranial portions of the caudal lobes. Necrotic lesions can vary from 1 to 2 mm to several centimeters in diameter and contain yellow caseous material (**Fig. 3**). They are distinct from typical lung abscesses in that they are not usually surrounded by a well-defined fibrous capsule.[158,164] Diffuse fibrinous or chronic fibrosing pleuritis are sometimes observed, and interlobular septae may contain edema fluid or linear yellow necrotic lesions.[10,46,136,157,158] Occasionally, chronic cases of *M bovis* pneumonia contain areas of lung sequestration.[10] Fibrinosuppurative tracheitis has been reported in calves with mycoplasmal lung infections.[76] Experimental and natural *M bovis*–associated respiratory disease is typically accompanied by hyperplasia of the lymphoid tissues in both the URT and LRT.[10,33] Foci of caseous necrosis in bronchial and mediastinal lymph nodes of affected calves have been observed.[10]

Histologically, lung lesions in naturally occurring *M bovis* infections are characterized by a subacute to chronic suppurative bronchopneumonia that is frequently necrotizing.[8,10,102,136,158,164,165] Mixed infections are common and often complicate characterization of lesions.[8,10,59,102,158,164] Bronchioles are filled with purulent exudate that contains abundant *M bovis* antigen on immunohistochemical staining, accompanied by varying degrees of peribronchiolar lympho-histiocytic cuffing, thickening of alveolar septa as a result of cellular infiltration, and atelectasis.

Two distinct types of necrotic lesions have been reported in *M bovis* pneumonia, the most common being multifocal pyogranulomatous inflammation with centers of caseous necrosis.[10,102,136,158,164,165] These well-delineated necrotic foci have centers of amorphous eosinophilic material in which degenerate neutrophils are sometimes visible, especially at the periphery, and are surrounded by a band of lymphocytes, plasma cells, macrophages, and fibroblasts. In many cases, it appears that foci of caseous necrosis are centered on obliterated bronchioles. Edema fluid, fibrin, and variable numbers of neutrophils and macrophages are often present in adjacent pulmonary parenchyma. The second, and less common, type of necrotic lesion described is fibrinopurulent broncho- or bronchointerstitial pneumonia accompanied by multifocal irregular areas of coagulative necrosis, surrounded by a dense zone of necrotic cells, especially neutrophils.[8,46,66,164,165] These types of lesions were reported to be the most common type observed in 6-month-old veal calves with mycoplasmal pneumonia.[165] Edema, fibrin deposition, and vascular and lymphatic

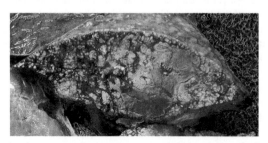

Fig. 3. *Mycoplasma bovis* pneumonia. Lungs may contain numerous foci of caseous necrosis.

thromboses in the interlobular septa may accompany these types of lesions.[136,164] Large amounts of *M bovis* antigen have been demonstrated in both caseous and co-agulative necrosis by immunohistochemical staining, especially at the periphery of lesions.[10,66,136,158,164] Whether the two distinct types of necrosis are a result of temporal events, co-infection with other pathogens, variation among strains of *M bovis*, or variation in the host response is unknown.

Lesions in the joints and tendon sheaths of calves after experimental inoculation of *M bovis* are characterized as necrotizing fibrinosuppurative arthritis or tenosynovitis.[32,33,63] Similar lesions have been reported in naturally occurring *M bovis* arthritis.[10,59,76,158] Gross lesions vary from minimal to severe, but chronically affected joints usually contain nonodorous, turbid, yellow, and fibrinous to caseous exudate accompanied by thickening of the joint capsule. Histologically, affected joints usually have severe erosion of articular cartilage, hyperplasia and caseous necrosis of synoviae, and thrombosis of subsynovial vessels.[10,63] Adjacent soft tissues, including ligaments and tendons, are frequently involved.[10,69,158] Large amounts of *M bovis* antigen in the periphery of necrotic lesions and within joint exudates have been demonstrated by immunohistochemical staining of the joints in cattle with natural and experimental *M bovis* arthritis.[10,33,59,158]

In calves with *M bovis*–associated otitis media, affected tympanic bullae are filled with fibrinosuppurative to caseous exudate.[65,66,68] Histologically, extensive fibrino-suppurative exudates fill the tympanic bullae and normal architecture may be obliterated.[65,66,68] The tympanic mucosa may have areas of ulceration and/or squamous metaplasia and is markedly thickened as a result of infiltrates of macrophages, neutrophils, and plasma cells, and proliferation of fibrous tissue. There is usually extensive osteolysis and/or remodeling of adjacent bone.[65,68,146] Lesions are accompanied by fibrinosuppurative eustachitis.[68] Large quantities of *M bovis* antigen have been observed within necrotic exudates, particularly at the margins of necrotic lesions within the tympanic bullae. This is similar to findings in calves with *M bovis* pneumonia.[66] In chronic cases, lesions frequently extend into the inner ear and include petrous temporal bone osteomyelitis.[66,68] Meningitis as a consequence of otitis interna is usually localized to the regions adjacent to the affected petrous temporal bone and characterized as fibrinous to fibrinosuppurative and sometimes necrotizing.[68,166] In addition, diffuse fibrinous meningitis was described in neonatal calves with *M bovis* meningitis, which likely originated from mycoplasmemia.[57]

M bovis–associated lesions have occasionally been identified in other body systems in both experimentally and naturally infected calves.[33,66,102,166] Ayling and colleagues[166] described a 10-month-old calf with a history of respiratory disease that had lesions of endocarditis and encephalitis from which *M bovis* was the only pathogen isolated. In another report, intratracheal inoculation of *M bovis* resulted in arthritis in one calf, and mycoplasma were isolated from the blood during the first week post-inoculation.[33] At necropsy, investigators observed perivascular mononuclear cell infiltration in portal areas of the liver, and immunohistochemical staining revealed *M bovis* in association with these lesions. Other investigators identified *M bovis* antigen within foci of mononuclear cell infiltrates in the liver and kidneys of two calves with chronic *M bovis* pneumonia.[102]

DIAGNOSIS

The occurrence of *M bovis* is generally underestimated for several reasons. *Mycoplasma* culture requires special equipment and expertise.[167] Although the role of mycoplasmas in disease of cattle has received increased recognition in the past decade, many laboratories will not routinely monitor for this organism unless *Mycoplasma* culture is specifically requested. In respiratory disease, multiple pathogens are often present. Because other bacteria such as *M hemolytica* and *P multocida* are easier to culture, the presence of *M bovis* may be missed.[10,99] Recent studies suggest that MbAD is underdiagnosed, perhaps because veterinarians and pathologists fail to recognize the infection during routine physical, gross, and microscopic examination.[10,88] *M bovis* is sometimes associated with a variety of unusual clinical presentations in which its involvement is not widely recognized, and so appropriate diagnostic tests may not be requested.

A history of respiratory disease that is poorly responsive to antibiotic therapy is suggestive of *M bovis* involvement, especially when accompanied by cases of arthritis and/or otitis media. Although the associated lung pathology can be variable, multiple nodular lesions of caseous necrosis are strongly suggestive of *M bovis* infections.[10,102] However, as there are no pathognomonic clinical or pathologic signs for MbAD, a definitive diagnosis is based on isolation of *M bovis* from the affected site, and/or by demonstration of its presence in affected tissues by polymerase chain reaction (PCR), capture enzyme-linked immunosorbent assay (ELISA), or immunohistochemistry (IHC).

The culture of bovine mycoplasmas requires the use of nutritionally complex media as well as a moist carbon dioxide–enriched atmosphere.[86,167–169] Growth of *M bovis* in appropriate media is typically apparent by 48 hours, but may take up to 10 days.[86,88,168] Mycoplasmal colonies on solid media are identified by their characteristic morphology (**Fig. 4**); growth in broth is indicated by turbidity, film formation, and by subculture onto solid media.[168] A number of pathogenic and nonpathogenic bovine mycoplasmas or other mollicutes (especially acholeplasmas) may be isolated from the URT or from sites of pathology, either alone or in mixed infections.[10,68,88] Many of these cannot be differentiated morphologically from *M bovis*, so speciation by immunologic methods (direct or indirect immunofluorescence or immunoperoxidase testing) or by PCR is necessary.[47,86,170]

In live calves with clinical signs of respiratory disease, mycoplasmal culture of transtracheal wash or broncho-alveolar lavage (BAL) fluids are suitable for the diagnosis of *M bovis* infections.[108,109,171] Comparisons of paired culture results from nasopharyngeal swabs and BAL samples in cattle with respiratory disease indicate that, in individual animals, isolation of *M bovis* from the URT is not well correlated with its presence in the LRT or with clinical disease.[108,109] For example, in one study,[109] nasal swabs had a sensitivity of only 21% for predicting *M bovis*–associated lung disease.

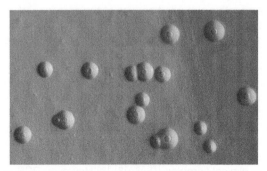

Fig. 4. Colonies of *Mycoplasma bovis* on solid media have the "fried egg" morphology that is typical of many mycoplasma species when viewed under a stereomicroscope (×40 magnification).

Nasopharyngeal swabs can be used at the group level to indicate the presence of M bovis within a calf facility,[31] although the sensitivity of this test has not been determined. In calves with arthritis or tenosynovitis, affected joints and tendon sheaths can be aspirated for culture.[61] Because of difficulties with access to the site of infection, samples are not usually collected from the tympanic bulla in live calves with otitis media. Meningitis secondary to otitis media-interna may be localized. In one report, cerebrospinal fluid samples collected for diagnostic purposes were more useful when collected from the atlanto-occipital rather than the lumbo-sacral space.[146]

Mycoplasma culture of necropsy specimens can be performed directly from homogenates of fresh tissues, aspirates, swabs collected from lesion sites, and lavage samples.[47,109,168] As for other infectious diseases, calves that are selected for necropsy to diagnose a herd problem should be representative of the cases seen in that herd. Culture of BAL samples collected at necropsy may be preferable to culture of lung tissue when tissues cannot be processed immediately. Mycoplasmas remain viable in BAL fluids for months at $-20°C$ or $-70°C$, for a few days at 4°C and for several hours at room temperature, whereas isolation rates from lung tissue decrease markedly over a few hours after collection because of release of mycoplasmal inhibitors from disrupted tissue.[169,172,173] Complete agreement between mycoplasmal cultures of paired BAL fluids collected at necropsy and corresponding lung tissue cultured immediately after collection from cattle euthanized for respiratory disease has been reported.[109] In the authors' experience, when there will be more than a few hours' delay until processing of tissue samples submitted to the diagnostic laboratory, it is advisable to also submit swabs of that tissue for Mycoplasma culture.

Sample handling and transport are particularly important to ensure the survival of M bovis. Swabs should be collected into transport media such as Ames (without charcoal) or Stuart's.[174] Swabs, lavage fluids, aspirates, milk, and colostrum samples should be refrigerated, and tissue samples should be collected as soon as possible after death and placed in sealed plastic bags on ice.[174] Samples should be transported to the laboratory within 24 hours.[174,175] If samples such as milk are stored frozen, they should still be submitted within 7 to 10 days of collection, as longer storage significantly decreases the isolation of M bovis.[175] Detection of mycoplasmas in clinical samples can potentially be improved by using enrichment techniques and large inoculum sizes.[87] Limitations of mycoplasma culture include the requirement for specialized equipment and expertise, the need to speciate any mycoplasmas that are isolated, the length of time before results are obtained, the overgrowth of slower growing species by other more rapidly growing mycoplasmas or other bacteria and fungi, the need to process samples rapidly after collection to maximize sensitivity, and the occurrence of false negative cultures because of the presence of antibiotics or other inhibitors in clinical samples.

In part to address frustrations with conventional culture techniques, a variety of PCR systems have been developed for the diagnosis of M bovis infections.[176–180] Three PCR systems have been widely adopted for clinical diagnostics, including (1) amplification of the 16SrRNA gene with species- or class-specific primers followed by digestion with various restriction enzymes to permit differentiation of several species of mollicutes within a single assay,[176,177] (2) amplification of the 16SrRNA gene with species-specific primers,[177,181] and (3) amplification of the housekeeping gene uvrC with species-specific primers.[177,179,182] PCR can be used for the speciation of mycoplasmas that have already been isolated by routine culture methods,[176,179,182] as well as for the direct detection of M bovis in clinical samples.[178,180,181,183] However, PCR performed directly from clinical samples can have variable sensitivity, and some authors report that samples containing fewer than 10^2 colony-forming units/mL were often detected as negative by PCR.[183] This detection level would be no better than standard culture procedures. Sensitivity has been improved by antigen capture before PCR using an *M bovis*–specific monoclonal antibody.[183] A nested PCR was slightly more sensitive than culture of fresh milk samples, but was much more sensitive than culture (100% compared with 27%) for detection of *M bovis* in milk after 2 years of frozen storage.[180]

Because of the very close genotypic relationship between *M bovis* and *Mycoplasma agalactiae* there has been considerable work invested in developing assays that accurately differentiate these two species.[177,179,181,182,184] However, because *M agalactiae* is a pathogen of small ruminants that is presumed to be absent from North America and is rarely isolated outside of its typical hosts, differentiation from *M bovis* is less of a concern on this continent than in regions where both pathogens exist.

A sandwich ELISA has been developed to capture *M bovis* antigen from culture medium or clinical samples, and is commercially available in Europe (Bio-X Diagnostics, Belgium).[185] The ELISA has a similar sensitivity to conventional culture when performed directly from clinical samples, but sensitivity is improved when samples are incubated in broth culture medium for a brief period before antigen capture.

Immunohistochemical demonstration of *M bovis* antigen within tissues is a sensitive and specific means of determining the involvement of *M bovis* in observed pathology.[6,8,10,66,136,158,164,165,186] Advantages of IHC are that it performs well using formalin-fixed, paraffin-embedded tissues, and can be performed retrospectively, especially when other findings suggest a *M bovis* infection but culture is negative. An additional advantage of IHC is that it reveals the location of *M bovis* within lesions. In one recent retrospective study,[10] 98% and 100% of cases of caseonecrotic bronchopneumonia from feedlot cattle submitted to a diagnostic laboratory were positive for *M bovis* by culture and IHC, respectively. In cases of fibrinosuppurative pneumonia where *M hemolytica* was isolated, *M bovis* was also isolated in 82% of cases, and was demonstrated by IHC in lesions of mixed infections (with *M hemolytica*) in 85% of cases.[10] The involvement of *M bovis* in lesions at a variety of other body sites has also been verified by IHC.[10,33,57,59,66,104,158] An indirect fluorescent antibody test using polyclonal antisera has been described for the detection of *M bovis* in fresh, frozen lung tissue.[72]

A variety of methods for the detection of *M bovis*–specific antibodies in serum and other body fluids have been described.[83,187–189] An indirect hemagglutination test (IHA) has been successfully used to demonstrate the presence of *M bovis*–specific antibody in serum, colostral whey, and joint fluid.[10,83,187] However, the most widely applied method to detect *M bovis*–specific antibodies is an indirect ELISA.[88,190] Most studies have used whole cell or membrane protein antigens derived from various reference or field strains of *M bovis*. Laboratory-grown strains of *M bovis* vary over time in their variable surface protein (Vsp) expression profiles, and it has been proposed that this may effect the reliability of immunologic assays[191]; however studies addressing whether this issue is of practical concern in diagnostic ELISA have not been published. Le Grand and colleagues[190] developed an indirect ELISA using membrane proteins derived from a phenotypic clonal variant of the *M bovis* type strain PG45 with a high level of expression of Vsp A. The assay performed well in experimentally and naturally infected cattle populations, although whether or not the antigen was superior to traditional antigens was not determined. A variety of ELISA tests for serologic detection of *M bovis* antibodies are now commercially available in Canada and Europe. For example, Biovet in Canada, Bio-X Diagnostics in Belgium, and Bommelli in Switzerland currently manufacture ELISA kits that detect *M bovis* antibodies.

M bovis–specific serum immunoglobulin is detectable as early as 6 (IgM) to 10 days (IgG) after experimental inoculation of *M bovis* into the respiratory tract.[188,190] Specific serum immunoglobulin concentrations remain elevated for months to years after *M bovis* infection, so a high titer does not necessarily indicate very recent exposure.[88,192] Maternal antibody can also result in high antibody levels in young calves, although with a half-life of 12 to 16 days, this typically wanes by a few months of age.[7] Virtala and colleagues[171] reported that of 75 pneumonic dairy calves younger than 3 months of age in which *M bovis* was isolated from tracheal wash samples, only 57% had a fourfold or greater increase in *M bovis* serum antibody titers by IHA.[171] The authors concluded that paired serum samples were not a good predictor of *M bovis*–associated respiratory disease, possibly because of the presence of maternal antibody titers. Other investigators also failed to find a correlation between serum antibody titers to *M bovis* and *M bovis*–associated respiratory disease in naturally infected individual animals.[83,193] However, calves with severe chronic respiratory disease caused by *M bovis* generally have high serum IgG titers.[165] On a group level, seroconversion has been predictive of *M bovis*–associated respiratory disease.[8,50] Therefore, serology is of limited diagnostic value in individual animals and is really most useful in epidemiologic surveillance.[83,190] Serology has also been effective as a biosecurity tool to screen new groups of cattle before introduction into a herd, but this would be applicable only to animals more than a few months of age, after maternal antibodies have waned.[88]

TREATMENT

The fact that *Mycoplasma* species lack a cell wall has important implications for treatment, as it means the beta-lactam antibiotics are ineffective.[194] *Mycoplasma* species are also naturally resistant to sulfonamides. Currently, only one product containing the triamilide antibiotic tulathromycin (Draxxin; Pfizer, Inc.) is approved for treatment of *Mb*AD in dairy calves in the United States. Other antimicrobials that have a theoretic basis for efficacy against *M bovis*, and that are approved in the United States for treatment of respiratory disease in dairy heifers younger than 20 months of age, include enrofloxacin, florfenicol, oxytetracycline, spectinomycin, tilmicosin, and tylosin. Recent evidence suggests that antimicrobial resistance to antibiotics traditionally used for treatment of *Mycoplasma* infections is increasing in field isolates of *M bovis* in North America[195,196] and Europe.[197,198] Isolates from both continents show widespread resistance to tetracyclines and tilmicosin, and European isolates show increasing resistance to spectinomycin. Although in vitro antibiotic susceptibility profiles of *M bovis* may be useful in making broad generalizations about antibiotic resistance, data have not been published on the relevance of these profiles to clinical efficacy on an individual or a herd level. The antibiotic susceptibility profiles of paired *M bovis* isolates obtained from nasal swabs and BAL samples in calves with respiratory disease were found to differ considerably within animals, suggesting that if susceptibility profiles are used, they need to be based on isolates obtained from the site of infection.[109] Methodology for and application of antimicrobial sensitivity testing of *M bovis* has been recently reviewed.[12]

In spite of the limited choice of potentially effective antibiotics available, antibiotics are widely used to treat *Mb*AD. However, treatment is frequently unrewarding, with affected cattle requiring a long duration of treatment or failing to respond to therapy.[3,49,53,57,59,65,67,103,146,159,199] Calves with chronic and/or multisystemic disease are reported to have a particularly poor response to treatment.[57,59,103,159,199] There are few controlled clinical trials evaluating the efficacy of various antibiotics available for treatment of *Mb*AD, and the few efficacy studies published must be interpreted with caution because most use experimentally infected calves and treatment is often started early in the disease course.[49,200,201] In an industry-sponsored study, tulathro-mycin was an effective treatment for respiratory disease in dairy calves that had been experimentally infected with *M bovis*, when treatment was initiated at 3 or 7 days after inoculation.[201] Likewise, tilmicosin administered 6 hours before inoculation or at the on-set of clinical disease was effective in reducing lung colonization by *M bovis* in calves that had been experimentally infected with *M hemolytica* and *M bovis*.[200] However, treatment with spectinomycin did not alter the clinical course of disease in calves with *M bovis* and *P multocida* pneumonia when treatment was started 6 days after in-oculation, although the numbers of *M bovis* in the lung were reduced in treated calves.[49]

Scant information is available regarding treatment of MbAD in field situations, and most studies have come from Europe. Marbofloxacin, a fluoroquinolone antibiotic, was an effective treatment for naturally occurring *M bovis*–associated respiratory dis-ease,[202] but this antibiotic cannot be used in cattle in the United States. Enrofloxacin, another fluorquinolone, recently has been approved for the treatment of respiratory disease in dairy heifers under 20 months of age in the US; however extra-label use (eg, for treatment of otitis media) is prohibited. Available therapies that have resulted in clinical improvement in calves with *M bovis*–associated respiratory disease in field trials include oxytetracycline, tilmicosin, or a combination of lincomycin and spectino-mycin.[92,203] However, given the recent evidence that resistance against these drugs is increasing, these antibiotics may no longer be appropriate choices. Without other data to guide choice of an antibiotic, selection of a specific treatment regimen from the list of potentially effective antibiotics based on past performance in the affected herd is frequently recommended.[103,157]

In addition to antibiotics, short-term use of anti-inflammatory drugs can be benefi-cial in the treatment of bovine respiratory disease.[204] Although these therapeutic agents have not been specifically evaluated for the treatment of MbAD, there is a log-ical basis for their use, as the inflammatory response may contribute significantly to the pathology of *M bovis* infections.[39,47] Nonspecific supportive therapy including oral or intravenous fluids and nutritional support may be indicated in specific animals.[146]

Irrigation of the middle ear after the tympanic membrane has ruptured has been rec-ommended for treatment of undifferentiated otitis media in calves.[34] Puncture of the tympanic membrane (myringotomy) followed by insertion of tympanostomy tubes is commonly used in the treatment of children with chronic or recurrent otitis me-dia,[205,206] and some veterinarians have promoted blind myringotomy using a sharp object such as a knitting needle in the treatment of otitis media in calves.[207] To the best of the authors' knowledge, studies on the risks and efficacy of this procedure in clinical cases have not been published. The potential benefit of myringotomy is the relief of pain and pressure caused by the buildup of exudate in the middle ear, as well as access to the middle ear for irrigation. Whether the procedure might provide relief for calves that have the thick, caseous exudate characteristic of chronic *M bovis* otitis media is not clear. In a recent study using calf cadavers, investigators reported that blind insertion of a 3.5-mm diameter straight knitting needle approximately 3 cm into the ear canal to perforate the ear drum was anatomically feasible.[208]

Surgical treatment of *M bovis*–associated otitis media/interna has been de-scribed.[146] A bilateral tympanic bulla osteotomy was performed on a 4-week-old calf with severe, chronic *M bovis*–associated otitis media-interna that had failed to re-spond to antibiotic treatment. Postsurgically, the tympanic bullae were lavaged daily with warm saline for 3 days, and antibiotics were continued for 16 days. Surgery co-incided with a dramatic improvement in clinical signs and the calf was reported to be clinically normal at 1 year of age. Because of the cost and complexity associated with this procedure, as well as the requirement for general anesthesia, its application is probably limited to refractory cases of otitis media in valuable calves without concurrent respiratory disease.

To summarize, antibiotic treatment of MbAD is often unrewarding, especially in calves with chronic or multisystemic infections. Improved efficacies are reported in experimental infection studies when treatment is initiated early in the disease course, suggesting that early intervention or, perhaps, metaphylactic therapy in high-risk calves (discussed later in this article) may be more rewarding. For example, when dealing with otitis media it is likely that initiation of treatment at the earliest onset of clinical signs (such as ear scratching or head shaking accompanied by fever) will be more successful than waiting until disease is more advanced and an obvious ear droop is present. Extended duration of antimicrobial therapy is frequently recommended for MbAD. Given the lack of data on the efficacy of antimicrobials or other treatment options (such as middle ear lavage) for MbAD that are specific to North American calves, together with concerns regarding antimicrobial use in today's livestock industries, controlled clinical trials to evaluate current therapeutic and metaphylactic antibiotic regimens are needed.

CONTROL AND PREVENTION
Biosecurity

Results of epidemiologic studies of mycoplasmal mastitis suggest that the best way to prevent M bovis infection is to maintain a closed herd or to screen and quarantine purchased animals.[2,117,209] Results of such studies also suggest that M bovis–associated mastitis can be effectively eliminated from dairy herds through aggressive surveillance and culling of infected cows.[4,210] In feedlot cattle, where these types of biosecurity measures are not practical, recommendations for the control and prevention of M bovis–associated respiratory disease and arthritis focus on limiting stress, vaccinating to reduce the incidence of other respiratory pathogens, and segregating affected groups of calves from new arrivals to reduce exposure of high-risk animals to M bovis.[157,159] Dairies that are expanding and calf ranches that rear animals from multiple sources obviously cannot maintain closed herds, and calf ranches are not usually able to screen new calves before introduction into the facility. However, calf ranches do have the ability to be selective in purchasing calves, and animals could be screened on arrival to determine if a particular supplier is consistently providing M bovis–infected calves. Prevention of MbAD is hampered in dairy calf operations by the extremely limited understanding of its epidemiology and risk factors.

Management of Calves in Mycoplasma bovis-Infected Herds

Current recommendations for prevention of MbAD in calf-rearing facilities are based on reducing exposure to M bovis (**Box 1**). Potential sources of exposure that could be controlled include unpasteurized bulk tank or waste milk, colostrum, and indirect or direct contact with respiratory aerosols from infected calves. Exposure to M bovis in milk could be limited by culling infected cows or avoiding the feeding of milk from infected cows in herds where the M bovis status of the lactating cows is monitored. A more widely applicable method of reducing exposure to M bovis is by pasteurizing milk before feeding, or by feeding milk replacer.[60,65,211] On-farm batch pasteurization of waste milk to 65°C for 1 hour or 70°C for 3 minutes,[60] or the use of a high-temperature short-time pasteurizer[211] will inactivate Mycoplasma species. Frequent monitoring by culture of pasteurized milk samples to ensure that pasteurization has been effective is important in any on-farm pasteurization program.[212] Pasteurization of

Box 1
Proposed strategies for the control of *Mb*AD in pre-weaned calves

Reduce the level of exposure to Mycoplasma bovis

1. Reduce exposure in milk

   a. Pasteurize whole milk

   b. Feed milk replacer

2. Reduce potential exposure in colostrum

   a. Avoid pooling

   b. Consider pasteurization

3. Reduce potential airborne exposure

   a. Provide adequate ventilation in calf housing

   b. Consider the impact of pen design on air quality

   c. Consider ways to reduce stocking density

4. Reduce exposure to sick calves

   a. Considering segregation of calves with clinical *Mb*AD

   b. Promptly treat clinical cases

5. Prevent fomite transmission

   a. Sanitize pens, hutches, buckets, and other equipment between uses

   b. Wear gloves when handling sick calves and change them between calves. Wear gloves when assisting calves to drink.

   c. Handle the youngest calves first

6. Consider "all-in, all-out" practices, or segregate older and younger calves at the earliest possible opportunity

7. Where *M bovis* is not already present, use biosecurity practices appropriate to the particular operation and monitor for *Mb*AD

Maximize calf defenses against Mycoplasma bovis

1. Use nonspecific measures to maximize respiratory and immune system health

   a. Provide good air quality

   b. Control other pathogens, and in particular address any deficiencies in the vaccination and monitoring programs for respiratory viruses and BVDV

   c. Provide good nutrition

   d. Address any colostrum management issues

   e. Minimize other sources of stress such as transport, heat and cold stress, and overcrowding

2. Consider metaphylactic antimicrobial use when high morbidity and mortality caused by *Mb*AD are being sustained

3. There are insufficient data on the efficacy of currently available vaccines to recommend their use in neonatal calves at this time

colostrum is also possible. Some recent studies have reported that on-farm batch pasteurization at 60°C for 30 minutes eliminated viable M bovis while immunoglobulin concentration and colostral consistency were not significantly affected.[213,214] Pasteurization methods that use higher temperatures have resulted in reduced colostral quality and unacceptable feeding characteristics.[211,213,214] If colostrum is not pasteurized, it has been recommended that it should not be pooled to minimize potential exposure of calves to M bovis.[47]

Large numbers of M bovis are shed in the respiratory secretions of calves with clinical MbAD.[3,31] It has therefore been recommended to segregate affected and healthy calves, although this is frequently impractical.[157] Other recommendations that have been made include taking appropriate precautions to prevent potential transfer of M bovis between calves by personnel or equipment.[88] Nipples, bottles, tube feeders, and buckets should be adequately sanitized, and pens disinfected between calves. As discussed earlier, M bovis survives surprisingly well in the environment, but it is highly susceptible to heat and to most commonly used chlorine-, chlorhexidine-, acid-, or iodine-based disinfectants.[215] Personnel should wear gloves when feeding calves (especially when feeding newborns or assisting sick calves to nurse), and change them between animals. Wherever possible, consideration should be given to "all-in, all-out" practices to prevent older animals from infecting younger ones,[88] or to segregation of older and younger animals within the facility if "all-in, all-out" is not practical.

Management practices that help control other respiratory diseases by maximizing the ability of the calf's respiratory system to resist and control infection have been recommended for M bovis, although none of these have been specifically evaluated with respect to this pathogen.[47,99,157] Such measures include providing proper nutrition and adequate ventilation at the pen level, and reducing environmental stressors such as overcrowding and heat and cold stress. Because viral respiratory pathogens, especially BVDV, may predispose to M bovis infection,[99,141] herd vaccination protocols for infectious bovine rhinotracheitis virus (IBR), parainfluenza type 3 virus (PI₃), BVDV, and bovine respiratory syncytial virus (BRSV), as well as the herd BVDV monitoring program, should be evaluated to ensure that they are appropriate. Although the role of passive transfer of M bovis–specific antibodies in protection of calves from MbAD is unclear, a sound colostrum feeding program can reduce the risk of infection with other respiratory pathogens,[99] and may therefore decrease the risk of secondary M bovis infections. Readers are referred to the article on respiratory disease in this issue for more discussion of respiratory disease control practices.

The prophylactic or metaphylactic use of antibiotics is generally undesirable but may be justified when high levels of morbidity and mortality are occurring. Strategic antibiotic treatment of calves that are deemed to be at high risk for respiratory disease upon arrival at feedlots has clearly been demonstrated to reduce the incidence and severity of respiratory disease.[216,217] In addition, feeding metaphylactic levels of antibiotics in milk replacer to dairy calves on calf ranches reduces disease incidence and delays the onset of clinical disease during the preweaning period.[218] For MbAD, the response to treatment when antibiotics are given before, or early in the course of experimentally induced disease, is often better than the response rates reported in field cases. This suggests that metaphylactic treatment might be more successful than initiating treatment after disease is clinically apparent. In one European study, investigators found that valnemulin added to the milk from 4 days of age for 3 weeks was effective in limiting MbAD in calves.[45] Animals in the treated group had fewer clinical signs and reduced clinical scores; however, disease was not eliminated and calves still required a considerable number of individual treatments. Nagatomo and colleagues[219] treated calves that were at high risk of MbAD with chloramphenicol.

Untreated calves had high mortality rates (up to 41%), while the onset of clinical disease was delayed in treated calves and all treated calves survived. Prophylaxis or metaphylaxis with antibiotics that are approved for use in US cattle has not been evaluated with respect to *Mb*AD in young calves.

Vaccination

From studies of the immune response to respiratory mycoplasmal infections in other species, it can be concluded that adaptive responses in place at the time of mycoplasmal exposure contribute to the control or prevention of new mycoplasmal infections.[38] It is therefore not surprising that under some circumstances, vaccination can at least partly protect calves from *Mb*AD. For example, in an experimental study, 1- to 5-month-old beef calves were vaccinated subcutaneously with live *M bovis*, intraperitoneally with live *M bovis*, or subcutaneously with a formalin-inactivated bacterin.[62] Two boosters were given at 10-day intervals and animals were challenged by intravenous inoculation of *M bovis*. Clinical arthritis was seen in 100% of nonvaccinated as compared with only 13% of vaccinated calves, and lesion severity was decreased in vaccinated calves that did develop arthritis.

In another study of an apparently efficacious vaccine in young calves, Nicholas and colleagues[220] vaccinated 3-week-old dairy calves with a single dose of saponin-inactivated bacterin. Calves received an aerosol challenge with live *M bovis* 3 weeks after vaccination. Vaccinated calves had fewer numbers of *M bovis* at colonized sites, fewer numbers of body sites colonized by *M bovis*, and reduced severity and incidence of clinical disease and lesions compared with control calves. There was also a significant decrease in body weight gain in control calves compared with vaccinates. Additionally, no vaccinated calves as compared with two of seven control calves developed arthritis. Vaccinated calves produced a strong IgG response before challenge, but IgG subtypes were not reported. No adverse events associated with vaccination were noted.

In another report of an apparently efficacious vaccine, a killed vaccine against four bovine respiratory pathogens (BRSV, PI$_3$, *M bovis*, and *M dispar*) was evaluated for protection against naturally occurring respiratory disease in beef calves.[135,221] Calves were vaccinated subcutaneously and received two boosters at 3-week intervals. In one study, three groups of beef calves aged 12, 7, and 3 weeks at the time of first vaccination were used, and calves were followed for 6 months.[221] Respiratory disease occurred in a significantly higher ($P < .05$) proportion of the control calves (27%) than vaccinated calves (16.3%). In a second study using the same vaccination protocol, *M bovis* and BRSV were implicated in outbreaks of respiratory disease during the trial period.[135] Morbidity as a result of respiratory disease was significantly reduced in vaccinated calves (25%) compared with controls (32%), and mortality in the vaccinated group was similarly reduced (2% and 9% for vaccinates and controls, respectively). No adverse effects of vaccination were observed.

In a report of *M bovis* vaccination of feedlot cattle, a bacterin consisting of autogenous formalin-inactivated strains of *M bovis* and *M hemolytica* was used in 3000 cattle at arrival.[222] The feedlot had a history of *Mb*AD. The vaccine was reported to be efficacious for the prevention of respiratory disease in newly introduced cattle, but, unfortunately, comparisons were made to a historical control group. No adverse effects of vaccination were noted.

Despite the promise shown in some of the studies discussed previously, other vaccine trials have been less successful. Rosenbusch vaccinated 2-month-old dairy calves with a formalin-inactivated bacterin prepared from two strains of *M bovis*.[223] Calves received a single booster at 3 weeks postvaccination, and were challenged by transthoracic inoculation of *M bovis*. Vaccination exacerbated disease, with four of five vaccinated calves as compared with only one of five control calves developing severe respiratory disease. A similar exacerbation of disease was seen in calves vaccinated with partially purified membrane proteins from *M bovis,* as clinical disease and pathology following aerosol challenge were more severe in vaccinated calves than in controls.[224] In a field trial using 330 neonatal dairy calves in two north-central Florida herds with endemic *M bovis* disease, calves were vaccinated at 3, 14, and 35 days of age using a commercially available *M bovis* bacterin.[37] The vaccine was not efficacious in reducing morbidity or mortality caused by respiratory disease, otitis media, or arthritis in these herds. The response to vaccination was herd-dependent, with a higher rate of otitis media associated with vaccination in one herd. Most calves in the study became colonized with *M bovis* in the first 2 weeks of life, and most clinical disease occurred between 3 and 6 weeks of age. A humoral immune response to vaccination was not detected until approximately 2 weeks after the third vaccine booster at approximately 7 weeks of age. The early age at which calves can become infected with *M bovis* in endemically infected facilities and represents perhaps the biggest challenge to the development of an effective *M bovis* vaccine for use in young calves. Other challenges to vaccination of neonatal calves are discussed in an article on neonatal vaccination in this issue.

Even where *M bovis* vaccines have been associated with clinical benefits, they often fail to induce an immune response that clears infection.[62,220] For example, intramuscular injection with formalin-killed *M bovis* with adjuvant followed after 14 days by intratracheal inoculation with killed organisms resulted in reduced *M bovis* in the lungs compared with control calves after intratracheal challenge, however significant numbers of mycoplasmas were still present in vaccinated calves.[225] Induction of protective immune responses against *M bovis* by vaccination is also complex. For example, in the aforementioned study, a vaccination protocol of three subcutaneous injections also induced protective responses, but two intramuscular or two intratracheal inoculations did not.[225] In these studies, the number of *M bovis* bacteria isolated from the lungs of calves was negatively correlated with IgG concentrations in BAL fluid, and different vaccination regimens were more or less effective at inducing an IgG response in the respiratory tract.

Despite very limited data on the field efficacy of *M bovis* vaccines, a number of bacterin-based vaccines for *M bovis* are licensed for marketing in the United States. To the best of the authors' knowledge, one vaccine is currently licensed for reducing the duration and severity of mycoplasmal mastitis in adult dairy cattle (Mycomune; Biomune, Lenexa, Kansas), and at least three vaccines are licensed for prevention of *M bovis*–associated respiratory disease in cattle. One product (Myco-B Bac; Texas Vet. Labs, Inc., San Angelo, Texas), is aimed at stocker and feeder cattle. Another product (Pulmo-Guard MbP; Boehringer Ingelheim Vetmedica, Inc., St. Joseph, Missouri) is licensed for vaccination of cattle older than 45 days of age and is primarily marketed to the beef industry. A third vaccine (Mycomune R; Biomune, Lenexa, Kansas) recently has been approved for use in calves 3 weeks of age or older as an aid in the prevention of *M bovis*-associated respiratory disease. In addition to these vaccines, a number of US companies are licensed to produce custom autogenous bacterins using strains of *M bovis* isolated from the target herds.

In conclusion, vaccination against *M bovis*, at least in older calves, is possible. However the vaccines reported to date do not prevent colonization of the URT with *M bovis* and vaccination can also induce harmful effects. The very young age at which calves often become infected with *M bovis* is perhaps the greatest challenge to the development of a successful vaccine. A better understanding of the immunology of the neonatal calf, especially with respect to ability to respond to different antigens, the types of responses that are produced, and modulation of these responses by mucosal and systemic adjuvants may improve our ability to produce efficacious *M bovis* vaccines, if indeed vaccination of the very young calf against *M bovis* is possible. Ongoing research is continually leading to a better understanding of *M bovis* antigens (for example, see Perez-Casal and Prysliak[226]) and this may lead to the development of more targeted vaccine approaches. In addition to research into new vaccination strategies, critical evaluation of currently marketed *M bovis* vaccines and autogenous bacterins in well-designed, independent efficacy studies that include a valid control group, blinding, adequate power, and relevant clinical outcomes, and that are conducted in an appropriate age group are clearly required. The paucity of such studies is a major gap in understanding the potential of currently available vaccines as a management strategy to control *M bovis* infections in young calves.

SUMMARY

M bovis has emerged as an important pathogen of young intensively reared calves in North America. A variety of clinical diseases are associated with *M bovis* infections of calves, including respiratory disease, otitis media, arthritis, and some other less common presentations. Clinical disease associated with *M bovis* is often chronic, debilitating, and poorly responsive to antimicrobial therapy. Current control measures are centered on reducing exposure to *M bovis* through contaminated milk or other sources, as well as nonspecific control measures to maximize the respiratory defenses of the calf; however, these management strategies often fail to control clinical mycoplasmal disease. The development of improved preventive, control, and treatment strategies for *Mycoplasma*–associated disease in young calves is hampered by a lack of understanding of the epidemiology of *M bovis* infections in young calves and of the host-pathogen interactions involved in the establishment of infection and development of clinical disease.

REFERENCES

1. Hale HH, Helmboldt CF, Plastridge WN, et al. Bovine mastitis caused by a *Mycoplasma* species. Cornell Vet 1962;52:582–91.
2. Gonzalez RN, Sears PM, Merrill RA, et al. Mastitis due to *Mycoplasma* in the state of New York during the period 1972–1990. Cornell Vet 1992;82:29–40.
3. Pfutzner H, Sachse K. *Mycoplasma bovis* as an agent of mastitis, pneumonia, arthritis and genital disorders in cattle. Rev Sci Tech 1996;15:1477–94.
4. Fox LK, Hancock DD, Mickelson A, et al. Bulk tank milk analysis: factors associated with appearance of *Mycoplasma* sp. in milk. J Vet Med B Infect Dis Vet Public Health 2003;50:235–40.
5. Gonzalez RN, Wilson DJ. Mycoplasmal mastitis in dairy herds. Vet Clin North Am Food Anim Pract 2003;19:199–221.
6. Haines DM, Martin KM, Clark EG, et al. The immunohistochemical detection of *Mycoplasma bovis* and bovine viral diarrhea virus in tissues of feedlot cattle with chronic, unresponsive respiratory disease and/or arthritis. Can Vet J 2001;42:857–60.
7. Tschopp R, Bonnemain P, Nicolet J, et al. [Epidemiological study of risk factors for *Mycoplasma bovis* infections in fattening calves]. Schweiz Arch Tierheilkd 2001;143:461–7 [in German].

8. Shahriar FM, Clark EG, Janzen E, et al. Coinfection with bovine viral diarrhea virus and *Mycoplasma bovis* in feedlot cattle with chronic pneumonia. Can Vet J 2002;43:863–8.

9. Thomas A, Ball H, Dizier I, et al. Isolation of mycoplasma species from the lower respiratory tract of healthy cattle and cattle with respiratory disease in Belgium. Vet Rec 2002;151:472–6.

10. Gagea MI, Bateman KG, Shanahan RA, et al. Naturally occurring *Mycoplasma bovis*-associated pneumonia and polyarthritis in feedlot beef calves. J Vet Diagn Invest 2006;18:29–40.

11. Fox L, Kirk JH, Britten A. *Mycoplasma* mastitis: a review of transmission and control. J Vet Med B Infect Dis Vet Public Health 2005;52:153–60.

12. Caswell JL, Archambault M. *Mycoplasma bovis* pneumonia in cattle. Anim Health Res Rev 2007;8:161–86.

13. Razin S, Yogev D, Naot Y. Molecular biology and pathogenicity of mycoplasmas. Microbiol Mol Biol Rev 1998;62:1094–156.

14. Rosengarten R, Citti C, Glew M, et al. Host-pathogen interactions in mycoplasma pathogenesis: virulence and survival strategies of minimalist prokaryotes. Int J Med Microbiol 2000;290:15–25.

15. Srikumaran S, Kelling CL, Ambagala A. Immune evasion by pathogens of bovine respiratory disease complex. Anim Health Res Rev 2007;8:215–29.

16. Vanden Bush TJ, Rosenbusch RF. Characterization of the immune response to *Mycoplasma bovis* lung infection. Vet Immunol Immunopathol 2003;94:23–33.

17. Vanden Bush TJ, Rosenbusch RF. *Mycoplasma bovis* induces apoptosis of bovine lymphocytes. FEMS Immunol Med Microbiol 2002;32:97–103.

18. Vanden Bush TJ, Rosenbusch RF. Characterization of a lympho-inhibitory peptide produced by *Mycoplasma bovis*. Biochem Biophys Res Commun 2004; 315:336–41.

19. Bennett RH, Jasper DE. Immunosuppression of humoral and cell-mediated responses in calves associated with inoculation of *Mycoplasma bovis*. Am J Vet Res 1977;38:1731–8.

20. Behrens A, Heller M, Kirchhoff H, et al. A family of phase- and size-variant membrane surface lipoprotein antigens (vsps) of *Mycoplasma bovis*. Infect Immun 1994;62:5075–84.

21. Lysnyansky I, Rosengarten R, Yogev D. Phenotypic switching of variable surface lipoproteins in *Mycoplasma bovis* involves high-frequency chromosomal rearrangements. J Bacteriol 1996;178:5395–401.

22. Beier T, Hotzel H, Lysnyansky I, et al. Intraspecies polymorphism of vsp genes and expression profiles of variable surface protein antigens (Vsps) in field isolates of *Mycoplasma bovis*. Vet Microbiol 1998;63:189–203.

23. Sachse K, Helbig JH, Lysnyansky I, et al. Epitope mapping of immunogenic and adhesive structures in repetitive domains of *Mycoplasma bovis* variable surface lipoproteins. Infect Immun 2000;68:680–7.

24. Nussbaum S, Lysnyansky I, Sachse K, et al. Extended repertoire of genes encoding variable surface lipoproteins in *Mycoplasma bovis* strains. Infect Immun 2002;70:2220–5.

25. Chambaud I, Wroblewski H, Blanchard A. Interactions between mycoplasma lipoproteins and the host immune system. Trends Microbiol 1999;7:493–9.

26. McAuliffe L, Ellis RJ, Miles K, et al. Biofilm formation by mycoplasma species and its role in environmental persistence and survival. Microbiology 2006;152: 913–22.

27. McAuliffe L, Kokotovic B, Ayling RD, et al. Molecular epidemiological analysis of *Mycoplasma bovis* isolates from the United Kingdom shows two genetically distinct clusters. J Clin Microbiol 2004;42:4556–65.

28. Poumarat F, Le Grand D, Solsona M, et al. Vsp antigens and vsp-related DNA sequences in field isolates of *Mycoplasma bovis*. FEMS Microbiol Lett 1999; 173:103–10.

29. Thomas A, Leprince P, Dizier I, et al. Identification by two-dimensional electrophoresis of a new adhesin expressed by a low-passaged strain of *Mycoplasma bovis*. Res Microbiol 2005;156:713–8.

30. Le Grand D, Solsona M, Rosengarten R, et al. Adaptive surface antigen variation in *Mycoplasma bovis* to the host immune response. FEMS Microbiol Lett 1996; 144:267–75.

31. Bennett RH, Jasper DE. Nasal prevalence of *Mycoplasma bovis* and IHA titers in young dairy animals. Cornell Vet 1977;67:361–73.

32. Chima JC, Wilkie BN, Nielsen KH, et al. Synovial immunoglobulin and antibody in vaccinated and nonvaccinated calves challenged with *Mycoplasma bovis*. Can J Comp Med 1981;45:92–6.

33. Thomas LH, Howard CJ, Stott EJ, et al. *Mycoplasma bovis* infection in gnotobiotic calves and combined infection with respiratory syncytial virus. Vet Pathol 1986;23:571–8.

34. Morin DE. Brainstem and cranial nerve abnormalities: listeriosis, otitis media/interna, and pituitary abscess syndrome. Vet Clin North Am Food Anim Pract 2004;20:243–73.

35. Morita T, Ohiwa S, Shimada A, et al. Intranasally inoculated *Mycoplasma hyorhinis* causes eustachitis in pigs. Vet Pathol 1999;36:174–8.

36. Morita T, Fukuda H, Awakura T, et al. Demonstration of *Mycoplasma hyorhinis* as a possible primary pathogen for porcine otitis media. Vet Pathol 1995;32:107–11.

37. Maunsell F. *Mycoplasma bovis* infection of dairy calves. Thesis (PhD) 2007; University of Florida.

38. Cartner SC, Lindsey JR, Gibbs-Erwin J, et al. Roles of innate and adaptive immunity in respiratory mycoplasmosis. Infect Immun 1998;66:3485–91.

39. Howard CJ, Thomas LH, Parsons KR. Immune response of cattle to respiratory mycoplasmas. Vet Immunol Immunopathol 1987;17:401–12.

40. Lu X, Rosenbusch RF. Endothelial cells from bovine pulmonary microvasculature respond to *Mycoplasma bovis* preferentially with signals for mononuclear cell transmigration. Microb Pathog 2004;37:253–61.

41. Jungi TW, Krampe M, Sileghem M, et al. Differential and strain-specific triggering of bovine alveolar macrophage effector functions by mycoplasmas. Microb Pathog 1996;21:487–98.

42. Gourlay RN, Thomas LH, Wyld SG. Increased severity of calf pneumonia associated with the appearance of *Mycoplasma bovis* in a rearing herd. Vet Rec 1989;124:420–2.

43. Brown MB, Dechant DM, Donovan GA. Association of *Mycoplasma bovis* with otitis media in dairy calves. IOM Lett 1998;12:104–5.

44. Stipkovits L, Ripley P, Varga J, et al. Clinical study of the disease of calves associated with *Mycoplasma bovis* infection. Acta Vet Hung 2000;48:387–95.

45. Stipkovits L, Ripley PH, Varga J, et al. Use of valnemulin in the control of *Mycoplasma bovis* infection under field conditions. Vet Rec 2001;148:399–402.

46. Bashiruddin JB, De Santis P, Varga E, et al. Confirmation of the presence of *Mycoplasma bovis* in Hungarian cattle with pneumonia resembling pleuropneumonia. Vet Rec 2001;148:743–6.

47. Rosenbusch R. Bovine mycoplasmosis. In: Proceedings of the 34th Annual Conference of the American Association of Bovine Practitioners. Vancouver (BC), September 13-15, 2001. p. 49–52.

48. Gourlay RN, Thomas LH, Howard CJ. Pneumonia and arthritis in gnotobiotic calves following inoculation with *Mycoplasma agalactiae* subsp *bovis*. Vet Rec 1976;98:506–7.

49. Poumarat F, Le Grand D, Philippe S, et al. Efficacy of spectinomycin against *Mycoplasma bovis* induced pneumonia in conventionally reared calves. Vet Microbiol 2001;80:23–35.

50. Martin SW, Bateman KG, Shewen PE, et al. A group level analysis of the associations between antibodies to seven putative pathogens and respiratory disease and weight gain in Ontario feedlot calves. Can J Vet Res 1990;54:337–42.

51. Van Donkersgoed J, Ribble CS, Boyer LG, et al. Epidemiological study of enzootic pneumonia in dairy calves in Saskatchewan. Can J Vet Res 1993;57:247–54.

52. Springer WT, Fulton RW, Hagstad HV, et al. Prevalence of *Mycoplasma* and *Chlamydia* in the nasal flora of dairy calves. Vet Microbiol 1982;7:351–7.

53. Allen JW, Viel L, Bateman KG, et al. Changes in the bacterial flora of the upper and lower respiratory tracts and bronchoalveolar lavage differential cell counts in feedlot calves treated for respiratory diseases. Can J Vet Res 1992;56:177–83.

54. Virtala AMK, Mechor GD, Grohn YT, et al. Epidemiologic and pathologic characteristics of respiratory tract disease in dairy heifers during the first three months of life. J Am Vet Med Assoc 1996;208:2035–42.

55. Allen JW, Viel L, Bateman KG, et al. Cytological findings in bronchoalveolar lavage fluid from feedlot calves: associations with pulmonary microbial flora. Can J Vet Res 1992;56:122–6.

56. Stalheim OH, Page LA. Naturally occurring and experimentally induced mycoplasmal arthritis of cattle. J Clin Microbiol 1975;2:165–8.

57. Stipkovits L, Rady M, Glavits R. Mycoplasmal arthritis and meningitis in calves. Acta Vet Hung 1993;41:73–88.

58. Rosenbusch R. Acute feedlot arthritis associated with distinct strains of *Mycoplasma bovis*. In: Proceedings of the 27th Annual Conference of the American Association of Bovine Practitioners. Pittsburgh (PA), September 22–25, 1994. p. 191.

59. Adegboye DS, Halbur PG, Nutsch RG, et al. *Mycoplasma bovis*-associated pneumonia and arthritis complicated with pyogranulomatous tenosynovitis in calves. J Am Vet Med Assoc 1996;209:647–9.

60. Butler JA, Sickles SA, Johanns CJ, et al. Pasteurization of discard mycoplasma mastitic milk used to feed calves: thermal effects on various mycoplasma. J Dairy Sci 2000;83:2285–8.

61. Byrne W, Fagan J, McCormack M. *Mycoplasma bovis* arthritis as a sequel to respiratory disease in bought-in weanling cattle in the Republic of Ireland. Ir Vet J 2001;54:516–9.

62. Chima JC, Wilkie BN, Ruhnke HL, et al. Immunoprophylaxis of experimental *Mycoplasma bovis* arthritis in calves—protective efficacy of live organisms and formalinized vaccines. Vet Microbiol 1980;5:113–22.

63. Ryan MJ, Wyand DS, Hill DL, et al. Morphologic changes following intraarticular inoculation of *Mycoplasma bovis* in calves. Vet Pathol 1983;20:472–87.

64. Dechant DM, Donovan GA. Otitis media in dairy calves: a preliminary case report. In: Proceedings of the 28th Annual Conference of the American Association of Bovine Practitioners. San Antonio (TX), September 14–17, 1995. p. 237.

65. Walz PH, Mullaney TP, Render JA, et al. Otitis media in preweaned Holstein dairy calves in Michigan due to *Mycoplasma bovis*. J Vet Diagn Invest 1997;9:250–4.
66. Maeda T, Shibahara T, Kimura K, et al. *Mycoplasma bovis*-associated suppurative otitis media and pneumonia in bull calves. J Comp Pathol 2003;129:100–10.
67. Francoz D, Fecteau G, Desrochers A, et al. Otitis media in dairy calves: a retrospective study of 15 cases (1987 to 2002). Can Vet J 2004;45:661–6.
68. Lamm CG, Munson L, Thurmond MC, et al. Mycoplasma otitis in California calves. J Vet Diagn Invest 2004;16:397–402.
69. Jensen R, Maki LR, Lauerman LH, et al. Cause and pathogenesis of middle-ear infection in young feedlot cattle. J Am Vet Med Assoc 1983;182:967–72.
70. Henderson JP, McCullough WP. Otitis media in suckler calves. Vet Rec 1993; 132:24.
71. Ayling RD, Bashiruddin SE, Nicholas RA. *Mycoplasma* species and related organisms isolated from ruminants in Britain between 1990 and 2000. Vet Rec 2004;155:413–6.
72. Knudtson WU, Reed DE, Daniels G. Identification of mycoplasmatales in pneumonic calf lungs. Vet Microbiol 1986;11:79–91.
73. Tegtmeier C, Uttenthal A, Friis NF, et al. Pathological and microbiological studies on pneumonic lungs from Danish calves. Zentralbl Veterinarmed B 1999;46: 693–700.
74. Friis NF. *Mycoplasma dispar* as a causative agent in pneumonia of calves. Acta Vet Scand 1980;21:34–42.
75. Bryson DG, McFerran JB, Ball HJ, et al. Observations on outbreaks of respiratory disease in housed calves–(1) epidemiological, clinical and microbiological findings. Vet Rec 1978;103:485–9.
76. Hewicker-Trautwein M, Feldmann M, Kehler W, et al. Outbreak of pneumonia and arthritis in beef calves associated with *Mycoplasma bovis* and *Mycoplasma californicum*. Vet Rec 2002;151:699–703.
77. ter Laak EA, Tully JG, Noordergraaf HH, et al. Recognition of *Mycoplasma canis* as part of the mycoplasmal flora of the bovine respiratory tract. Vet Microbiol 1993;34:175–89.
78. Hirose K, Kobayashi H, Ito N, et al. Isolation of mycoplasmas from nasal swabs of calves affected with respiratory diseases and antimicrobial susceptibility of their isolates. J Vet Med B Infect Dis Vet Public Health 2003;50:347–51.
79. Alexander PG, Slee KJ, McOrist S, et al. Mastitis in cows and polyarthritis and pneumonia in calves caused by *Mycoplasma* species bovine group 7. Aust Vet J 1985;62:135–6.
80. Hum S, Kessell A, Djordjevic S, et al. Mastitis, polyarthritis and abortion caused by *Mycoplasma* species bovine group 7 in dairy cattle. Aust Vet J 2000;78:744–50.
81. Howard CJ, Thomas LH, Parsons KR. Comparative pathogenicity of *Mycoplasma bovis* and *Mycoplasma dispar* for the respiratory tract of calves. Isr J Med Sci 1987;23:621–4.
82. Thomas LH, Howard CJ, Parsons KR, et al. Growth of *Mycoplasma bovis* in organ cultures of bovine foetal trachea and comparison with *Mycoplasma dispar*. Vet Microbiol 1987;13:189–200.
83. Rosendal S, Martin SW. The association between serological evidence of mycoplasma infection and respiratory disease in feedlot calves. Can J Vet Res 1986; 50:179–83.
84. USDA. Mycoplasma in bulk tank milk on U.S. dairies. Fort Collins (CO): USDA:APHIS:VS: CEAH, National Animal Health Monitoring System; 2003. N395.0503.

85. Kirk JH, Glenn K, Ruiz L, et al. Epidemiologic analysis of *Mycoplasma* spp isolated from bulk-tank milk samples obtained from dairy herds that were members of a milk cooperative. J Am Vet Med Assoc 1997;211:1036–8.

86. Jasper DE. Bovine mycoplasmal mastitis. Adv Vet Sci Comp Med 1981;25: 121–59.

87. Biddle MK, Fox LK, Hancock DD. Patterns of mycoplasma shedding in the milk of dairy cows with intramammary mycoplasma infection. J Am Vet Med Assoc 2003;223:1163–6.

88. Nicholas RA, Ayling RD. *Mycoplasma bovis*: disease, diagnosis, and control. Res Vet Sci 2003;74:105–12.

89. USDA. Dairy 2007, Part I: Reference of dairy cattle health and management practices in the United States. Fort Collins (CO): USDA:APHIS:VS CEAH, National Animal Health Monitoring System; 2007. N480.1007.

90. Wells SJ, Garber LP, Hill GW. Health status of preweaned dairy heifers in the United States. Prev Vet Med 1997;29:185–99.

91. Donovan GA, Dohoo IR, Montgomery DM, et al. Associations between passive immunity and morbidity and mortality in dairy heifers in Florida, USA. Prev Vet Med 1998;34:31–46.

92. Musser J, Mechor GD, Grohn YT, et al. Comparison of tilmicosin with long-acting oxytetracycline for treatment of respiratory tract disease in calves. J Am Vet Med Assoc 1996;208:102–6.

93. Rosengarten R, Citti C. The role of ruminant mycoplasmas in systemic infection. In: Stipkovits L, Rosengarten R, Frey J, editors. Mycoplasmas of ruminants: pathogenicity, diagnostics, epidemiology and molecular genetics. Brussels: European Commission; 1999. p. 14–7.

94. Kaneene JB, Hurd HS. The National Animal Health Monitoring System in Michigan. 3. Cost estimates of selected dairy-cattle diseases. Prev Vet Med 1990;8: 127–40.

95. Esslemont RJ, Kossaibati MA. The cost of respiratory diseases in dairy heifer calves. Bovine Practitioner 1999;33:174–8.

96. Waltner-Toews D, Martin SW, Meek AH. The effect of early calfhood health status on survivorship and age at first calving. Can J Vet Res 1986;50:314–7.

97. Warnick LD, Erb HN, White ME. Lack of association between calf morbidity and subsequent first lactation milk production in 25 New York Holstein herds. J Dairy Sci 1995;78:2819–30.

98. Virtala AM, Mechor GD, Grohn YT, et al. The effect of calfhood diseases on growth of female dairy calves during the first 3 months of life in New York State. J Dairy Sci 1996;79:1040–9.

99. Ames TR. Dairy calf pneumonia—the disease and its impact. Vet Clin North Am Food Anim Pract 1997;13:379–91.

100. Warnick LD, Erb HN, White ME. The relationship of calfhood morbidity with survival after calving in 25 New York Holstein herds. Prev Vet Med 1997;31: 263–73.

101. Donovan GA, Dohoo IR, Montgomery DM, et al. Calf and disease factors affecting growth in female Holstein calves in Florida, USA. Prev Vet Med 1998;33: 1–10.

102. Adegboye DS, Hallbur PG, Cavanaugh DL, et al. Immunohistochemical and pathological study of *Mycoplasma bovis*-associated lung abscesses in calves. J Vet Diagn Invest 1995;7:333–7.

103. Apley MD, Fajt VR. Feedlot therapeutics. Vet Clin North Am Food Anim Pract 1998;14:291–313.

104. Kinde H, Daft BM, Walker RL, et al. *Mycoplasma bovis* associated with decubital abscesses in Holstein calves. J Vet Diagn Invest 1993;5:194–7.
105. ter Laak EA, Noordergraaf JH, Dieltjes RP. Prevalence of mycoplasmas in the respiratory tracts of pneumonic calves. Zentralbl Veterinarmed B 1992;39: 553–62.
106. Goltz JP, Rosendal S, McCraw BM, et al. Experimental studies on the pathogenicity of *Mycoplasma ovipneumoniae* and *Mycoplasma arginini* for the respiratory tract of goats. Can J Vet Res 1986;50:59–67.
107. Friis NF, Ahrens P, Larsen H. *Mycoplasma hyosynoviae* isolation from the upper respiratory tract and tonsils of pigs. Acta Vet Scand 1991;32:425–9.
108. Allen JW, Viel L, Bateman KG, et al. The microbial flora of the respiratory tract in feedlot calves: associations between nasopharyngeal and bronchoalveolar lavage cultures. Can J Vet Res 1991;55:341–6.
109. Thomas A, Dizier I, Trolin A, et al. Comparison of sampling procedures for isolating pulmonary mycoplasmas in cattle. Vet Res Commun 2002;26:333–9.
110. Wiggins MC, Woolums AR, Sanchez S, et al. Prevalence of *Mycoplasma bovis* in backgrounding and stocker cattle operations. J Am Vet Med Assoc 2007;230: 1514–8.
111. Boothby JT, Jasper DE, Zinkl JG, et al. Prevalence of mycoplasmas and immune responses to *Mycoplasma bovis* in feedlot calves. Am J Vet Res 1983;44:831–8.
112. Bocklisch H, Pfutzner H, Martin J, et al [*Mycoplasma bovis* abortion of cows following experimental infection]. Arch Exp Veterinarmed 1986;40:48–55 [in German].
113. Thomas CB, Willeberg P, Jasper DE. Case-control study of bovine mycoplasmal mastitis in California. Am J Vet Res 1981;42:511–5.
114. Lago A, McGuirk SM, Bennett TB, et al. Calf respiratory disease and pen microenvironments in naturally ventilated calf barns in winter. J Dairy Sci 2006;89: 4014–25.
115. Jasper DE, Alaubaid JM, Fabrican J. Epidemiologic observations on mycoplasma mastitis. Cornell Vet 1974;64:407–15.
116. Bushnell RB. Mycoplasma mastitis. Vet Clin North Am Large Anim Pract 1984;6: 301–12.
117. Step DL, Kirkpatrick JG. Mycoplasma infection in cattle. II. Mastitis and other diseases. Bovine Practitioner 2001;35:171–6.
118. Bray DR, Brown MB, Donovan GA. Mycoplasma again. In: Proceedings of the 38th Annual Florida Dairy Production Conference. Gainesville (FL), May 1–2, 2001. p. 52–60.
119. Woldehiwet Z, Mamache B, Rowan TG. Effects of age, environmental temperature and relative humidity on the colonization of the nose and trachea of calves by *Mycoplasma* spp. Br Vet J 1990;146:419–24.
120. Reinhold P, Elmer S. Consequences of changing ambient temperatures in calves—part 2: changes in the health status within three weeks after exposure. Dtsch Tierarztl Wochenschr 2002;109:193–200.
121. Bayoumi FA, Farver TB, Bushnell B, et al. Enzootic mycoplasmal mastitis in a large dairy during an eight-year period. J Am Vet Med Assoc 1988;192:905–9.
122. Thomas LH, Swann RG. Influence of colostrum on the incidence of calf pneumonia. Vet Rec 1973;92:454–5.
123. Davidson JN, Yancey SP, Campbell SG, et al. Relationship between serum immunoglobulin values and incidence of respiratory disease in calves. J Am Vet Med Assoc 1981;179:708–10.

124. Corbeil LB, Watt B, Corbeil RR, et al. Immunoglobulin concentrations in serum and nasal secretions of calves at the onset of pneumonia. Am J Vet Res 1984;45:773–8.

125. Bryson DG. Calf pneumonia. Vet Clin North Am Food Anim Pract 1985;1:237–57.

126. Barrington GM, Parish S. Bovine neonatal immunology. Vet Clin North Am Food Anim Pract 2001;17:463–76.

127. Foote MR, Nonnecke BJ, Fowler MA, et al. Effects of age and nutrition on expression of CD25, CD44, and L-selectin (CD62L) on T-cells from neonatal calves. J Dairy Sci 2005;88:2718–29.

128. Howard CJ. Comparison of bovine IgG1, IgG2 and IgM for ability to promote killing of *Mycoplasma bovis* by bovine alveolar macrophages and neutrophils. Vet Immunol Immunopathol 1984;6:321–6.

129. Uribe HA, Kennedy BW, Martin SW, et al. Genetic parameters for common health disorders of Holstein cows. J Dairy Sci 1995;78:421–30.

130. Abdel-Azim GA, Freeman AE, Kehrli ME Jr, et al. Genetic basis and risk factors for infectious and noninfectious diseases in US Holsteins. I. Estimation of genetic parameters for single diseases and general health. J Dairy Sci 2005;88: 1199–207.

131. Davis JK, Thorp RB, Maddox PA, et al. Murine respiratory mycoplasmosis in F344 and LEW rats: evolution of lesions and lung lymphoid cell populations. Infect Immun 1982;36:720–9.

132. Hickman-Davis JM, Michalek SM, Gibbs-Erwin J, et al. Depletion of alveolar macrophages exacerbates respiratory mycoplasmosis in mycoplasma-resistant C57BL mice but not mycoplasma-susceptible C3H mice. Infect Immun 1997;65: 2278–82.

133. Yancey AL, Watson HL, Cartner SC, et al. Gender is a major factor in determining the severity of mycoplasma respiratory disease in mice. Infect Immun 2001; 69:2865–71.

134. Wilkie B, Mallard B. Selection for high immune response: an alternative approach to animal health maintenance? Vet Immunol Immunopathol 1999;72: 231–5.

135. Howard CJ, Stott EJ, Thomas LH, et al. Protection against respiratory disease in calves induced by vaccines containing respiratory syncytial virus, parainfluenza type 3 virus, *Mycoplasma bovis* and *M dispar*. Vet Rec 1987;121:372–6.

136. Rodriguez F, Bryson DG, Ball HJ, et al. Pathological and immunohistochemical studies of natural and experimental *Mycoplasma bovis* pneumonia in calves. J Comp Pathol 1996;115:151–62.

137. Mosier DA. Bacterial pneumonia. Vet Clin North Am Food Anim Pract 1997;13: 483–93.

138. Vogel G, Nicolet J, Martig J, et al [Pneumonia in calves: characterization of the bacterial spectrum and the resistance patterns to antimicrobial drugs]. Schweiz Arch Tierheilkd 2001;143:341–50 [in German].

139. Houghton SB, Gourlay RN. Synergism between *Mycoplasma bovis* and *Pasteurella hemolytica* in calf pneumonia. Vet Rec 1983;113:41–2.

140. Kapil S, Basaraba RJ. Infectious bovine rhinotracheitis, parainfluenza-3, and respiratory coronavirus. Vet Clin North Am Food Anim Pract 1997;13:455–69.

141. Shahriar FM, Clark EG, Janzen E, et al. *Mycoplasma bovis* and primary bovine virus diarrhea virus co-association in chronic pneumonia of feedlot cattle: a histopathological and immunohistochemical study. In: Proceedings of the 33rd Annual Conference of the American Association of Bovine Practitioners. Rapid City (SD), September 21–23, 2000. p. 146–7.

142. Gourlay RN, Houghton SB. Experimental pneumonia in conventionally reared and gnotobiotic calves by dual infection with *Mycoplasma bovis* and *Pasteurella haemolytica*. Res Vet Sci 1985;38:377–82.

143. Lopez A, Maxie MG, Ruhnke L, et al. Cellular inflammatory response in the lungs of calves exposed to bovine viral diarrhea virus, *Mycoplasma bovis*, and *Pasteurella hemolytica*. Am J Vet Res 1986;47:1283–6.

144. Bakaletz LO, Daniels RL, Lim DJ. Modeling adenovirus type 1-induced otitis media in the chinchilla: effect on ciliary activity and fluid transport function of eustachian tube mucosal epithelium. J Infect Dis 1993;168: 865–72.

145. Eskola J, Hovi T. Respiratory viruses in acute otitis media. N Engl J Med 1999; 340:312–4.

146. Van Biervliet J, Perkins GA, Woodie B, et al. Clinical signs, computed tomographic imaging, and management of chronic otitis media/interna in dairy calves. J Vet Intern Med 2004;18:907–10.

147. Friis NF, Kokotovic B, Svensmark B. *Mycoplasma hyorhinis* isolation from cases of otitis media in piglets. Acta Vet Scand 2002;43:191–3.

148. Faden H, Duffy L, Wasielewski R, et al. Relationship between nasopharyngeal colonization and the development of otitis media in children. Tonawanda/Williamsville pediatrics. J Infect Dis 1997;175:1440–5.

149. Kennedy BJ, Novotny LA, Jurcisek JA, et al. Passive transfer of antiserum specific for immunogens derived from a nontypeable *Haemophilus influenzae* adhesin and lipoprotein D prevents otitis media after heterologous challenge. Infect Immun 2000;68:2756–65.

150. Miles K, McAuliffe L, Persson A, et al. Insertion sequence profiling of UK *Mycoplasma bovis* field isolates. Vet Microbiol 2005;107:301–6.

151. Poumarat F, Solsona M, Boldini M. Genomic, protein and antigenic variability of *Mycoplasma bovis*. Vet Microbiol 1994;40:305–21.

152. Kusiluka LJ, Kokotovic B, Ojeniyi B, et al. Genetic variations among *Mycoplasma bovis* strains isolated from Danish cattle. FEMS Microbiol Lett 2000; 192:113–8.

153. Butler JA, Pinnow CC, Thomson JU, et al. Use of arbitrarily primed polymerase chain reaction to investigate *Mycoplasma bovis* outbreaks. Vet Microbiol 2001; 78:175–81.

154. Biddle MK, Fox LK, Evans MA, et al. Pulsed-field gel electrophoresis patterns of mycoplasma isolates from various body sites in dairy cattle with mycoplasma mastitis. J Am Vet Med Assoc 2005;227:455–9.

155. Gonzalez RN, Jayarao BM, Oliver SP, et al. Pneumonia, arthritis and mastitis in dairy cows due to *Mycoplasma bovis*. In: Proceedings of the 32nd Annual Meeting of the National Mastitis Council. Kansas City (MO), February 15–17, 1993. p. 178–85.

156. Stipkovits L, Ripley PH, Tenk M, et al. The efficacy of valnemulin (Econor) in the control of disease caused by experimental infection of calves with *Mycoplasma bovis*. Res Vet Sci 2005;78:207–15.

157. Step DL, Kirkpatrick JG. Mycoplasma infection in cattle. I. Pneumonia-arthritis syndrome. Bovine Practitioner 2001;35:149–55.

158. Clark T. Relationship of polyarthritis and respiratory disease in cattle. In: Proceedings of the 35th Annual Conference of the American Association of Bovine Practitioners. Madison (WI), September 26–28, 2002. p. 26–9.

159. Stokka GL, Lechtenberg K, Edwards T, et al. Lameness in feedlot cattle. Vet Clin North Am Food Anim Pract 2001;17:189–207.

160. Alberti A, Addis MF, Chessa B, et al. Molecular and antigenic characterization of a *Mycoplasma bovis* strain causing an outbreak of infectious keratoconjunctivitis. J Vet Diagn Invest 2006;18:41–51.

161. Jack EJ, Moring J, Boughton E. Isolation of *Mycoplasma bovis* from an outbreak of infectious bovine kerato conjunctivitis. Vet Rec 1977;101:287.

162. Kirby FD, Nicholas RA. Isolation of *Mycoplasma bovis* from bullocks' eyes. Vet Rec 1996;138:552.

163. Levisohn S, Garazi S, Gerchman I, et al. Diagnosis of a mixed mycoplasma infection associated with a severe outbreak of bovine pinkeye in young calves. J Vet Diagn Invest 2004;16:579–81.

164. Khodakaram-Tafti A, Lopez A. Immunohistopathological findings in the lungs of calves naturally infected with *Mycoplasma bovis*. J Vet Med A Physiol Pathol Clin Med 2004;51:10–4.

165. Radaelli E, Luini M, Loria GR, et al. Bacteriological, serological, pathological and immunohistochemical studies of *Mycoplasma bovis* respiratory infection in veal calves and adult cattle at slaughter. Res Vet Sci 2008;85:282–90.

166. Ayling R, Nicholas R, Hogg R, et al. *Mycoplasma bovis* isolated from brain tissue of calves. Vet Rec 2005;156:391–2.

167. Waites KB, Taylor-Robinson D. Mycoplasmas and ureaplasmas. In: Murray PR, Baron EJ, Pfeller MA, editors. Manual of clinical microbiology. 7th edition. Washington, DC: American Society for Microbiology; 1999. p. 782–94.

168. Gourlay RN, Howard CJ. Recovery and identification of bovine mycoplasmas. In: Tully JG, Razin S, editors. Methods in mycoplasmology. New York: Academic Press Inc.; 1983. p. 81–90.

169. Nicholas R, Baker S. Recovery of mycoplasmas from animals. Methods Mol Biol 1998;104:37–43.

170. Poumarat F, Perrin B, Longchambon D. Identification of ruminant mycoplasmas by dot immunobinding on membrane filtration (MF dot). Vet Microbiol 1991;29:329–38.

171. Virtala AM, Grohn YT, Mechor GD, et al. Association of seroconversion with isolation of agents in transtracheal wash fluids collected from pneumonic calves less than three months of age. Bovine Practitioner 2000;34:77–80.

172. Gourlay RN. Lavage techniques for recovery of animal mycoplasmas. In: Tully JG, Razin S, editors. Methods in mycoplasmology. New York: Academic Press Inc.; 1983. p. 149–51.

173. Taylor-Robinson D, Chen TA. Growth inhibitory factors in animal and plant tissues. In: Razin S, Tully JG, editors. Methods in mycoplasmology. New York: Academic Press Inc.; 1983. p. 109–14.

174. Clyde WA, McCormack WM. Collection and transport of specimens. In: Razin S, Tully JG, editors. Methods in mycoplasmology. New York: Academic Press Inc.; 1983. p. 103–7.

175. Biddle MK, Fox LK, Hancock DD, et al. Effects of storage time and thawing methods on the recovery of *Mycoplasma* species in milk samples from cows with intramammary infections. J Dairy Sci 2004;87:933–6.

176. Ayling RD, Nicholas RA, Johansson KE. Application of the polymerase chain reaction for the routine identification of *Mycoplasma bovis*. Vet Rec 1997;141:307–8.

177. Bashiruddin JB, Frey J, Konigsson MH, et al. Evaluation of PCR systems for the identification and differentiation of *Mycoplasma agalactiae* and *Mycoplasma bovis*: a collaborative trial. Vet J 2005;169:268–75.

178. Hotzel H, Sachse K, Pfutzner H. Rapid detection of *Mycoplasma bovis* in milk samples and nasal swabs using the polymerase chain reaction. J Appl Bacteriol 1996;80:505–10.
179. Subramaniam S, Bergonier D, Poumarat F, et al. Species identification of *Mycoplasma bovis* and *Mycoplasma agalactiae* based on the *uvr*C genes by PCR. Mol Cell Probes 1998;12:161–9.
180. Pinnow CC, Butler JA, Sachse K, et al. Detection of *Mycoplasma bovis* in preservative-treated field milk samples. J Dairy Sci 2001;84:1640–5.
181. Chavez Gonzalez YR, Ros BC, Bolske G, et al. In vitro amplification of the 16S rRNA genes from *Mycoplasma bovis* and *Mycoplasma agalactiae* by PCR. Vet Microbiol 1995;47:183–90.
182. Thomas A, Dizier I, Linden A, et al. Conservation of the *uvr*C gene sequence in *Mycoplasma bovis* and its use in routine PCR diagnosis. Vet J 2004;168: 100–2.
183. Hotzel H, Heller M, Sachse K. Enhancement of *Mycoplasma bovis* detection in milk samples by antigen capture prior to PCR. Mol Cell Probes 1999;13:175–8.
184. Foddai A, Idini G, Fusco M, et al. Rapid differential diagnosis of *Mycoplasma agalactiae* and *Mycoplasma bovis* based on a multiplex-PCR and a PCR-RFLP. Mol Cell Probes 2005;19:207–12.
185. Ball HJ, Finlay D. Diagnostic application of monoclonal antibody (MAb)-based sandwich ELISAs. Methods Mol Biol 1998;104:127–32.
186. Adegboye DS, Rasberry U, Halbur PG, et al. Monoclonal antibody-based immunohistochemical technique for the detection of *Mycoplasma bovis* in formalin-fixed, paraffin-embedded calf lung tissues. J Vet Diagn Invest 1995;7: 261–5.
187. Boothby JT, Jasper DE, Rollins MH. Characterization of antigens from mycoplasmas of animal origin. Am J Vet Res 1983;44:433–9.
188. Brank M, Le Grand D, Poumarat F, et al. Development of a recombinant antigen for antibody-based diagnosis of *Mycoplasma bovis* infection in cattle. Clin Diagn Lab Immunol 1999;6:861–7.
189. Ghadersohi A, Fayazi Z, Hirst RG. Development of a monoclonal blocking ELISA for the detection of antibody to *Mycoplasma bovis* in dairy cattle and comparison to detection by PCR. Vet Immunol Immunopathol 2005;104:183–93.
190. Le Grand D, Calavas D, Brank M, et al. Serological prevalence of *Mycoplasma bovis* infection in suckling beef cattle in France. Vet Rec 2002;150: 268–73.
191. Rosengarten R, Yogev D. Variant colony surface antigenic phenotypes within *Mycoplasma* strain populations: implications for species identification and strain standardization. J Clin Microbiol 1996;34:149–58.
192. Le Grand D, Philippe S, Calavas D, et al. Prevalence of *Mycoplasma bovis* infection in France. In: Poveda JB, Fernandez A, Frey J, editors. Mycoplasmas of ruminants: pathogenicity, diagnostics, epidemiology and molecular genetics. Brussells: European Commission; 2001. p. 106–9.
193. Martin SW, Bateman KG, Shewen PE, et al. The frequency, distribution and effects of antibodies, to seven putative respiratory pathogens, on respiratory disease and weight gain in feedlot calves in Ontario. Can J Vet Res 1989;53:355–62.
194. Taylor-Robinson D, Bebear C. Antibiotic susceptibilities of mycoplasmas and treatment of mycoplasmal infections. J Antimicrob Chemother 1997;40:622–30.
195. Francoz D, Fortin M, Fecteau G, et al. Determination of *Mycoplasma bovis* susceptibilities against six antimicrobial agents using the E test method. Vet Microbiol 2005;105:57–64.

196. Rosenbusch RF, Kinyon JM, Apley M, et al. In vitro antimicrobial inhibition profiles of *Mycoplasma bovis* isolates recovered from various regions of the United States from 2002 to 2003. J Vet Diagn Invest 2005;17:436–41.

197. Ayling RD, Baker SE, Peek ML, et al. Comparison of in vitro activity of danofloxacin, florfenicol, oxytetracycline, spectinomycin and tilmicosin against recent field isolates of *Mycoplasma bovis*. Vet Rec 2000;146:745–7.

198. Thomas A, Nicolas C, Dizier I, et al. Antibiotic susceptibilities of recent isolates of *Mycoplasma bovis* in Belgium. Vet Rec 2003;153:428–31.

199. Stalheim OH, Stone SS. Isolation and identification of *Mycoplasma agalactiae* subsp. *bovis* from arthritic cattle in Iowa and Nebraska. J Clin Microbiol 1975;2:169–72.

200. Gourlay RN, Thomas LH, Wyld SG, et al. Effect of a new macrolide antibiotic (tilmicosin) on pneumonia experimentally induced in calves by *Mycoplasma bovis* and *Pasteurella hemolytica*. Res Vet Sci 1989;47:84–9.

201. Godinho KS, Rae A, Windsor GD, et al. Efficacy of tulathromycin in the treatment of bovine respiratory disease associated with induced *Mycoplasma bovis* infections in young dairy calves. Vet Ther 2005;6:96–112.

202. Thomas E, Madelenat A, Davot JL, et al. Clinical efficacy and tolerance of marbofloxacin and oxytetracycline in the treatment of bovine respiratory disease. Rec Med Vet Ec Alfort 1998;174:21–7.

203. Picavet T, Muylle E, Devriese LA, et al. Efficacy of tilmicosin in treatment of pulmonary infections in calves. Vet Rec 1991;129:400–3.

204. Bednarek D, Zdzisinska B, Kondracki M, et al. Effect of steroidal and non-steroidal anti-inflammatory drugs in combination with long-acting oxytetracycline on non-specific immunity of calves suffering from enzootic bronchopneumonia. Vet Microbiol 2003;96:53–67.

205. Lous J, Burton MJ, Felding JU, et al. Grommets (ventilation tubes) for hearing loss associated with otitis media with effusion in children. Cochrane Database Syst Rev 2005;(1):CD001801.

206. Poetker DM, Ubell ML, Kerschner JE. Disease severity in patients referred to pediatric otolaryngologists with a diagnosis of otitis media. Int J Pediatr Otorhinolaryngol 2006;70:311–7.

207. Schnepper R. Practice tips. In: Proceedings of the 35th Annual Conference of the American Association of Bovine Practitioners. Madison (WI), September 26–28, 2002. p. 26–8.

208. Villarroel A, Heller M, Lane VM. Imaging study of myringotomy in dairy calves. Bovine Practitioner 2006;40:14–7.

209. AABP. Special report from the AABP mastitis committee: mycoplasma fact sheet. Opelika (AL): American Association of Bovine Practitioners; 2005.

210. Brown MB, Shearer JK, Elvinger F. Mycoplasmal mastitis in a dairy herd. J Am Vet Med Assoc 1990;196:1097–101.

211. Stabel JR, Hurd S, Calvente L, et al. Destruction of *Mycobacterium paratuberculosis, Salmonella* spp., and *Mycoplasma* spp. in raw milk by a commercial on-farm high-temperature, short-time pasteurizer. J Dairy Sci 2004;87:2177–83.

212. Godden SM, Fetrow JP, Feirtag JM, et al. Economic analysis of feeding pasteurized nonsaleable milk versus conventional milk replacer to dairy calves. J Am Vet Med Assoc 2005;226:1547–54.

213. Godden S, McMartin S, Feirtag J, et al. Heat-treatment of bovine colostrum. II: effects of heating duration on pathogen viability and immunoglobulin G. J Dairy Sci 2006;89:3476–83.

214. McMartin S, Godden S, Metzger L, et al. Heat treatment of bovine colostrum. I: effects of temperature on viscosity and immunoglobulin G level. J Dairy Sci 2006;89:2110–8.

215. Boddie RL, Owens WE, Ray CH, et al. Germicidal activities of representatives of five different teat dip classes against three bovine mycoplasma species using a modified excised teat model. J Dairy Sci 2002;85:1909–12.

216. Galyean ML, Gunter SA, Malcolmcallis KJ. Effects of arrival medication with tilmicosin phosphate on health and performance of newly received beef cattle. J Anim Sci 1995;73:1219–26.

217. Thomson DU, White BJ. Backgrounding beef cattle. Vet Clin North Am Food Anim Pract 2006;22:373–98.

218. Berge AC, Lindeque P, Moore DA, et al. A clinical trial evaluating prophylactic and therapeutic antibiotic use on health and performance of preweaned calves. J Dairy Sci 2005;88:2166–77.

219. Nagatomo H, Shimizu T, Higashiyama Y, et al. Antibody response to *Mycoplasma bovis* of calves introduced to a farm contaminated with the organism. J Vet Med Sci 1996;58:919–20.

220. Nicholas RA, Ayling RD, Stipkovits LP. An experimental vaccine for calf pneumonia caused by *Mycoplasma bovis*: clinical, cultural, serological and pathological findings. Vaccine 2002;20:3569–75.

221. Stott EJ, Thomas LH, Howard CJ, et al. Field trial of a quadrivalent vaccine against calf respiratory disease. Vet Rec 1987;121:342–7.

222. Urbaneck D, Liebig F, Forbrig T, et al. Experiences with herd-specific vaccines against respiratory infections with *M. bovis* in a large feedlot. Prakt Tierarzt 2000;81:756–63.

223. Rosenbusch RF. Test of an inactivated vaccine against *Mycoplasma bovis* respiratory disease by transthoracic challenge with an abscessing strain. IOM Lett 1998;5:185.

224. Bryson DG, Ball HJ, Brice N, et al. Pathology of induced *Mycoplasma bovis* calf pneumonia in experimentally vaccinated animals. In: Stipkovits L, Rosengarten R, Frey J, editors. Mycoplasmas of ruminants: pathogenicity, diagnostics, epidemiology and molecular genetics. Brussels: European Commission; 1999. p. 128–32.

225. Howard CJ, Gourlay RN, Taylor G. Immunity to *Mycoplasma bovis* infections of the respiratory tract of calves. Res Vet Sci 1980;28:242–9.

226. Perez-Casal J, Prysliak T. Detection of antibodies against the *Mycoplasma bovis* glyceraldehyde-3-phosphate dehydrogenase protein in beef cattle. Microb Pathog 2007;43:189–97.

Respiratory Distress Syndrome in Calves

Ulrich Bleul, DMV

KEYWORDS

- Neonate • Calf • Preterm • Respiratory distress • Surfactant

Perinatal mortality, defined as the percentage of calves that die shortly before, during, and within 48 hours after birth, ranges from 3% to 10.3% in most countries.[1,2] The most common causes are respiratory and metabolic disorders, trauma, hypogamma-globulinemia, congenital infection, congenital anomalies, and umbilical infection.[3] Respiratory and metabolic disorders are by far the most important cause of death in this time period. Mixed respiratory and metabolic acidosis attributable to hypoxia or anoxia during parturition is the most common disorder in calves that are born after a normal gestation length.

Calves that are born prematurely, however, suffer predominantly from disorders caused by incomplete organ development. This can be life threatening in calves with immaturity of the brain, locomotor system, gastrointestinal tract, or lungs. Often, premature calves are unable to breath normally, regulate body temperature, and nurse because the corresponding centers in the brain are not fully developed. These calves are unable to stand and have tendon laxity and incomplete bone ossification. Intestinal motility is impaired, and absorption of immunoglobulins and nutrients is reduced. In most cases, the first clinical sign of prematurity is progressive respiratory difficulty.[4] Although there is no uniform definition,[5,6] these clinical signs appear as tachypnea and expiration accentuated by an abdominal lift and expiratory grunt, and in association with characteristic blood gas changes, are called respiratory distress syndrome (RDS), similar to the disorder seen in human neonatology. RDS is sometimes referred to as "neonatal asphyxia" because it is only seen after birth. This is in contrast to fetal asphyxia, which is caused by inadequate supply of oxygen to the fetus in utero or during parturition.

This article focuses on establishment of respiration post natum along with the production and function of surfactant. The clinical findings and results of blood gas analysis in calves with RDS are described and treatment options discussed.

PATHOPHYSIOLOGY OF RESPIRATION POST NATUM
The First Breath

Successful transition from an intrauterine life in amniotic fluid, with gas exchange by the umbilical cord, to extrauterine life depends on establishment of postnatal

Clinic of Reproductive Medicine, Department of Farm Animals, Vetsuisse-Faculty, University of Zurich, Winterthurerstrasse 260, CH-8057 Zurich, Switzerland
E-mail address: ubleul@vetclinics.uzh.ch

Vet Clin Food Anim 25 (2009) 179–193
doi:10.1016/j.cvfa.2008.10.002
0749-0720/08/$ – see front matter © 2009 Elsevier Inc. All rights reserved.

respiration by the lungs. This requires that all parts of the respiratory system begin to function properly in a very short period of time. Irregular respiratory movements occur in the fetal period, and they progress to continuous periodic movements to transport air in and out of the lungs in the postnatal period.

It is still unknown what triggers the first breath. Studies in lambs and human infants strongly suggest that a multitude of stimuli can initiate respiration. These include external factors, such as tactile, visual, or thermal stimuli.[7] Stimulation of thermoreceptors in the skin by a cold stimulus was shown to initiate respiration in fetal lambs.[8] Changes in Pa_{O_2} and Pa_{CO_2} can also stimulate respiration. Increased Pa_{CO_2}, caused by reduced elimination from the circulation or an increase in the rate of metabolism, results in respiration. Paradoxically, in the fetus, an increase in P_{O_2} stimulates respiratory movements, whereas hypoxia results in inhibition of respiratory movements.[9]

A simultaneous increase in pulmonary circulation must also occur to accommodate the dramatic increase in gas exchange requirements. Less than 10% of cardiac output goes to the lungs in the fetal period, whereas after birth almost all of the blood volume flows to the lungs because the pulmonary circulation is in series, and not parallel, to the systemic circulation. This is achieved by a marked decrease in vascular resistance of the lungs and blood pressure in the pulmonary artery. In calves, the pressure decreases from 80 mm Hg to 30 mm Hg within the first 12 hours of birth.[10]

The replacement of pulmonary fluid from the fetal period with air is equally as important as the changes in circulation. Studies in lambs have shown that fluid is continually produced and secreted in the lungs.[11] The fluid content of the lungs decreases in the fetal period by about 35% before birth. Some of the fluid is pressed out of the lungs and the upper airways by compression of the thorax in the birth canal during parturition. Approximately one third of the fluid remains in the lungs immediately after birth; however, most of it is rapidly resorbed, and a smaller fraction is expelled during respiration.[9,11]

The first breath should be the most powerful breath ever taken in a newborn. It requires a great deal of energy because the first breath must overcome a pressure that is 6 to 20 times higher than subsequent breaths. The elasticity of the lungs, surface tension, and high viscosity of the pulmonary fluid must be overcome, the latter constituting the greatest resistance. Incoming air fills only a few areas of lung, whereas other regions remain collapsed. With subsequent breaths, air is retained in the lungs after expiration, thereby opening more and more areas of lung. Air remains in the lungs mainly because of higher alveolar stability, which in turn results from reduced alveolar surface tension by surfactant.[9]

Surfactant

The word "surfactant" was created from the term "surface active agent," which describes its function in the lungs. Surfactant is not a single pure substance but rather a combination of 90% lipids and 10% proteins. The lipid portion is primarily phospholipids, most of which are phosphatidylcholines. Phospholipids are the critical component of surfactant to reduce surface tension in the lungs. Type-II pneumocytes produce, store, secrete, and resorb phospholipids,[12] which form a monolayer in the alveoli and distal bronchioli.

Type II pneumocytes also produce surfactant proteins (SP). Four types of SP have been described for humans, cattle, and a few other species.[12,13] SP-A is the most common type in mature neonates. It regulates the secretion of phospholopids and their inclusion in the surfactant monolayer, along with resorption into type II pneumocytes. Together with SP-D it also plays an important role in pulmonary immunodefense. These proteins bind pathogens and promote their removal.[14] The other two

SP, SP-B and SP-C, enhance rapid inclusion of phospholipids in the air-fluid interface of the monolayer and have a key function in surfactant metabolism. Reduced amounts or absence of SP-B in newborn human infants leads to terminal RDS.[12]

PATHOPHYSIOLOGY OF RESPIRATORY DISTRESS SYNDROME

The pathophysiology of RDS in human infants and lambs (which provide a research model for human RDS) has been intensely investigated,[12,15,16] although studies in cattle are limited.[17–20] Based on the similarity of clinical signs and pathologic findings, it is thought that the underlying mechanisms of RDS in infants and calves are very similar.[19–21]

Approximately 50% of premature human infants born at 26 to 28 weeks of gestation develop signs of RDS. After this time, the rate of RDS decreases with increasing duration of gestation.[22] Various pulmonary developments that are critical for lung function occur in the last quarter of gestation. There is an increase in the pool of surfactant lipids in pneumocytes, and the structure of the lung changes such that the distance for diffusion of respiratory gases becomes shorter and the surface for gas exchange larger.[23] Lambs also have increased production of surfactant in this time period. The surfactant system is completely developed when 86% to 90% of the average gestational length has been reached.[24] Comparative studies have not been done in cattle. Calves that are born before 90% of the normal gestation length have an increased incidence of RDS, however, which is probably caused by insufficient amounts of surfactant.[21,25]

A varying degree of atelectasis can be seen in premature calves, lambs, foals, and infants.[20] In lambs, the extent of atelectasis correlates with the length of gestation and the amount of pulmonary surfactant.[22] Insufficient surfactant leads to end-expiratory collapse of lung regions that are inadequately or not aerated afterward. These atelectatic regions result in inadequate surface area for gas exchange, and the neonate increases its respiratory rate to maintain adequate ventilation. If this is not achieved, hypoxia ensues. Hypoxia has two main negative effects: it damages surfactant-producing pneumocytes, and it causes vasoconstriction of pulmonary vessels, which results in decreased pulmonary circulation. This in turn causes damage to various pulmonary cells and possibly leads to alveolar and interstitial edema.[26] In addition, there may be exudation of protein, which together with cell debris forms hyaline membranes in the alveoli. Hyaline membranes not only impair alveolar structure but also inactivate surfactant,[27] which exacerbates the surfactant deficiency. This vicious circle is depicted in **Fig. 1**.

The effects of RDS may be aggravated by cardiovascular disturbances. There is a substantial change in the cardiovascular system of mature neonates. The initiation of respiration results in a dramatic reduction in pulmonary pressure and increased blood flow into the pulmonary capillaries. This reduces the pressure in the right atrium compared with the left, which results in closure of the foramen ovale between the two chambers. In addition, severing of the umbilical cord leads to an increase in peripheral resistance in the systemic circulation. Blood that used to flow mainly from the pulmonary trunk into the aorta by the ductus arteriosus (right-to-left shunt) in the fetus now flows by a left-to-right shunt into the lungs. In the following hours to days, there is progressive closure of the ductus arteriosus caused by the high Po_2 in the aortic blood.[28] In neonates with RDS, hypoxia caused by surfactant deficiency causes vasoconstriction of the pulmonary vessels. This results in an increase in the pulmonary circulation pressure, causing partial or complete right-to-left shunting.[26] This leads to further reduction of the oxygen content of the blood and life-threatening hypoxia.

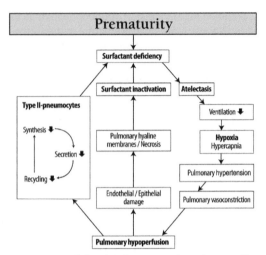

Fig. 1. Schematic representation of the development of respiratory distress syndrome.

Another cause of RDS in newborn human infants is aspiration of meconium.[12] Meconium impairs the function of surfactant in several ways. Incorporation of phospholipids from the meconium inhibits the production of a stable monolayer. In addition, the formation of surfactant and protein aggregates from the meconium prevents the incorporation of surfactant phospholipids in the monolayer. Meconium also causes an inflammatory reaction in the lungs, which most likely has a direct effect on type II pneumocyte function.[12] The functional result of meconium aspiration is similar to insufficient production and availability of surfactant. In contrast to surfactant deficiency, meconium aspiration is more likely to occur in full-term human infants. Meconium aspiration also occurs in calves, because meconium may be passed before or during birth of the calf. Schuijt[29] observed passage of meconium or discoloration of the hair with meconium in 16% of calves born by caesarian section. Components of meconium have been found in the lungs of calves and were associated with inflammatory lesions.[30] Postmortem examination of calves that had clinical signs of RDS revealed hair and phagocytosed meconium in the bronchi.[31] Studies on the effect of these lesions on respiration have not been performed in calves.

There are very few systematic studies on the relationship between surfactant deficiency and histologic lung lesions in newborn calves. Danlois and colleagues[17,18] investigated the composition of surfactant and its physical characteristics in healthy Belgian White and Blue calves, and those with RDS. Healthy Belgian White and Blue calves had lower concentrations of SP-B and SP-C than healthy Holstein-Friesian calves.[17] Belgian White and Blue calves with clinical and histologic signs of RDS had no SP-C or only very small amounts.[18] The study did not determine whether this factor alone was responsible for the signs of RDS, however, or whether there is an association between RDS and SP-C deficiency in calves of other breeds. There is an urgent need for further investigation of the causes and pathophysiology of RDS in premature calves.

CLINICAL PRESENTATION
Incidence

There are no data on the incidence of RDS in calves. The morbidity rate of RDS in human infants and horses is also unknown; however, it is one of the leading causes of death in these two species.[32,33] RDS is the fourth most common cause of human neonatal death in the United States. It is important to note that most infants affected by RDS are premature babies born before 35 weeks of gestation. Similarly, except for rare exceptions, the risk of RDS is highest in premature calves, particularly those born before 270 days of gestation.[25] In two experimental studies in which calves were born after 258 to 270 days of gestation by caesarian section, 32% and 60% had clinical signs of RDS.[5,6] In two clinical studies of premature calves with RDS that were born naturally, or because of emergency slaughter of the dam, the mean gestational length was 262 days.[34,35] Occasionally, calves born after a normal gestation period are affected by RDS.[34,36] Hypothyroidism was thought to be the cause of RDS in one calf,[36] because thyroid hormones together with other hormones are involved in lung maturation.[37]

Clinical Findings

RDS is a group of signs caused by a deficiency of surfactant.[26,38] Premature birth and blood gas abnormalities are also associated with RDS.[5,20] Calves that develop RDS have no respiratory abnormalities immediately after birth.[19] Many of the affected calves have signs of immaturity, however, because of a shorter than normal gestation. A rounded head, silky short hair, short umbilical hair, and eruption of no or only a few incisors are common.[39] These calves are usually underweight and have flexor tendon laxity. Approximately 10 to 15 minutes after birth, signs of progressive respiratory difficulty occur and reach a peak after the first hour of life. Affected calves have inspiratory and expiratory dyspnea.[39] During inspiration, the thorax is drawn in, especially the caudal part, and the abdomen bulges outward. In premature calves, respiratory effort is afforded primarily by the diaphragm, which contracts markedly during inspiration to facilitate a high intrathoracic pressure and expansion of poorly compliant lungs. During this process the abdominal organs are displaced caudally causing the abdomen to bulge ventrally. Because of weak intercostal musculature and the very pliable thorax of premature calves, the tensed diaphragm pulls the thoracic walls inward. This process is called "intercostal retraction." The opposite occurs during expiration; the ventral abdomen moves dorsally and the thorax expands. In calves with severe dyspnea, a rocking movement between the thorax and abdomen becomes apparent.[40] Grunting, caused by partial closure of the glottis, is often heard during expiration. It is thought that partial closure of the glottis serves to increase the amount of retained air in the lungs to maintain the functional residual capacity during expiration. Affected calves also develop progressive tachypnea to achieve adequate gas exchange.[41] The mucous membranes of these calves are often pale initially and become increasingly cyanotic.

DIAGNOSTIC METHODS

Other than physical examination, blood gas analysis is the most important tool in the diagnosis of RDS. Just as there are no clinical signs of RDS immediately after birth, so too are there no blood gas or acid-base abnormalities at this time. In both premature and mature calves, gas exchange before and during partuition occurs by the umbilical cord. Immediately after severance of the cord, adequate gas exchange begins in calves with normal alveolar ventilation and pulmonary perfusion. With alveolar ventilation and pulmonary perfusion mismatch, however, which occurs in neonates with surfactant deficiency, there is inadequate uptake of oxygen and removal of carbon dioxide. Depending on the severity of atelectasis, it takes minutes to hours for pathognomonic changes in blood gas values to become apparent.

Venous or arterial blood can be used to measure changes in blood gases. There are good correlations between the partial pressure of carbon dioxide in arterial ($Paco_2$) and venous blood.[5] Arterial blood is required for determination of the Pao_2, however, because the Po_2 of venous blood does not correlate with that of arterial blood, and calves with RDS-related hypoxia have few changes in venous blood Po_2.[5,42] Arterial blood can be collected from various arteries.[42,43] Collection of blood from the medial intermediate branch of the caudal auricular artery is probably the easiest method because it can be performed in standing or recumbent calves with little restraint (**Fig. 2**). Furthermore, puncture of this artery is not associated with complications, such as hematoma or arteritis. In human infants and foals, an arterial Pao_2 of less than 60 mm Hg is considered a sign of RDS.[32,38] In calves with RDS, the Pao_2 was considerable lower than 60 mm Hg.[5,34] The calves in these two studies had a Pao_2 of 29.7 $\pm$ 12.9 and 38.4 $\pm$ 8.8 mm Hg 1 hour after birth. Because healthy calves had a mean Pao_2 of 47.8 $\pm$ 17.8 mm Hg to 58.1 $\pm$ 13.1 mm Hg 30 to 60 minutes after birth, the cut-off point of 60 mm Hg established for foals seems to be too high for calves.[5,42] Partial pressures under 45 mm Hg together with pertinent clinical signs are most likely pathognomonic for RDS.

In calves with RDS, marked hypercapnia with values between 58.2 $\pm$ 11 mm Hg and 80.7 $\pm$ 31.1 mm Hg are regularly seen.[5,20,42] Because of the wide range, however, this variable has less diagnostic potential. In addition to hypoxia and hypercapnia, calves with RDS have progressive acid-base abnormalities in both venous and arterial blood.

Immediately after birth almost all calves have mild metabolic and respiratory acidosis.[1] Typically, the initial pH and base excess values do not differ between healthy calves and those that subsequently develop RDS.[5,20] In the first 30 to 60 minutes after birth, there is a decrease in both pH and base excess, which is more pronounced in calves with RDS. After this time, the values normalize in healthy calves but not in calves with RDS. The decrease in pH is caused by accumulation of carbon dioxide (CO_2) in the blood because it cannot be adequately eliminated. Carbon dioxide, which is a weak acid in blood, can only be eliminated by the lungs.[44] Because of the high $Paco_2$, part of the CO_2 in blood is transported as bicarbonate. This is why the bicarbonate concentration, and the base excess, does not decrease to the same extent as the pH. Calves with RDS primarily have a respiratory acidosis at the beginning.[34] Because of the developing tissue hypoxia and reduced perfusion of peripheral tissues caused by circulatory centralization to vital organs, the production of lactate from anaerobic metabolism increases.[5,45] Blood gas analysis and determination of base

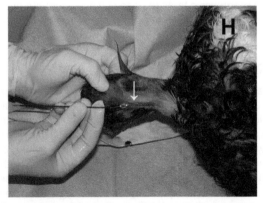

Fig. 2. Collection of arterial blood from the medial intermediate branch of the caudal auricular artery. H, head; ↓, artery.

excess and lactate concentration reveals that calves with RDS have mixed respiratory and metabolic acidosis.

In human infants and foals in intensive care because of RDS, radiographic examination of the lungs 24 to 48 hours after birth is an important tool to determine the presence and severity of atelectasis.[32,46,47] Affected patients have reduced lung volume, increased lung density, diffuse infiltrates, and air bronchograms.[32,47–49] Although systematic radiographic studies of the lungs of neonatal calves with RDS are lacking, similar radiographic findings were described in a cloned calf with severe RDS.[50]

Another diagnostic test in humans is the determination of lecithin and sphingomyelin concentrations (the two surfactant phospholipids) in amniotic fluid by thin-layer chromatography, a test that has also been investigated in calves.[6,20,51] Sphingomyelin occurs in amniotic fluid in a relatively constant concentration in the last trimester of pregnancy, whereas lecithin is produced by the lungs in increasing amounts toward the end of pregnancy and released into the amniotic fluid.[52] A ratio of lecithin to sphingomyelin greater than 2 indicates a mature surfactant system in the calf.[20] This test has not become routine in veterinary medicine because it is expensive and complicated.

THERAPY

In principle, early treatment intervention is desired to prevent the sequelae of ventilation and perfusion abnormalities, such as acidosis or right-to-left shunt. The problem is that healthy calves and those that subsequently develop RDS cannot be differentiated by physical examination or blood gas analysis immediately after birth. Neonatal calves that are identified as high-risk patients based on history or the initial physical examination should be closely monitored. Risk factors are a gestation length of less than 270 days, caesarian section performed before stage I of labor, and clinical signs of immaturity.

General Management of Calves Immediately After Birth

In calves with risk factors for RDS, resuscitation methods similar to those for fetal asphyxia are indicated. These entail clearing the upper airways, stimulating respiration, and minimizing heat loss.[53] Because of poor lung compliance in calves with RDS, the workload of respiration is high, and reducing upper airway resistance becomes critical. A tube can be used to remove mucus from the nose, mouth, and pharyngeal region. An electric or hand-powered vacuum pump is very useful for this procedure.[34,53] Simple methods that can be used in the barn include suctioning with a hand-powered pump and a well-sealed face mask or suspension of the calf by the hind legs (for a maximum of 60 seconds) so that gravity allows the secretions to drain. These measures were shown to have a positive effect on postnatal gas exchange in healthy neonatal calves.[53,54] As discussed previously, the workload of respiration in premature neonates is afforded mainly by the diaphragm because the intercostal muscles are not fully developed. If these calves are suspended by the hind legs, the abdominal viscera pushes against the diaphragm, which may interfere with the respiratory mechanics and exacerbate the ventilatory disturbances. Stimulation of respiration in calves at risk for RDS is rarely required. Exceptions are severely premature calves, in which failure to breathe or delayed onset of breathing may occur, presumably because of an immature respiratory center. Respiratory stimulation can be attempted with application of cold water to the back of the head (thermal stimulation) or by administration of drugs (eg, doxapram hydrochloride).[39,53] The use of drugs to stimulate respiration is described in greater detail by Nagy elsewhere in this issue.

Calves expend a great deal of energy to maintain a normal body temperature after birth. This is particularly true in premature calves, because they have less brown fat than mature calves. They are unable to maintain their body temperature in the same manner as mature calves[55] and often suffer from marked hypothermia.[34,56] To conserve energy and prevent life-threatening hypothermia, cold ambient temperatures and drafts should be avoided. Supplemental heat using an infrared heater can be provided. Calves warmed with a heat lamp after birth had improved ventilation with slower and deeper breathing.[53] Placing the calf in sternal recumbency also improves gas exchange substantially.[54] Compared with mature calves in lateral recumbency, those in sternal recumbency had better oxygen and carbon dioxide exchange, which is likely because of better alveolar ventilation and a change in the shape of and stress on the thorax, diaphragm, and lungs.[54] The positive effects of sternal recumbency are also expected in calves with RDS, and placing the patient in this position with lateral support is recommended. If this is not possible, the calf should be turned from side to side frequently to prevent mechanical compression of the down lung.

Ventilatory Support

There are numerous studies and reports on different ventilatory support systems in human and equine neonatology.[26,57–59] They range from oxygen administration to mechanical respiration, and all of them have substantial personnel and equipment requirements. It is a good idea to assess the chosen therapy regularly based on clinical signs and blood gas analysis so that unnecessary lengthy treatments are avoided when they are no longer required. Alternatively, it may be necessary to institute more involved therapy if the patient's condition does not improve or if it starts to deteriorate.

Oxygen Therapy

Although intranasal insufflation of oxygen in calves has been repeatedly reported to be minimally effective,[60–62] intranasal oxygen administration in 20 calves with clinical signs of RDS resulted in an increase in the Pao_2 from 38.4 ± 8.8 mm Hg to 58.7 ± 17.8 mm Hg within 3 hours, in the absence of other treatments.[34] Humidified oxygen at a flow rate of 5 to 6 L per minute was administered by a plastic catheter (size 10F), which was introduced into one nostril and advanced to the level of the medial canthus of the eye (**Fig. 3**). After a maximum of 3 hours, the flow rate was reduced to 3 to 4 L/min. In calves that require oxygen insufflation for long periods, tube placement should be alternated between nostrils every 48 hours and secretions cleared from the nares. Oxygen therapy only increases the availability of oxygen; it has no effect on the proportion of aerated and atelectatic lung. Not all treated calves have an adequate increase in the Pao_2 and oxygen saturation. Calves that do not have a Pao_2 greater than 55 mm Hg within 12 hours of therapy have a poor prognosis,[34] and may require mechanical ventilation to survive. An oxygen saturation of 70% to 90% should be the target in calves that respond to oxygen administration. A higher saturation is not necessary and increases the risk of toxic (free radical) changes caused by oxygen.[34,63]

Ventilation Techniques

There are few reports on mechanical ventilation of calves with respiratory disorders post natum. In two cases reports, mechanical ventilation was described in cloned calves that had hypoventilation, hypercapnia, hypoxemia, and pulmonary hypertension.[50,64] The calves did not respond to oxygen insufflation and were mechanically ventilated. All methods of mechanical ventilation require nasotracheal or orotracheal intubation.[58] Depending on the size of the calf, endotracheal tubes with an inner

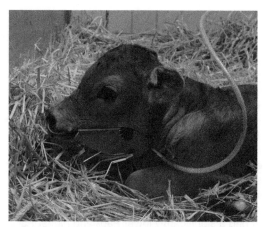

Fig. 3. A premature calf with an intranasal catheter for oxygen administration.

diameter of 6 to 10.5 mm can be used by an orotracheal route.[65] A rebreathing bag can be used temporarily for intermittent ventilation using room air or oxygen. To avoid overinflation of the lungs, it is useful to incorporate a safety valve that prevents the ventilatory pressure from exceeding 30 to 40 mm Hg.[21,58] The rate of ventilation should be 15 to 25 breaths per minute.

Continuous mechanical ventilation is only feasible with constant monitoring by a trained nursing team. It is well known from equine neonatology that mechanical ventilation requires meticulous monitoring of vital functions and of inspired oxygen and expired carbon dioxide concentrations, and serial blood gas analyses.[58] There are various settings for the ventilator mode, which depend on the condition of the calf. Because experience with respect to mechanical ventilation of calves with RDS is limited, the guidelines from equine neonatology may be used.[48,58,59]

The use of positive end-expiratory pressure is particularly useful in mechanical ventilation of neonates with surfactant deficiency because they frequently have hypoxia caused by atelectasis, with resulting intrapulmonary shunting and mismatching of alveolar ventilation and pulmonary perfusion. The use of positive end-expiratory pressure leads to an increase in the amount of air in the lungs at end expiration, which prevents collapse of the alveoli, stabilizes the weak thorax, and improves the ventilation-to-perfusion ratio.[59] Other areas of atelectasis are opened and stabilized with each breath. In foals, a positive end-expiratory pressure of 4 to 5 cm H_2O is recommended, but this should be confirmed based on lung compliance and the Pao_2. A positive end-expiratory pressure that is too high can cause overexpansion of the lungs and have negative effects on the cardiovascular system.[59] Continuous positive airway pressure is based on a similar principle and is a newer technique used in human medicine. With continuous positive airway pressure, patients are fitted with a respiration mask or intranasal prongs and are not intubated.[23,38] Investigation of the effects of continuous positive airway pressure in ruminants is limited to an experimental study in premature lambs.[23] Although the lambs treated with continuous positive airway pressure had lower Pao_2 and higher $Paco_2$ values than mechanically ventilated lambs, they had less lung damage.[23] Studies on the side effects of ventilatory support in animals are very limited. Damage caused by excessive pressure or oxygen therapy can negate the positive effects of the treatment.[59,66] This must be considered in view of the fact that surfactant, which can prevent alveolar damage caused by mechanical ventilation,[41] is rarely used in veterinary neonatology.

Surfactant Therapy

Based on the clinical, pathologic, and laboratory findings, it can be assumed that RDS in calves is caused by surfactant deficiency. The administration of surfactant, which is standard procedure in premature human infants, seems to be a useful therapy in calves with RDS. Commercially available surfactant products for use in human medicine contain surfactant from calf or porcine lung or synthetic components, and are very expensive. In two studies involving surfactant administration to calves with RDS, the surfactant was collected and processed from slaughterhouse specimens of bovine lungs by the authors themselves.[50,56] In one of the studies, the phospholipid concentration was determined and 100 mg/kg surfactant was administered into the trachea of the premature calves by an endotracheal tube. Afterward, the calves were moved from sternal into right and then left lateral recumbency to improve distribution of the surfactant. The calves also received intranasal oxygen. The premature calves of the control group, which were not treated with surfactant, also received oxygen insufflation but had a significantly lower Pa_{O_2} and higher Pa_{CO_2} after 12 hours of treatment compared with the calves that had received surfactant. All the calves in the control group died, whereas the mortality rate in the premature calves treated with surfactant was 40%.[56] Although these data seem promising, the cost of commercially available surfactant products makes their use virtually impossible in calves. For example, prices were calculated for administering a 100 mg/kg dose of two leading surfactant products available world-wide. In a 40-kg calf, therapy with Curosurf (Chiesi Farmaceutici, Parma, Italy) is about $12,000 dollars, whereas a single treatment with Survanta (Abbott Laboratories, Abbott Park, Illinois) is approximately $16,000 in the United States.

Supportive Therapy

Premature calves with clinically diagnosed RDS often have disorders of other organ systems and diseases that result from impaired ventilation. Respiratory and metabolic acidosis predominates in the first hours of life.[5,34] A blood pH of greater than or equal to 7.2 is adequate but calves with lower values must be treated.[32,67] Respiratory acidosis is treated by improving gas exchange. The most common treatment for metabolic acidosis in newborn calves is intravenous administration of sodium bicarbonate ($NaHCO_3$).[39,68] Because the bicarbonate anion (HCO_3^-) reacts with the hydrogen ion (H^+) to form water and carbon dioxide, one must first determine whether the calf is able to expire carbon dioxide adequately; most calves with RDS do not and instead accumulate carbon dioxide in the blood. Tris buffer and Carbicarb, which buffer hydrogen ions without the formation of additional carbon dioxide, are alternatives to $NaHCO_3$. Carbicarb is an equimolar mixture of $NaHCO_3$ and sodium carbonate (Na_2CO_3). The carbonate anion (CO_3^{2-}) reacts with a hydrogen ion to form bicarbonate (HCO_3^-). Hydrogen ions are derived from blood proteins or from dissolved CO_2. Because CO_3^{2-} is a stronger base than HCO_3^-, the protons are buffered mainly by CO_3^{2-}. With the plasma HCO_3^- concentration close to the normal range, only a small proportion of the newly formed HCO_3^- ions produce CO_2.[39,69] A Carbicarb solution containing 0.33 M $NaHCO_3$ and 0.33 M Na_2CO_3 is administered using the following formula: body weight $\times$ (−base excess) $\times$ 0.4.[67] Tris buffer, which also reacts with hydrogen ions without producing CO_2, has side effects that include vascular irritation and accumulation of hydrogen-laden Tris molecules in patients with renal insufficiency. Because renal dysfunction with anuria or oliguria is common in patients with RDS,[32] adequate intravenous fluid therapy is indicated regardless of whether or not Tris buffer is used.

Glucocorticoids are sometimes administered to calves with suspected RDS to aid in postnatal lung maturation. In contrast to prenatal administration, however, postnatally administered glucocorticoids have not been shown to affect the production of surfactant and lung maturation.[39] Administration of a bronchodilator, such as the β_2-sympathomimetic drug clenbuterol, has also been recommended in neonates with RDS.[32] In a study involving double-muscled calves with RDS, however, the drug had no positive effect.[70] Furthermore, the use of this drug in calves is prohibited in the United States.

CONTROL

Generally, calves born before 270 days of gestation have a high risk of developing RDS. Procedures that may result in premature birth (eg, foot trimming using mechanical chutes, sedation with $\alpha2$ agonists, and transport) should be avoided in this critical time period. When this is not possible, RDS may be avoided by induction of parturition by the administration of glucocorticoids and prostaglandin $F_{2\alpha}$ to the dam after 260 days of gestation. Calves born 30 hours after the administration of a prostaglandin $F_{2\alpha}$ analog or flumethasone had significantly higher venous pH values than calves of untreated dams.[6] The same study found that treatment of the dams resulted in an increase in the lecithin-to-sphyngomyelin ratio in the calves. These results are in agreement with clinical and experimental studies in human medicine, which found that there was stimulation of type II pneumocytes and subsequent synthesis of surfactant phospholipids by glucocorticoids.[12] In cattle, the efficacy of this treatment decreases with a decreasing length of gestation and treatment is not effective before 260 days of gestation.[39] When a pregnant cow must be euthanized before 260 days without hormonal induction of parturition, it is unlikely that the calf is viable. Cows that are between 230 to 260 days of gestation, however, in which a modified 7-day regime for induction of parturition is possible, usually produce a premature but viable calf that does not develop RDS. Each case must be viewed individually to determine whether keeping the dam alive for the induction procedure is humane. Induction begins with administration of 5 mg dexamethasone intramuscularly every 12 hours for 4 days. On day 5, the dose of dexamethasone is doubled to 10 mg every 12 hours. In some cows, parturition occurs on day 6; in the remainder, 40-mg dexamethasone and an abortigenic dose of prostaglandin $F_{2\alpha}$ is given once on day 6.[39]

SUMMARY

Although the exact cause of RDS in premature calves is not fully understood, it is probably attributable to lung immaturity. Pulmonary atelectasis results in decreased gas exchange, and neonates have progressive dyspnea and hypoxia. Diagnosis is based on the clinical findings and results of blood gas analysis. Depending on the severity of the respiratory abnormalities, supportive respiratory therapy, oxygen administration, or mechanical ventilation may be required. Prevention of RDS is achieved by the administration of glucocorticoids to the dam in planned induction of parturition.

REFERENCES

1. Bleul U. Peripartales Monitoring des Rinderfetus und Konsequenzen für die Therapie der Asphyxie [Peripartal monitoring of the bovine fetus and consequences for therapy of asphyxia]. Habilitation Thesis, Clinic of Reproductive Medicine. Zurich, Switzerland 2008.
2. Johanson JM, Berger PJ. Birth weight as a predictor of calving ease and perinatal mortality in Holstein cattle. J Dairy Sci 2003;86:3745–55.

3. Mee JF. Newborn dairy calf management. Vet Clin North Am Food Anim Pract 2008;24:1–17.

4. Berchtold M, Zaremba W, Grunert E. Kälberkrankheiten. In: Walser K, Bostedt H, editors. Neugeborenen- und Säuglingskunde. Stuttgart (Germany): Enke; 1990. p. 266–71.

5. Pickel M, Zaremba W, Grunert E. Comparison of arterial and venous blood gas and acid-base values in prematurely born healthy calves or calves with a late asphyxia. Zentralbl Veterinarmed A 1989;36:653–63.

6. Zaremba W, Grunert E, Aurich JE. Prophylaxis of respiratory distress syndrome in premature calves by administration of dexamethasone or a prostaglandin F2 alpha analogue to their dams before parturition. Am J Vet Res 1997;58:404–7.

7. Adamson SL. Regulation of breathing at birth. J Dev Physiol 1991;15:45–52.

8. Gluckman PD, Gunn TR, Johnston BM. The effect of cooling on breathing and shivering in unanaesthetized fetal lambs in utero. J Physiol 1983;343: 495–506.

9. Mortola JP. Gestation and birth. In: Mortola JP, editor. Respiratory physiology of newborn mammals: a comparative perspective. Baltimore (MD): John Hopkins University Press; 2001. p. 4–42.

10. Reeves JT, Leathers JE. Circulatory changes following birth of the calf and the effect of hypoxia. Circ Res 1964;15:343–54.

11. Harding R, Sigger JN, Wickham PJD, et al. The regulation of flow of pulmonary fluid in fetal sheep. Respir Physiol 1984;57:47–59.

12. Zimmermann LJI, Janssen DJMT, Tibboel D, et al. Surfactant metabolism in the neonate. Neonatology 2005;87:296–307.

13. Takahashi A, Waring AJ, Amirkhanian J, et al. Structure-function relationships of bovine pulmonary surfactant proteins: SP-B and SP-C. Biochim Biophys Acta 1990;1044:43–9.

14. Crouch EC. Collectins and pulmonary host defense. Am J Respir Cell Mol Biol 1998;19:177–201.

15. Ainsworth SB. Pathophysiology of neonatal respiratory distress syndrome: implications for early treatment strategies. Treat Respir Med 2005;4:423–37.

16. Finer NN. Surfactant use for neonatal lung injury: beyond respiratory distress syndrome. Paediatr Respir Rev 2004;5:S289–97.

17. Danlois F, Zaltash S, Johansson J, et al. Pulmonary surfactant from healthy Belgian white and blue and Holstein Friesian calves: biochemical and biophysical comparison. Vet J 2003;165:65–72.

18. Danlois F, Zaltash S, Johansson J, et al. Very low surfactant protein C contents in newborn Belgian white and blue calves with respiratory distress syndrome. Biochem J 2000;351(Pt 3):779–87.

19. Eigenmann UJ, Grunert E, Koppe U. Delayed asphyxia of calves (delivered prematurely by caesarean section). Berl Munch Tierarztl Wochenschr 1981;94: 249–54.

20. Eigenmann UJ, Schoon HA, Jahn D, et al. Neonatal respiratory distress syndrome in the calf. Vet Rec 1984;114:141–4.

21. Vestberg J. Respiratory problems of newborn calves. Vet Clin North Am Food Anim Pract 1997;13:411–24.

22. Reynolds EOR, Jacobson HN, Motoyama EK, et al. The effect of immaturity and prenatal asphyxia on the lungs and pulmonary function of newborn lamb: the experimental production of respiratory distress. Pediatrics 1965;35: 382–92.

23. Jobe AH, Kramer BW, Moss TJ, et al. Decreased indicators of lung injury with continuous positive expiratory pressure in preterm lambs. Pediatr Res 2002;52: 387–92.
24. Mescher EJ, Platzker AC, Ballard PL, et al. Ontogeny of tracheal fluid, pulmonary surfactant, and plasma corticoids in the fetal lamb. J Appl Phys 1975;39: 1017–21.
25. Varga J. Cardiopulmonary adaptation to the extra uterine life in newborn calves during the first 24 hours PhD Thesis, Department and Clinic of Obstetrics and Reproduction, Budapest 2000.
26. Wauer RR. Das atemnotsyndrom (ANS). In: Wauer RR, editor. Surfactanttherapie Grundlagen, Diagnostik, Therapie. 2nd edition. Stuttgart (Germany): Thieme; 1997. p. 2–20.
27. Jobe A. Respiratory distress syndrome: new therapeutic approaches to a complex pathophysiology. Adv Pediatr 1983;30:93–130.
28. Kajimoto H, Hashimoto K, Bonnet SN, et al. Oxygen activates the Rho/Rho-kinase pathway and induces RhoB and ROCK-1 expression in human and rabbit ductus arteriosus by increasing mitochondria-derived reactive oxygen species: a newly recognized mechanism for sustaining ductal constriction. Circulation 2007;115: 1777–88.
29. Schuijt G. Aspects of obstetrical perinatology in cattle. Utrecht (The Netherlands): Proefschrift Universiteit Utrecht; 1992.
30. Lopez A, Bildfell R. Pulmonary inflammation associated with aspirated meconium and epithelial cells in calves. Vet Pathol 1992;29:104–11.
31. Schoon HA, Kikovic D. Morphological demonstration and pathogenetic evaluation of amniotic fluid aspiration to confirm the diagnosis of pulmonary asphyxia of newborn calves and foals. Dtsch Tierarztl Wochenschr 1987;94:73–6.
32. Knottenbelt D, Holdstock N, Madigan JE. Equine neonatology. London: Elsevier; 2004.
33. National Center for Health Statistics. Advance report of final mortality statistics, 1991. In: Public Health Service C, vol 42. Hyattsville (MD): US Department of Health and Human Services; 1993.
34. Bleul UT, Bircher BM, Kahn WK. Effect of intranasal oxygen administration on blood gas variables and outcome in neonatal calves with respiratory distress syndrome: 20 cases (2004–2006). J Am Vet Med Assoc 2008;233:289–93.
35. Pirie HM, Selman IE. Acute respiratory distress syndrome in a premature calf. Vet Rec 1969;85:293–4.
36. Grunert E, Schoon HA, Bölting D. Case report of respiratory distress syndrome (late asphyxia) and hypothyreosis in a newborn calf. Tierarztl Umsch 1992;47: 344–51.
37. Clements JA, Avery ME. Lung surfactant and neonatal respiratory distress syndrome. Am J Respir Crit Care Med 1998;157:S59–66.
38. Verder H, Albertsen P, Ebbesen F, et al. Nasal continuous positive airway pressure and early surfactant therapy for respiratory distress syndrome in newborns of less than 30 weeks' gestation. Pediatrics 1999;103:e24.
39. Zerbe H, Zimmermann DK, Bendix A. Neonatal asphyxia in calves: diagnosis, therapy and prophylaxis. Tierarztl Prax Ausg G Grosstiere Nutztiere 2008;36:163–9.
40. Fok T-F. Respiratory distress syndrome. In: Yu VYH, Feng Z, Tsang RC, et al, editors. Textbook of neonatal medicine. Hong Kong: Hong Kong University Press; 1996. p. 265–74.
41. Jobe AH. Pharmacology review: why surfactant works for respiratory distress syndrome. NeoReviews 2006;7:e95–106.

42. Bleul U, Lejeune B, Schwantag S, et al. Blood gas and acid-base analysis of arterial blood in 57 newborn calves. Vet Rec 2007;161:688–91.
43. Nagy O, Kovac G, Seidel H, et al. The effect of arterial blood sampling sites on blood gases and acid-base balance parameters in calves. Acta Vet Hung 2001;49:331–40.
44. Mayfeldt BK. Der Säure-Basen-Haushalt. In: Die Blutgasfibel. 3rd edition. Copenhagen (Denmark): Radiometer; 2004. p. 51–82.
45. Deshpande SA, Platt MPW. Association between blood lactate and acid-base status and mortality in ventilated babies. Arch Dis Child Fetal Neonatal Ed 1997;76:F15–20.
46. Bedenice D. Prognose und Risikofaktoren der röntgenologischen Lungenveränderungen neonataler Fohlen [Risk factors and prognostic variables of radiographic pulmonary disease in neonatal foals]. Dissertation Thesis, Clinical for Animal Reproduction, Faculty of Veterinary Medicine, Freie Universität Berlin, Germany 2004.
47. Verma RP. Respiratory distress syndrome of the newborn infant. Obstet Gynecol Surv 1995;50:542–55.
48. Koterba AM. Respiratory disease: approach to diagnosis. In: Koterba AM, Drummond WH, editors. Equine clinical neonatology. Philadelphia: Lippincott Williams and Wilkins; 1990. p. 153–76.
49. Lamb CR, O'Callaghan MW, Paradis MR. Thoracic radiography in the neonatal foal: a preliminary report. Vet Radiol Ultrasound 1990;31:11–6.
50. Hill JR, Roussel AJ, Cibelli JB, et al. Clinical and pathologic features of cloned transgenic calves and fetuses (13 case studies). Theriogenology 1999;51:1451–65.
51. Toulova M, Vojtisek B, Tomsik F. Lecithin and sphingomyelin in the amniotic fluid of cows in late pregnancy. Vet Med (Praha) 1981;26:129–34.
52. Gluck L, Kulovich MV. Lecithin-sphingomyelin ratios in amniotic fluid in normal and abnormal pregnancy. Am J Obstet Gynecol 1973;115:539–46.
53. Uystepruyst CH, Coghe J, Dorts TH, et al. Effect of three resuscitation procedures on respiratory and metabolic adaptation to extra uterine life in newborn calves. Vet J 2002;163:30–44.
54. Uystepruyst C, Coghe J, Dorts T, et al. Sternal recumbency or suspension by the hind legs immediately after delivery improves respiratory and metabolic adaptation to extra uterine life in newborn calves delivered by caesarean section. Vet Res 2002;33:709–24.
55. Lammoglia MA, Bellows RA, Grings EE, et al. Effects of feeding beef females supplemental fat during gestation on cold tolerance in newborn calves. J Anim Sci 1999;77:824–34.
56. Karapinar T, Dabak M. Treatment of premature calves with clinically diagnosed respiratory distress syndrome. J Vet Intern Med 2008;22:462–6.
57. Greenough A, Donn SM. Matching ventilatory support strategies to respiratory pathophysiology. Clin Perinatol 2007;34:35–53.
58. Kahn W, Palmer J, Vaala W. Assisted respiration techniques for foals in a unit for intensive care of newborn large animals. Tierarztl Prax 1992;20:492–502.
59. Palmer JE. Ventilatory support of the critically ill foal. Vet Clin North Am Equine Pract 2005;21:457–86.
60. Berchtold M, Zaremba W, Grunert E. Störungen im perinatalen Zeitraum. In: Walser K, Bostedt H, editors. Neugeborenen- und Säuglingskrankheiten. Stuttgart (Germany): Ferdinand Enke Verlag; 1990. p. 265–71.

61. Kesting K. Postpartum care of cow and calf. In: Youngquist RS, Threlfall WR, editors. Current therapy in large animal theriogenology. 2nd edition. Philadelphia: Elsevier Saunders; 2006. p. 324–9.

62. Noakes DE, Arthur GH. The newborn and its care. In: Noakes DE, Parkinson T, England G, et al, editors. Arthur's veterinary reproduction and obstetrics. 8th edition. London: W.B. Saunders; 2001. p. 198–202.

63. Tin W, Milligan DW, Pennefather P, et al. Pulse oximetry, severe retinopathy, and outcome at one year in babies of less than 28 weeks gestation. Arch Dis Child 2001;84:F106–10.

64. Buczinski S, Boysen SR, Fecteau G. Mechanical ventilation of a cloned calf in respiratory failure. Journal of Veterinary Emergency and Critical Care 2007;17: 179–83.

65. Brunson DB. Ventilatory support of the newborn calf. Compendium on Continuing Education for the Practicing Veterinarian 1981;3:S47–52.

66. Manning AM. Oxygen therapy and toxicity. Vet Clin North Am Small Anim Pract 2002;32:1005–20.

67. Bleul U, Bachofner C, Stocker H, et al. Comparison of sodium bicarbonate and carbicarb for the treatment of metabolic acidosis in newborn calves. Vet Rec 2005;156:202–6.

68. Bleul UT, Schwantag SC, Kahn WK. Effects of hypertonic sodium bicarbonate solution on electrolyte concentrations and enzyme activities in newborn calves with respiratory and metabolic acidosis. Am J Vet Res 2007;68:850–7.

69. Bachofner C. Die Behandlung metabolischer Azidosen bei neugeborenen Kälbern mit Carbicarb [Carbicarb for the treatment of metabolic acidosis in newborn calves]. Dissertation Thesis, Zurich, Switzerland; 2003.

70. Genicot B, Close R, Lindsey JK, et al. Pulmonary function changes induced by three regimens of bronchodilating agents in calves with acute respiratory distress syndrome. Vet Rec 1995;137:183–6.

Septicemia and Meningitis in the Newborn Calf

Gilles Fecteau, DMV [a],*, Bradford P. Smith, DVM [b],
Lisle W. George, DVM, PhD [c]

KEYWORDS

- Neonatal sepsis • Bacteremia • Sepsis
- Failure of passive transfer
- Systemic inflammatory response syndrome
- Multiple organ dysfunction syndromes • Meningitis

Neonatal septicemia, bacteremia, and sepsis are terms that have been used to describe newborn calves with a systemic infection. There are slight differences in the definition of each term. "Bacteremia" refers to a laboratory finding where a bacterium has been detected in the blood of a patient by culture methods. In general, the term does not necessarily imply a systemic effect of the bacteria. One may compare the term with leukopenia that describes a laboratory finding but does not necessarily imply that the patient is suffering from any specific disease. "Septicemia" is a term referring to a systemic disease associated with the presence and to some extent the persistence of pathogenic microorganisms or their toxins in the blood. The term implies that the patient is ill. It also includes all microorganisms, and is not limited to bacteria. "Sepsis" is defined as a combination of an infection (or suspected infection) and a systemic inflammatory response. The infection source can be focal or generalized and can be identified or at least suspected. In many cases the calf's immune defense mechanisms are able to control the invading bacteria, but in other cases this does not occur efficiently. There is a balance between an effective immune response and an immune response that cascades and results in adverse effects, such as shock. The systemic inflammatory response syndrome is the host inflammatory cascade initiated when the host defense system either fails to recognize or to clear the infection. The identification of systemic inflammatory response syndrome in human medicine requires four criteria: (1) core temperature abnormality (increase or decrease); (2) heart rate abnormality (tachycardia or bradycardia); (3) tachypnea; and (4) leukocyte count abnormality (leucopenia or leukocytosis). Septic shock is the aggravation of the septic

[a] Faculté de Médecine Vétérinaire, Université de Montréal, 3200 Rue Sicotte, CP 5000, St. Hyacinthe, QC J2S 7C6, Québec, Canada
[b] School of Veterinary Medicine, University of California, Davis, Davis, CA 95616, USA
[c] St. Matthews University, Grand Cayman, British West Indies
* Corresponding author.
E-mail address: gilles.fecteau@umontreal.ca (G. Fecteau).

Vet Clin Food Anim 25 (2009) 195–208
doi:10.1016/j.cvfa.2008.10.004
0749-0720/08/$ – see front matter © 2009 Elsevier Inc. All rights reserved.

vetfood.theclinics.com

state to a point where hypotension or hypoperfusion develops. Septic shock is a combination of variable degrees of hypovolemic (fluid losses through capillary leakage), cardiogenic (from myocardial depressant effects of sepsis), and distributive shock (decreased systemic vascular resistance). In between sepsis and septic shock, there is also a definition of severe sepsis implying that organ dysfunction progressively develops. Multiple organ dysfunction syndrome refers to a clinical situation where a critically ill patient is so severely affected by a primary pathologic condition that several organs fail. The definitions that are used in human medicine were accepted at an international pediatric sepsis consensus conference.[1] In view of the considerable new information regarding pathogenesis of sepsis and potentially useful therapeutic agents, the need for a rigorous definition becomes evident. Without appropriate and universal terminology and case definition, scientific evaluation of any treatment regimen becomes virtually impossible. Although the definitions are necessary and useful for research purposes, when treating a patient, they may not fall clearly into the proposed categories no matter how well they are defined.

For purposes of developing a clinical scoring system, the authors have proposed and used the definition presented in **Table 1**.[2] The clinician is often faced with making decisions as to whether or not to treat the calf for bacteremia without benefit of laboratory results. Neonatal septicemia in calves is a condition that has been described for more than 100 years. In North America, it is traditionally described as disease affecting young dairy calves under 2 weeks of age and suffering from failure of passive transfer. Most are exposed to a virulent bacterium, such as *Escherichia coli* or *Salmonella*, and develop systemic infections. The disease is reported to be sporadic or epidemic if management practices result in a high prevalence of failure of passive transfer calves or high exposure of calves to bacterial pathogens. Septicemia can also occur in calves up to 10 or 12 weeks of age with apparently normal passive transfer when they encounter virulent *Salmonella sp* or *Mannheimia hemolytica*.

ETIOLOGY

Escherichia coli have long been incriminated as the principle microbial agent responsible for neonatal septicemia in the bovine. "Colisepticemia" has been used to refer to a vast array of clinical presentations. Several studies have shown the diversity of bacteria associated with the disease. **Table 2** lists various isolates and their relative frequency as presented in studies from different research groups. Clearly, although *E coli* are the most frequent etiologic agent, it is certainly not the only agent.

Table 1 Definition of septicemia		
Criteria	Positive	Negative
1. Blood culture growth (rapidity)	<48 h	>48 h
2. Bacteria cultured	Pathogen	Contaminant
3. Complete blood count (2 of 3)	Yes	No
White cell count	Elevated/reduced	Normal
Fibrinogen concentration	>5 g/L (>500 mg/dL)	<5 g/L (<500 mg/dL)
Bands neutrophils (%)	>2%	<2%

When 2 out of the 3 criteria were met the animal was considered septicemic.
From Fecteau G, Paré J, Van Metre DC, et al. Use of a clinical sepsis score for predicting bacteremia in neonatal dairy calves on a calf rearing farm. Can Vet J 1997;38:101–4; with permission.

Table 2
Bacteria cultured from the blood of septicemic calves from four different studies

	Fecteau et al[15] n (%)	Lofstedt et al[22] n (%)	Hariharan et al[37] n (%)	Aldridge et al[38] n (%)
Gram-negative enterics				
Escherichia coli	26 (50)	29 (55)	17 (65)	4 (57)
Klebsiella pneumoniae	4 (8)	–	–	–
Klebsiella spp	2 (4)	–	–	–
Klebsiella oxytoca	1 (2)	–	–	–
Salmonella dublin	2 (4)	–	–	–
Salmonella typhimurium	2 (4)	–	–	–
Salmonella spp	–	–	–	1 (14)
Campylobacter spp	–	8 (16)	–	–
Campylobacter fetus subsp fetus	1 (2)	–	2 (8)	–
Enterobacter cloacae	1 (2)	–	–	–
Hafnia spp	–	–	–	1 (14)
Citrobacter spp	–	–	1 (4)	–
Gram-positive cocci				
Staphylococcus spp	1 (2)	5 (10)	–	–
Staphylococcus aureus	1 (2)	–	–	–
Staphylococcus hyicus	1 (2)	–	–	–
Staphylococcus simulans	1 (2)	–	–	–
Group D Streptococci	–	–	3 (12)	–
Nonhemolytic Streptococcus spp	1 (2)	–	–	1 (14)
Aerococcus viridans	1 (2)	–	–	–
Enterococcus spp	–	1 (2)	–	–
Gram-negative non enterics				
Pseudomonas aeruginosa	–	2 (4)	–	–
Mannheimia haemolytica	–	1 (2)	1 (4)	–
Acinetobacter spp	–	1 (2)	–	–
Gram-positive rods				
Arcanobacterium pyogenes	–	1 (2)	1 (4)	–
Bacillus spp	2 (4)	1 (2)	1 (4)	–
Listeria spp	1 (2)	–	–	–
Anaerobes				
Bacteroides eggerthii	1 (2)	–	–	–
Bacteroides thetaiomicron	1 (2)	–	–	–
Prevotella bivia	1 (2)	–	–	–
Prevotella loescheii	1 (2)	–	–	–
Clostridium spp	–	1 (2)	–	1 (14)
Total	51	50	26	7

Salmonella, Campylobacter, Klebsiella, and different Staphylococcus have also been isolated from the blood of calves.

The relative importance of the different invasive (as opposed to enteropathogenic) E coli groups varies between the geographic regions studied, but the literature specifically recognizes the significance of groups O78, O137, and O153.[3] The bacteria that successfully causes septicemia must first invade the host by an entry point, survive the host's specific and nonspecific immune response mechanisms, and finally spread through the body ultimately to cause damage. Adhesion capacity, serum resistance, production of aerobactin, and the synthesis of toxins are all recognized as potential virulence factors. Once in tissues or blood, bacterial cell wall lipopolysaccharide, also called "endotoxin," causes a number of profound physiologic responses including anorexia, abnormal thermoregulation, leukopenia, altered heart rate, reduced cardiac output and blood pressure, and ultimately collapse and death.[4]

PATHOGENESIS

Newborn calves are particularly at risk for developing septicemia because they are dependent on colostral antibodies and cells (passive transfer of immunity) for ultimate protection. Calves lack a normal adult intestinal flora and when born in a heavily contaminated environment, colonization with virulent pathogens may occur before the establishment of normal competitive flora. Septicemia may also be associated with a primary site of infection (umbilical infection or any other primary focus of infection).

The association between passively acquired immunoglobulins and neonatal septicemia is well established in the bovine. Colostral leukocytes enhance humoral immunity.[5,6] Neutrophil function in neonatal calves is less effective as compared with adults.[7-9] Elevated cortisol during the first 7 to 10 days of age may play a role in the neutrophil depletion function.[10] Competence of the immune system is dependent on age of the calf and antigen.[11] Colostrum may suppress the humoral response to specific antigens.[12]

The source of pathogenic bacteria is most likely the contaminated environment. Infection may also be acquired in utero through the placenta or during parturition. The feeding of contaminated colostrum can also be an important source of infection in dairy calves.[13] The contagious nature of neonatal septicemia in calves has not been investigated thoroughly. From a few studies performed in the 1960s and 1970s, it was postulated that clusters or outbreaks of E coli septicemia occur when the bacteria was present in the environment. Pathogenic bacteria can be isolated from nasal secretions and saliva of sick calves.[3] A large number of bacteria can also be excreted in the urine, and can contribute to the dissemination of pathogenic agents in the environment.[3] The bacteria isolated from blood may also sometimes be isolated from the intestine of the same subject, but not in all cases.[14] In one study, a cluster of septicemia associated with the same O serogroups was observed in a large calf operation.[15] Bacteriologic survey of the farm indicated that the pathogenic bacteria were located in specific areas of the farm rather than being disseminated. These results suggest that a common source of virulent isolates could contribute to the incidence of the disease.

A primary entry site for bacteria is the intestine. In the first postnatal hours, nonspecific pinocytosis may allow the bacteria and immunoglobulins to enter the systemic circulation. In older calves with enteritis (bacterial, viral, or protozoal), the loss of integrity of the intestinal wall may allow bacteria to gain access to the circulation. The nasal mucosa, nasopharynx, and the oropharynx are also possible entry points, particularly for invasive organisms, such as Salmonella. The umbilicus and the related internal structures remain an important infection site. In older calves (second and third week of age), a primary site of infection (septic joint, septic growth plate, pneumonia, or

meningitis) could also be the source of septicemia or it may represent the consequences of septicemia.

Infection and the host inflammatory responses need to be differentiated. The immune response, in combination with the reticuloendothelial system, prevents the development of sepsis from an opportunistic or pathogenic invasion. This initiates an
inflammatory cascade involving highly toxic mediators, which if uncontrolled eventually lead to systemic inflammatory response syndrome and subsequent multiple organ
dysfunction syndrome. There is a balance between an appropriate, yet effective, immune response and an overzealous response to the bacteria or their toxins.[4]

Endotoxin (lipopolysaccharide), mannose, and glycoprotein components of the cell
wall of gram-negative bacteria bind to macrophages, leading to activation and expression of inflammatory genes. Superantigens or toxins associated with gram-positive
bacteria may also activate circulating macrophages and lymphocytes, which release
cytokines and initiate an inflammatory mediator cascade. Consequences of the initiation of the cascade include the production of arachidonic acid metabolites, release of
myocardial depressant factors and endogenous opiates, activation of the complement system, and the production and release of many other mediators of sepsis.

The following mediators are known to be involved in the inflammatory cascade:
tumor necrosis factor; interleukins-1, -2, -4, -6, and -8; platelet-activating factor;
interferon-γ; eicosanoids (leukotrienes B_4, C_4, D_4, and E_4; thromboxane A_2; prostaglandins E_2 and I_2); granulocyte-macrophage colony-stimulating factor; endothe-
lium-derived relaxing factor; endothelin-1; complement fragments C3a and C5a;
toxic oxygen radicals; proteolytic enzymes from polymorphonuclear neutrophils;
platelets; transforming growth factor-β; vascular permeability factor; macrophage-de-
rived procoagulant and inflammatory cytokine; bradykinin; thrombin; coagulation
factors; fibrin; plasminogen activator inhibitor; myocardial depressant substance;
β-endorphin; heat shock proteins; and adhesion molecules (endothelin-derived adhesion molecule [E-selectin]; intercellular adhesion molecule-1; vascular adhesion
molecule-1).[16]

All mediators have numerous effects, which if uncontrolled may lead to the systemic
ultimately clinical signs of sepsis. Increased endothelial permeability, myocardial depression, and intermediary metabolism disruption are important complications that
eventually lead to hypovolemia, hypotension, and respiratory failure.

CLINICAL MANIFESTATIONS

Septicemia should be included in the differential diagnosis of many conditions affecting the calf. Septicemia should be seriously considered whenever there is multiple organ dysfunction, or when severe cardiorespiratory signs are encountered. Classic
septicemia is described as a condition affecting newborn calves between 2 and 6
days of age. The progression is rapid and most often fatal. Very early in the disease,
the clinical signs are vague, nonspecific, and likely attributed to other disease. An alteration in mental status ranging from a mild depression to coma is commonly observed. Lack of suckling ability or enthusiasm toward nursing is an early nonspecific
clinical sign. Abnormal rectal temperature (fever or hypothermia) is not consistent;
however, sustained tachycardia and eventually tachypnea develop. Hyperemia of
the mucous membranes and scleral injection are frequently observed. Capillary fragil-
ity may initiate petechiation of the mucous membranes. Eventually, hypotension and
clinical signs that are associated with poor cardiac output (slow capillary refill, diminished peripheral pulse, cold extremities, and decreased urine output) become prominent. Hypovolemia usually develops. Diarrhea is not present in all cases but is

common in the terminal stages of septicemia. Immunoglobulin-deficient calves may be predisposed to both enteric and nonenteric infections, so concurrent gastrointestinal diseases can lead to diarrhea.

A less fulminant form of septicemia may occur in slightly older calves (7–28 days) in which localized infection is evident (arthritis, growth plate infection, hypopyon, meningitis, pneumonia). Some of these calves may also have diarrhea. Possible explanations for this subacute form of septicemia are partial failure of passive transfer or exposure to less virulent bacteria. The meningitis complication is discussed later as a separate clinical entity.

DIAGNOSIS

The early diagnosis of septicemia remains a challenge in veterinary medicine and in human perinatology. Neonatal calves may be assigned to two clinical groups: those presented with clinical signs compatible with septicemia, and those presented without clinical signs but considered at risk based on the history. Because of the rapid deterioration seen in many cases of septicemia and the most likely success of early treatment, most clinicians institute antimicrobial treatment based on a presumptive diagnosis without laboratory confirmation.

Early clinical signs of septicemia can be subtle and nonspecific. The presence of focal infection or a clinical picture consistent with infection increases the suspicion of sepsis. The definitive diagnosis of septicemia/bacteremia, however, is based on a blood culture. The jugular vein should be clipped, shaved, scrubbed, and disinfected before sampling. Two samples of 5 to 10 mL of whole blood (label on the blood culture bottle indicates the precise quantity of blood to add) are drawn using a sterile syringe and needle (60-minute interval between the two samples). The blood is then transferred into the blood culture bottle using a new sterile needle. The purpose of taking two samples is to increase the chances of isolating the bacteria and to facilitate the interpretation of results if opportunistic or contaminating bacteria are found in one sample. The bottle is then submitted to the laboratory for culture and susceptibility testing. If the bottle is not submitted immediately, it should be stored at room temperature or at 37°C. A negative result must be interpreted with caution because many factors may interfere with bacterial isolation from a blood culture. These include prior antibiotic therapy, presence of opsonizing antibodies, number of bacteria, and course of the diseases. Cultures of other body fluids, such as joint, cerebrospinal, peritoneal, or pleural fluids, may be helpful for bacteriologic diagnosis whenever the blood culture is negative.

Some laboratory findings may increase the suspicion of septicemia. Hematologic abnormalities of septicemia vary with the severity of the disease. Abnormal neutrophil count (neutrophilia and neutropenia) and increased immature forms (bands, myelocytes, metamyelocytes) are frequently seen. Vacuolation, toxic granules, and Döhle bodies may be observed in neutrophils. Fibrinogen concentration is often elevated. Thrombocytopenia may be present in severe cases. One observational study of suspected septic shock in calves found that 8 out of 12 calves had at least three abnormal coagulation parameters. Activated partial thromboplastin time, prothrombin time, thrombin time, fibrinogen, and fibrinogen degradation products were included in the coagulation profile. The most common abnormal parameters were activated partial thromboplastin time and prothrombin time in seven cases.[17] Hypoglycemia, or less often hyperglycemia, may be observed. A metabolic acidosis is also frequently present in septic calves. Lactic acidosis occurs as the disease progresses, resulting from increased tissue L-lactate production and a decreased hepatic clearance, and intestinal production and absorption of bacterial D-lactic acid. Renal and liver parameters and the laboratory tests to assess them are often abnormal in severe cases. Some calves develop respiratory disease (respiratory distress syndrome) or pneumonia, and suffer from hypoxemia or hypoventilation. Medical imaging of the chest (radiograph and ultrasound) can also be valuable ancillary tests if economics permit. Thoracic radiographs of septicemic calves may show increased interstitial patterns. Analysis of centesis fluid from the pleura (or peritoneum) may show purulent inflammation with or without bacteria. Septicemic calves have low serum proteins, caused by low globulins. Plasma IgG concentrations that are below 500 mg/dL are consistent with a diagnosis of failure of passive transfer.[18]

Diagnostic markers for neonatal sepsis could be helpful if they have a well-defined cut-off value to allow differentiation between the infected and noninfected patient and would aid early detection of the disease. In general, markers belong to one of the following categories: cell surface markers (CD11b, CD64, and CD69); chemokines and cytokines (interleukin-6 and -8); or acute-phase reactants (C-reactive proteins, procalcitonin, and serum amyloid A).[19]

SCORING SYSTEM TO HELP EARLY DIAGNOSIS OF SEPSIS AND SEPTICEMIA

The most important indicators to aid in the diagnosis of septicemia have been studied in human infants and foals.[20,21] In calves, Lofstedt and colleagues[22] presented two models for predicting septicemia based on all possible predictors studied. Fecteau and colleagues[2] described a clinical score intended to be used on the farm and a more complete scoring system intended to be used in patients on which ancillary tests were performed. Predictors included in the different models are presented in **Table 3**.

RELATED COMPLICATIONS TO SEPSIS: NEONATAL BACTERIAL SUPPURATIVE MENINGITIS

The collective role of the meninges is to support, protect, and contribute to the irrigation and nourishment of the central nervous system. Meningitis is defined as the inflammation of one or more of the three covering layers of the meninges (dura mater, arachnoid, pia mater) in the central nervous system. The spaces that form between the arachnoid and the pia mater contain the cerebrospinal fluid (CSF). The CSF protects and nourishes the central nervous system. The two most clinically important cisternae are the cisterna magna and the lumbosacral cistern, both of which may be used to collect CSF on living animals.

Etiologic Agents

Neonatal bacterial suppurative meningitis and bacterial sepsis are often linked, and the same types of bacteria are responsible. Gram-negative bacteria, *E coli* in particular, are reported to be the most common meningeal pathogens in calves.[23–26] Some *E coli* virulence factors may be of importance in the development of neonatal bacterial suppurative meningitis because the successful meningeal pathogen must overcome sequential host defense mechanisms to reach the CSF and replicate. *E coli* that are found in meningitic calves are nonhemolytic; synthesize hydroxymate and colicin V; and express the 31a surface antigen, antibody resistance, aerobactin production, and fimbriation.[27]

Pathogenesis

The means of pathogen entry into the meninges is poorly understood. Specific mechanisms may include the development of a sustained and high-grade bacteremia in the

Table 3
Parameters included in the predictive model for septicemia by two different research groups

Parameters	Lofstedt et al[22]	Fecteau et al[2]
Clinical (only)		
Age	<5 d	>7 d
Focal infection	Yes	Yes
Posture	Recumbent	–
Suckling reflex	Weak to absent	–
Summation of five clinical signs including: hydration, scleral injection, ability to stand (attitude), umbilicus, and fecal appearance	–	Total score
Laboratory and clinical		
Glucose	–	<5.6 mmol/L (<101 mg/dL)
Creatinine (moderate increase)	176–500 mmol/L (1–2 mg/dL)	–
Creatinine (marked increase)	>500 mmol/L (>2 mg/dL)	–
Neutrophil toxic changes	>1%	–
Immature neutrophils (bands)	–	>1%
Fibrinogen	–	<3 g/L or >8 g/L (<300 mg/dL or >800 mg/dL)
Serum proteins	–	>55 g/L (5.5 g/dL) >45 g/L and <55 g/L (>4.5 g/dL and <5.5 g/dL) <45 g/L (4.5 g/dL)
Failure of passive transfer	Yes	–
Age	–	>7 d
Heart rate	–	<100 or >160
Respiratory rate	–	>65
Focal infection	Yes	Yes
Posture (ability to stand)	Recumbent	0: standing to 3: recumbent
Suckling reflex	Weak to absent	–

Values in parenthesis are in American units.
— means that this parameter was not used for the final model. The variable may or may not have been available to study depending of the study design.

highly perfused dural venous system and choroid plexuses, adherence of S fimbriae from some strains of E coli, or the phagocytosis of the pathogens by circulating monocytes and endocytosis through the microvascular endothelial cells.[28] Bacteria survive and proliferate in the poorly defended CSF. Complement is essentially nonexistent in CSF, which when combined with low numbers of specific antibodies leads to inadequate opsonization of meningeal pathogens. Despite an early influx of leukocytes into the CSF in bacterial meningitis, the host defense system remains suboptimal because opsonic activity is deficient.[29] The sequelae of meningitis are associated with the release of cytokines and the direct effects of bacterial invasion. Bacteria may release endotoxins, which lead to inflammatory infiltrates that cause thromboses of the arachnoidal or subependymal veins. Congestion or hemorrhagic infarction may follow with subsequent necrosis of nerve cells.[30] Inflammatory changes in the subarachnoid space may affect the choroid plexus, decreasing the absorption of fluid and potentially creating hypertensive hydrocephalus.

Clinical Manifestations

Calves suffering from neonatal bacterial suppurative meningitis are often presented because they have lost their suckle reflex and appear lethargic. Previous treatment for undifferentiated diarrhea is common. Fever is often present, unless nonsteroidal anti-inflammatory drugs have been administered or if the animal is in an extremely cold environment. The calves may have an extended head and neck (**Fig. 1**). Attempts to flex or reposition the neck often result in a tonic extension and thrashing of the limbs. Hyperesthesia is common. With time, a profound depression develops and eventually the animal becomes comatose and nonresponsive, or may develop tonic-clonic seizures. Spinal reflexes are described to be exaggerated.

Diagnosis

The presumptive diagnosis of bacterial meningitis is based on demonstration of failure of passive transfer; presence of a septic focus, such as omphalophlebitis or septic arthritis; and the presence of the clinical signs described previously. The definitive diagnosis, however, is based on an abnormal CSF analysis. Collection of CSF from the lumbosacral space is easy and safe in ruminants. Suppurative CSF can be obtained from the lumbosacral cistern of animals with neonatal bacterial suppurative meningitis (**Fig. 2**). The fluid must be handled carefully to preserve cellular integrity, and rapidly cooled and transported to the laboratory. Normal values and standard techniques for CSF collection have been described.[31] Microscopic examination of CSF is essential for accurate diagnosis of neonatal bacterial suppurative meningitis. The number of nucleated cells and the protein concentration is markedly increased. The proportion of neutrophils may reach as high as 80%.[23–25] The ratio of CSF to plasma glucose

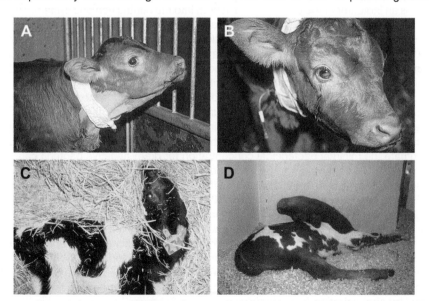

Fig. 1. Calves exhibiting clinical signs of meningitis secondary to septicemia. (*A*) The calf is depressed and maintains an extended neck when manipulated. (*B*) The presence of fibrin and white blood cells in the anterior chamber of the eye (hypopyon) is suspected. (*C, D*) Calves with more advanced meningitis.

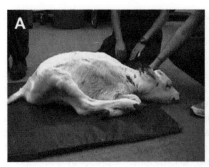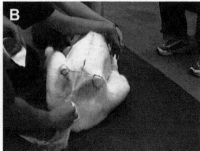

Fig. 2. (*A*) This figure demonstrates one technique for performing a lumbosacral CSF tap. Others prefer the standing position or lateral recumbency. Note that the legs are brought forward to widen the lumbosacral space. (*B*) Proper location to attempt collection of CSF fluid. (*Courtesy of* Geoff W. Smith, DVM, MS, PhD, Raleigh, NC.)

concentration is less than one in animals with bacterial meningitis because of bacterial metabolism of glucose in the CSF. Xanthochromia (yellow color) is considered abnormal but is inconsistent. Free or intracellular bacteria may be observed in some cases.

Treatment

Treatment of bacterial meningitis is difficult and the mortality rate is high. Antimicrobials are the most important therapeutic modality for treatment of bacterial meningitis in calves.

The physicochemical properties (lipid solubility, molecular weight, protein binding, and ionization) and the pharmacokinetics of a drug influence its penetration through the blood-brain barrier. The CSF to blood concentration ratio of an antibiotic at steady state is an indicator of the penetration of a drug into the central nervous system. These ratios are described for several antimicrobials used in human medicine and laboratory animals. In farm animals, however, very little is known about these values.[32] Another key factor to consider is the suboptimal immune response in the CSF (lack of complement and antibody), which implies that to be effective an antibiotic needs to reach the minimal bactericidal concentration. The antibiotic concentrations in the CSF should be compared with the minimal bactericidal concentration value for the targeted pathogens rather than using the standard minimum inhibitory concentration. A drug that diffuses relatively easily into the CSF (eg, aminoglycosides) may not be the best choice because with standard dosing regimens the concentrations achieved may only approximate the minimal bactericidal concentration for gram-negative bacteria causing meningitis.[32] Alternatively, the β-lactams diffuse less efficiently through the blood-brain barrier; however, they can reach effective therapeutic concentrations in the CSF because larger doses can be used without risk of toxicity.[32] The expected ratios of CSF antibiotic concentrations to bacterial minimum inhibitory concentration (minimal bactericidal concentration is better but those numbers are not always available) are part of the equation. The data available on this are lacking in farm animals. One study available in calves presents the pharmacokinetics of florfenicol. The maximum concentration of florfenicol achieved in the CSF after a single IV dose of 20 mg/kg was 4.67 ± 1.51 μg/mL. The concentration in the CSF remained above the minimum inhibitory concentration for *Histophilus somni* for 20 hours.[33]

Practically, the chosen antimicrobial to treat meningitis in ruminants should have a good spectrum against gram-negative and gram-positive pathogens. The availability, formulation, and approval of the antibiotic for use in cattle are also taken into consideration. The actual selection is often reduced to third- or fourth-generation cephalosporins (ceftiofur, 5–10 mg/kg one to three times a day IM or IV); sodium ampicillin (10–20 mg/kg three times a day IV); fluoroquinolones (enrofloxacin, 5 mg/kg IV twice a day) in countries where the drug is approved for use; and trimethoprim-sulfonamide (5 mg/kg based on the trimethoprim two or three times a day IV). A combination of drugs is routinely used to broaden the spectrum (ampicillin-ceftiofur or ampicillin-trimethoprim-sulfonamide). Note that all the antimicrobial regimens previously described are empiric and derived from comparative medicine and clinical experience. Solid scientific evidence to corroborate those regimens in the treatment of bacterial meningitis in ruminants is not available at this time. One should remember that the inflammation present in the meninges increases drug diffusion toward the CSF, and as the animal improves, diffusion decreases. Intrathecal treatment does not improve the prognosis in human medicine and seems too complicated for use in farm animals.[30] Duration of therapy is empiric; 14 days seems to be the minimum in human medicine.[29,30]

Anti-inflammatory drugs are indicated in patients suffering from meningitis to improve their attitude in general and also to control the secondary effects of sepsis. The choice between steroidals and nonsteroidal anti-inflammatory agents remains empiric, however, in calves. In human medicine, steroidal anti-inflammatory agents are indicated in cases of meningitis associated with *Haemophilus influenzae*. In all other situations, the questions remain unanswered.[29] Convulsions should be treated appropriately. Diazepam (0.1–0.2 mg/kg), IV every 30 minutes, should be administered until convulsions are controlled.

GENERAL TREATMENT OF SEPTICEMIA IN NEONATAL CALVES

Neonatal septicemia is a critical condition with a high mortality. Treatment goals aim to (1) control the infection, (2) modulate the inflammatory response, and (3) support the animal during the critical phase.

Appropriate cultures should be obtained if judged necessary. Legally permitted antibiotics should be administered as soon as possible to minimize the bacterial load. The choice and the dosage of antibiotic depend on several factors and personal preferences, along with past experience, are often determinant elements. When selecting antimicrobial agents, bacterial resistance patterns on a particular farm should be considered. It is generally accepted that the intravenous route is preferable whenever possible and the spectrum must cover gram-negative and gram-positive bacteria. In a practical situation, appropriate antimicrobial choices are third- or fourth-generation cephalosporins (ceftiofur, 5–10 mg/kg one to three times a day IM or IV); sodium ampicillin (10–20 mg/kg three times a day IV); and florfenicol, although even when given intravenously at the extralabel dosage of 20 mg/kg twice a day it only exceeds the MIC90 value in plasma for 1 hour.[33] Combinations of drugs can be used to broaden the spectrum of activity (eg, as ampicillin-ceftiofur or ampicillin-trimethoprim-sulfonamide). Fluoroquinolones can also be effective in countries where their use is permitted. Once the pathogen has been identified and the susceptibility pattern determined (on the individual or on the farm), the most appropriate antibiotic can be chosen.

If uncontrolled, the inflammatory response may cause harm. Consequently, steroidal and nonsteroidal anti-inflammatory drugs could be considered for ancillary treatment. Most clinicians prefer the use of nonsteroidal anti-inflammatory drugs for animals that are in septic shock. The authors most often use flunixin meglumine (0.25–0.33 mg/kg three times per day). Possible side effects of aggressive nonsteroidal anti-inflammatory drug treatment include abomasal ulcers and renal toxicity, particularly in dehydrated animals. The decision to use nonsteroidal anti-inflammatory drugs in any patient is based on the presence of hematologic evidence of left shift and neutrophilic toxic changes. The duration of nonsteroidal anti-inflammatory drug treatment is often limited to 2 to 3 days because of potential toxicity. Nonsteroidal anti-inflammatory drugs should not be continued for any longer than they are considered essential for survival.

Supportive treatments for septicemic patients include providing warmth and good bedding, correction of secondary problems, administration of intravenous fluids, plasma transfusion, oral or parenteral nutrition, and oxygen administration. Problems that must be addressed include hypovolemia, hypoglobulinemia, hypoglycemia, metabolic acidosis, electrolyte abnormalities, and hypoxia. Intravenous fluids (or oral as a compromise on the farm) should be administered. Dextrose (2.5%–5%) combined with normal saline (0.9%) should be administered at a rate of at least 50 mL/kg/24 hours. Plasma transfusion (1–2 L of plasma from an adult donor negative to Bovine Leukosis Virus [BLV]) may be used. Hypertonic sodium bicarbonate (5.4%) can be used to correct metabolic acidosis if the base deficit exceeds 10 mmol/L. Nutrition is important and septicemic neonates either nurse reluctantly or are inappetant. As a result, they do not ingest an adequate amount of milk. If the animal refuses to nurse, then tube feeding should be used to ensure that the calf ingests at least 10% to 15% of its bodyweight in milk per 24 hours. The feeding schedule may involve several feedings per day (three to five) and should start with small amounts and be gradually increased in amount to prevent abdominal distention. If the gastrointestinal system does not tolerate the tube-feeding regimen, parenteral nutrition should be considered. There is usually no need for total parenteral nutrition because most animals continue to nurse or tolerate tube feeding up to 5% of their bodyweight. Partial parenteral nutrition is less expensive, simpler to manage, and provides enteral nutrients to maintain gastrointestinal system functions. Calves suffering from hypoxia without hypercapnia may benefit from intranasal oxygen insufflation (5–10 L/h). If hypoventilation is present then mechanical ventilation becomes the treatment of choice. Ventilation of calves may not be feasible depending on the economics of the situation.[34]

Appropriate nursing care should be provided and emphasized to the client or the calf caretaker. Optimal temperature (not too cold or too warm) and ventilation are important. Septicemic newborns tend to lie down most of the time and appropriate bedding (heavy thickness of straw) is important to prevent ulceration of the skin around joint areas. Straw is superior bedding to shavings because it provides better insulation and tends to stay dry on the surface while watery feces or urine settle to the bottom of the pen. Fecal material needs to be washed from the perineum regularly to prevent accumulation and myiasis. Eyes of laterally recumbent animals should be checked repeatedly for corneal ulcers. Corneal irritation should be treated aggressively with antibiotics and postural changes of the calf.

PREVENTION

Adequate colostrum management is essential for the prevention of septicemia in calves. Adequate transfer of colostral immunoglobulins can be achieved by feeding at least 4 L of colostrum to a calf weighing 40 kg or more (proportionately less for lighter calves) as soon as possible after birth and certainly before 6 to 8 hours of age. Protection against colisepticemia is achieved with less than 25 g of immunoglobulins according to one study.[35] Hyperimmune serum directed against common serotypes of E coli and immunization of late pregnant cows have shown some benefit in experimental situations.[36] Finally, the environment and management practices on the farm should be investigated. Clusters of septicemia could be related to specific risk factors. As an example, feeding heavily contaminated colostrum could be the origin of septicemia on some farms. Prevention through excellent cleanliness and management practices is the most effective means of controlling and preventing neonatal sepsis.

REFERENCES

1. Goldstein B, Giroir B, Randolph A, et al. International consensus conference on pediatric sepsis. International Pediatric Sepsis Consensus Conference: definitions for sepsis and organ dysfunction in pediatrics. Pediatr Crit Care Med 2005;6:2–8.
2. Fecteau G, Paré J, Van Metre DC, et al. Use of a clinical sepsis score for predicting bacteremia in neonatal dairy calves on a calf rearing farm. Can Vet J 1997;38: 101–4.
3. Gay CC, Besser TE. *Escherichia coli* septicemia in calves. In: Gyles CL, editor. *Escherichia coli* in domestic animals and humans, 1st Edition. CAB International, Wallingford. p. 75–80.
4. Smith BP. Understanding the role of endotoxins in gram-negative septicemia. Vet Med 1986;81:1148–61.
5. Riedel-Caspari G. The influence of colostral leukocytes on the course of an experimental *Escherichia coli* infection and serum antibodies in neonatal calves. Vet Immunol Immunopathol 1993;35:275–88.
6. Liebler-Tenorio EM, Riedel-Caspari G, Pohlenz JF, et al. Uptake of colostral leukocytes in the intestinal tract of newborn calves. Vet Immunol Immunopathol 2002; 85:33–40.
7. Toman M, Psikal I, Mensík J, et al. Phagocytic activity of blood leukocytes in calves from birth to 3 months of age. Vet Med (Praha) 1985;30:401–8.
8. Hauser MA, Koob MD, Roth JA, et al. Variation of neutrophil function with age in calves. Am J Vet Res 1986;47:152–3.
9. Doré M, Slauson DO, Neilsen NR, et al. Decreased respiratory burst activity in neonatal bovine neutrophils stimulated by protein kinase C agonists. Am J Vet Res 1991;52:375–80.
10. Griebel PJ, Schoonderwoerd M, Babiuk LA. Ontogeny of the immune response: effect of protein energy malnutrition in neonatal calves. Can J Vet Res 1987;51: 428–35.
11. Da Roden L, Smith BP, Spier SJ, et al. Effect of calf age and *Salmonella* bacterin type on ability to produce immunoglobulins directed against *Salmonella* whole cells or lipopolysaccharide. Am J Vet Res 1992;53:1895–9.
12. Endsley JJ, Roth JA, Ridpath J, et al. Maternal antibody blocks humoral but not T cell responses to BVDV. Biologicals 2003;31:123–5.
13. Fecteau G, Baillargeon P, Higgins R, et al. Bacterial contamination of colostrum fed to newborn calves in Québec dairy herds. Can Vet J 2002;43:523–7.
14. Smith HW, Halls S. The experimental infection of calves with bacteriaemia-producing strains of *Escherichia coli*: the influence of colostrum. J Med Microbiol 1968;1:61–78.
15. Fecteau G, Metre DC, Pare J, et al. Bacteriological culture of blood from critically ill neonatal calves. Can Vet J 1997;38:95–100.
16. Kliegman RM, Behrman RE, Jenson HB, et al. Sepsis, septic shock, and systemic inflammatory response syndrome. In: Kliegman R, et al, editors. Nelson textbook of pediatrics. 18th edition. Saunders, Philadelphia; p.1094.

17. Irmak K, Sen I, Cöl R, et al. The evaluation of coagulation profiles in calves with suspected septic shock. Vet Res Commun 2006;30:497–503.
18. Roy JHB. The calf. 5th edition. Butterworths, Toronto (ON): p. 41.
19. Ng PC, Lam HS. Diagnostic markers for neonatal sepsis. Curr Opin Pediatr 2006; 18:125–31.
20. Brewer BD, Koterba AM. Development of a scoring system for the early diagnosis of equine neonatal sepsis. Equine Vet J 1988;20:18–22.
21. Philip AG, Hewitt JR. Early diagnosis of neonatal sepsis. Pediatrics 1980;65: 1036–41.
22. Lofstedt J, Dohoo IR, Duizer G, et al. Model to predict septicemia in diarrheic calves. J Vet Intern Med 1999;13:81–8.
23. Green SL, Smith LL. Meningitis in neonatal calves: 32 cases (1983–1990). J Am Vet Med Assoc 1992;201:125–8.
24. Scott PR, Penny CD. A field study of meningoencephalitis in calves with particular reference to analysis of cerebrospinal fluid. Vet Rec 1993;133:119–21.
25. Ferrouillet C, Fecteau G, Higgins R, et al. Analysis of cerebrospinal fluid for diagnosis of nervous system diseases in cattle [in French]. Le Point Veterinaire 1998; 29:783–8.
26. Cordy DR. Pathomorphology and pathogenesis of bacterial meningoventriculitis of neonatal ungulates. Vet Pathol 1984;21:587–91.
27. Contrepois M, Ribot Y. Study of Escherichia coli isolated from bovine septicaemia cases. 1. With meningitis symptoms. 2. With an immunodepression syndrome and purpura haemorrhagica [in French]. Bull Acad Vet Fr 1986;59:465–73.
28. Tunkel AR, Scheld WM. Acute meningitis. In: Mandell GL, Bennet JE, Dolin R, et al, editors. Mandell: principles and practice of infectious diseases. Philadelphia: Churchill Livingstone; 2000. p. 959–91.
29. Polin RA, Harris MC. Neonatal bacterial meningitis. Semin Neonatol 2001;6: 157–72.
30. Philip AG. Neonatal meningitis in the new millenium. NeoReviews 2003;4:e73–80.
31. Scott PR. Diagnostic techniques and clinicopathologic findings in ruminant neurologic disease. Vet Clin North Am Food Anim Pract 2004;20:215–30.
32. Lutsar I, Mccracken GH, Friedland IR, et al. Antibiotic pharmacodynamics in cerebrospinal fluid. Clin Infect Dis 1998;27:1117–27.
33. de Craene BA, Deprez P, D'Haese E, et al. Pharmacokinetics of florfenicol in cerebrospinal fluid and plasma of calves. Antimicrobial Agents Chemother 1997;41:1991–5.
34. Buczinski S, Boysen SR, Fecteau G, et al. Assisted ventilation in a conscious cloned calf suffering from acute respiratory distress syndrome: a case report. J Vet Emerg Crit Care 2007;17:179–83.
35. Hunt E, Hunt LD. Escherichia coli challenge in agammaglobulinemic calves fed colostrum supplements. Proceedings 9th American College Veterinary Internal Medicine Forum. 1991;543–5.
36. Fey H. Immunology of the newborn calf: its relationship to colisepticemia. Ann NY Acad Sci 1971;176:49–63.
37. Hariharan H, Bryenton J, St-Onge J, et al. Blood cultures from calves and foals. Can Vet J 1992;33:56–7.
38. Aldridge BM, Garry FB, Adams R, et al. Neonatal septicemia in calves: 25 cases (1985–1990). J Am Vet Med Assoc 1993;203:1324–9.

Abomasal Ulceration and Tympany of Calves

Tessa S. Marshall, BVSc, MS

KEYWORDS

- Abomasal ulcers • Bloat • Tympany • Calves
- *Clostridium perfringens* • Antacids

This article reviews the current knowledge on the pathophysiology of abomasal ulcer formation and abomasal tympany in calves. The development of ulcers and bloat has been attributed to many factors, including coarse feed, environmental stress, vitamin and mineral deficiencies, and bacterial infections. This article discusses various factors thought to play a role in development of these abomasal conditions in calves.

ABOMASAL ULCERATION

Abomasal ulcers and erosions are an economic concern for all types of calf-raising systems. Prevalence rates of 0.2% to 5.7% have been reported in beef calves,[1] 32% to 76% in healthy veal calves,[2,3] 1.0% to 2.6% in healthy dairy cows,[4,5] 1.8% in healthy beef cows,[6] and 1.6% in feedlot cattle.[7] The difficulty in managing abomasal ulcers lies in determining the underlying causes, of which several have been identified. Multiple theories have been suggested to explain the occurrence of ulcers in calves, such as trauma to the mucosa from the addition of coarse roughage feeds, pica secondary to enteritis, abomasal bezoars, environmental and physical stress, hyperacidity, vitamin E deficiency, lactic acidosis, mycotic infection, and low immune status associated with copper deficiency. Several microorganisms have been isolated from various cases of ulcers, including *Escherichia coli*, *Sarcina*-like spp, and *Clostridium perfringens*. However, unlike the relationship between *Helicobacter pylori* and gastric ulcers in humans, no infectious component has been confirmed in cattle.

Erosions and ulcers may both be found in the abomasum. Erosions are discrete mucosal defects that do not penetrate the muscularis mucosa. They are usually multiple, circular, and appear as small hyperemic indentations in the mucosa. In contrast, ulcers penetrate the entire thickness of the mucosa and may extend through the submucosa, muscularis externa, and serosa. These may be single or multiple and vary in size. Ulcers usually appear as irregular depressions in the abomasal surface. The

University of Missouri-Columbia, 900 East Campus Drive, Columbia, MO 65211, USA
E-mail address: marshallts@missouri.edu

Vet Clin Food Anim 25 (2009) 209–220
doi:10.1016/j.cvfa.2008.10.010
0749-0720/08/$ – see front matter © 2009 Elsevier Inc. All rights reserved.

central crater of the ulcer is covered with fibrinonecrotic material and is surrounded by raised, rounded edges. Four categories of abomasal ulcers are described:

Type 1. Nonperforating ulcer: The ulcer does not perforate the abomasal wall and intraluminal hemorrhage is minimal (**Fig. 1**).

Type 2. Nonperforating ulcer with severe blood loss: The ulcer does not perforate the abomasal wall, but erodes a major vessel in the submucosa, resulting in severe intraluminal hemorrhage (**Fig. 2**).

Type 3. Perforating ulcer with local peritonitis: The ulcer perforates the abomasal wall and abomasal contents leak into the peritoneal cavity or omental bursa. Peritonitis is localized by fibrin deposition and the abomasum becomes adhered to the peritoneum, omentum, or surrounding viscera (**Fig. 3**).

Type 4. Perforating ulcer with diffuse peritonitis: The ulcer perforates the abomasal wall and abomasal contents quickly leak into and spread throughout the peritoneal cavity, resulting in diffuse peritonitis (**Fig. 4**).[8]

An animal may have ulcers that simultaneously meet the criteria for more than one of these categories (eg, ulcers that both bleed and perforate).

In veal calves abomasal ulcers are typically found around the pylorus.[3,5,9,10] The presence of ulcers in this region has been attributed to several causes, including the alkalinization of the pyloric antrum by bile reflux from the duodenum.[11] However, the ductus choledochus and ductus pancreaticus enter the small intestine at a greater distance from the pylorus in cattle than in humans, thus decreasing the likelihood of bile reflux.[11] Also, the torus pyloricus in cattle may act as a ball valve preventing reflux. Mechanical trauma to the pyloric mucosa by coarse feedstuffs and tricobezoars has also been suggested as a cause for ulcers.[1,3,12]

Effects of Abomasal Ulcers

Abomasal ulcers are hard to diagnose antemortem because there are almost no signs or symptoms. Affected calves can be found dead, and these are usually calves of higher quality than those in the rest of the herd. Calves are often offspring of heavy-milking dams or can be among the most aggressive nursers in groups of bottle-fed calves. This behavior may allow spillover of milk into the reticulorumen, allowing bacterial fermentation and colonization of the abomasum. However, ulcers are a common incidental finding at slaughter for veal calves. Calves raised in loose housing have significantly higher ulcer-severity scores compared with crated calves.[3] However, the

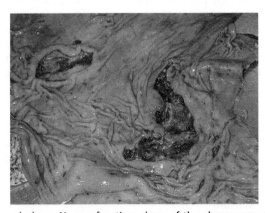

Fig. 1. Type I abomasal ulcers. Nonperforating ulcers of the abomasum of a calf.

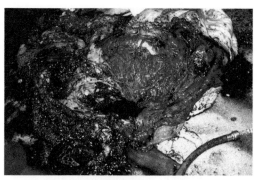

Fig. 2. Type II abomasal ulcers. Nonperforating ulcers of the abomasum with severe hemorrhage.

calves with the higher scores (more severe lesions) also have the greatest carcass weights. Thus the ulcers do not appear to have a significant effect on growth rates.[3]

Of interest is a trial looking at calves with abomasal ulcers and comparing their growth and food conversion rates. In this study, calves with abomasal lesions did not appear to have any significant decrease in their efficiency of fattening.[9]

Factors Related to Abomasal Ulcers

Age
Age distribution among calves with ulcers is fairly consistently divided into two groups: calves in the preruminant stage (<3 weeks) and calves in the transitional phase (3–8 weeks) when the abomasum is most susceptible to ulcer formation.[13] There is a reduction in cases around 2 months of age. Because these cases tend to occur in the spring and early summer, blame for the ulcers is sometimes placed on seasonal factors. However, seasonal factors probably do not play a role. In all likelihood, cases occur in mainly in spring and early summer because many calves are at a susceptible age during those seasons.

Weather
Outbreaks of abomasal ulcers and tympany often occur after periods of bad weather. During extreme weather, calves fail to nurse or nurse poorly, and may end up gorging themselves after the bad weather has passed, resulting in proliferation of bacteria that cause fermentation.[14] Ahmed and colleagues[15] suggest that a period of weather-induced inappetence leads to low abomasal luminal pH, thereby promoting the

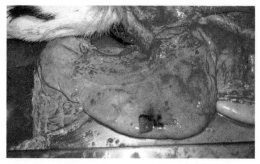

Fig. 3. Type III abomasal ulcers. Perforating ulcers of the body of the abomasum with local peritonitis.

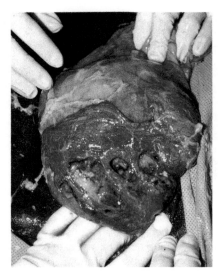

Fig. 4. Type IV abomasal ulcers. Perforating ulcers in the abomasum with diffuse peritonitis.

formation of ulcers. Suckling frequency has been proposed as a method for controlling abomasal pH in calves. Calves suckling cow's milk have been shown to have significantly lower mean abomasal luminal pH when compared with calves suckling either whey- or soy-protein milk replacers. Ahmed and colleagues[16] found that increasing the frequency of suckling increases the mean 24-hour abomasal luminal pH and the percentage of the 24-hour period that the pH is greater than 3.0.[15] This study found that suckling eight times per day (every 3 hours) increases the luminal pH to over 3.0 for the greatest percentage of the 24-hour recording period. The combined effects of decreased suckling frequency and increased volume suckled each feeding during periods of inclement weather might facilitate the development of abomasal ulceration.

Beef calves usually suckle three to six meals on average per 24 hours,[17,18] thus maintaining a higher average abomasal pH. Therefore an increase in the suckling frequency of dairy and veal calves to above the industry standard of every 12 hours more closely reflects the suckling behavior of beef calves and may decrease the frequency of ulceration by increasing the number of hours each day that the abomasal pH is greater than 3.0.[15]

Housing
Housing has been found to play a small part in the incidence of abomasal ulcers. Increased stocking density or an increase in the availability of dirt or hair in the environment may play a role. Calves housed on pasture have a significantly lower incidence of disease than those housed in pens or in stubble fields.[1]

Stress
Stress has been associated with ulcers in other species. Several of the factors mentioned above (housing, group mixing, and weather) have been thought to contribute to ulcer formation through the body's response to stress. Cortisone and corticotropin reduce gastric mucus secretion, which limits mucosal protection. Also, steroids decrease cell renewal in the gastric mucosa.[14]

Hair balls

Hair balls (trichobezoars) (**Fig. 5**) are thought to have an abrasive action on the abomasal mucosa, which may disrupt the normal mucosal defensive barriers and allow autodigestion to occur. In one study, calves less than 1 month of age that had died as a result of ulcers had a fourfold increase in the risk of having a hair ball in their abomasum as compared with calves dying of other causes.[13] However, in older calves, about 60% had abomasal hair balls regardless of the cause of death. Although the exact relationship between the presence of hair balls and the formation of abomasal ulcers is not well understood, they certainly don't appear to be necessary for the development of ulcers.

Mineral deficiencies

Mineral deficiencies, particularly copper or selenium deficiency, are often associated with ulceration and poor performance in calves. Low serum copper may result in derangement of elastin cross-linkages, thus compromising the abomasal mucosa and its microvasculature.[14] Copper deficiency may also cause decreased cytochrome oxidase activity of leukocytes, which contributes to decreased neutrophil function and increased susceptibility to infection.[19] The role played by copper deficiency in ulcer formation is questionable based on the research results currently available. Trace mineral deficiencies tend to be regional problems and may vary from year to year.[20]

Clostridium perfringens type A

C perfringens type A has been associated with many diseases in cattle. Experimental intraruminal inoculation of *C perfringens* type A results in varying degrees of depression, diarrhea, abdominal bloat, abomasitis, and abomasal ulceration.[19] However, the ulcers are frequently multiple, diffuse, never perforating, and associated with ecchymotic and petechial hemorrhage and with mucosal edema. In a study of 14 calves with fatal ulcers, Jelinski and colleagues[12] found that only 6 had a heavy growth of *C perfringens* type A. This suggests that this pathogen is not necessary in the formation of fatal ulcers. The ulcerative lesions usually seen in beef cattle differ in that they are typically singular and localized to a discrete region of the abomasum.[21]

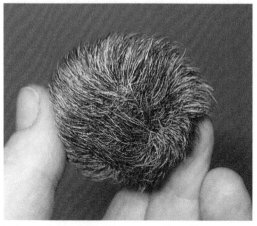

Fig. 5. Hair ball (trichobezoar) from the abomasum of a calf.

Clostridium perfringens *type D*

C perfringens type D has been isolated from at least one case of abomasitis and ulceration. Although this bacteria normally inhabitant the small intestine in ruminants, irregular feeding or hungry animals drinking excess milk may promote the overgrowth of *C perfringens* type D in calves. Affected calves were 6 weeks of age and showed signs of decreased appetite and lethargy. At necropsy, the abomasum contained dark fluid, and the mucosa was edematous and covered in many minute ulcers.[22]

Clinical Signs

A thorough physical examination is essential because of the many differential diagnoses for abdominal pain and distension in calves. Signs include lethargy, abdominal distension with tympany, colic, bruxism, fluid distension of the abomasum, diarrhea, and death. The hematocrit is usually low with type 2 ulcers. A fecal occult blood test may be positive with types 1 and 2. However, a single negative test does not rule out gastrointestinal bleeding (**Fig. 6**). The sensitivity increases when testing multiple samples. Plasma fibrinogen concentration is often high in types 3 and 4. A white blood cell count may show leukocytosis/neutrophilia with types 3 and 4. Abdominocentesis often indicates inflammation with type 4 and is sometimes supportive in type 3.

Exploratory laparotomy is the most definite way to diagnose ulcers antemortem. Laparotomy and necropsy are the only ways to definitively diagnose ulcers. Most ulcers are found on the greater curvature of the fundic region or in the pyloric region. Erosions are usually located on the edges (linear erosions) and sides (punctate erosions) of the abomasal folds. See **Box 1** for a partial list of differential diagnoses.

Diagnostic Tests

A diagnostic test that has been investigated is pepsinogen concentration. Pepsinogen is an inactive form of pepsin, an important proteolytic enzyme. Bovine pepsinogen is activated when the pH is 5.0 or less. As the luminal pH increases (>3.0), the proteolytic activity of pepsinogen decreases. Increased activation of pepsinogen to pepsin by enhanced acidity can cause ulcers.[23] Elevated pepsinogen has been found when there is a gastric or duodenal ulcer, but the specific role of serum pepsinogen in detecting abomasal ulcers in cattle has not been confirmed. At least one study has shown that a serum pepsinogen concentration of more than 5.0 U/L coincided with severe abomasal ulceration in cattle. However this test is nonspecific, as other diseases, such as

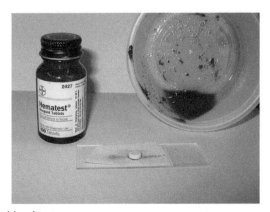

Fig. 6. Fecal occult blood test.

> **Box 1**
> **Differential diagnoses**
>
> Bleeding ulcers
>
>   Coccidiosis
>
>   Salmonellosis
>
>   Intussusception
>
>   Duodenal ulcer
>
>   Abomasal volvulus
>
>   Bovine virus diarrhea/mucosal disease
>
>   Malignant catarrhal fever
>
>   Winter dysentery
>
>   Mycotoxicosis
>
>   Heavy-metal poisoning
>
>   Coagulopathies
>
> Perforated ulcers
>
>   Traumatic reticuloperitonitis
>
>   Rupture of another abdominal organ (eg, uterus)
>
>   Other septic conditions (navel ill)
>
> Other differentials
>
>   Ruminal tympany
>
>   Uncomplicated left-side or right-side displacement of the abomasum
>
>   Indigestion
>
>   Internal parasitism
>
>   Dilatation and dislocation/torsion of the cecum
>
>   Peritonitis of other origins

telodorsagiasis (formerly ostertagiasis), also cause an elevation in pepsinogen concentration.[4,23,24]

Treatments and Control Recommendations

Normal preprandial abomasal pH in calves is between 1.0 and 2.0.[25] In adult cows, this pH is between 2.0 and 2.5. Suckling frequency has been suggested as a method for control of abomasal pH in calves. As stated earlier, increasing the frequency of suckling has been shown to increase the mean 24-hour abomasal luminal pH and the percentage of the 24-hour period that the pH is greater than 3.0.[15] Calves that suckled eight times per day (every 3 hours) had an increase in abomasal pH greater than 3.0 for the greatest percentage of the 24-hour recording period.

Beef calves usually suckle three to six meals per 24 hours,[17,18] thus maintaining a higher average abomasal pH as compared with dairy calves. Therefore increasing the feeding frequency of dairy and veal calves above the industry standard of every 12 hours more closely reflects the suckling behavior of beef calves and may decrease the frequency of ulceration by increasing the number of hours each day that the abomasal pH is greater than 3.0.[15]

In general, treatment is reserved for animals with bleeding ulcers or deep, nonperforated ulcers. Treatment of abomasal ulcers has historically included blood transfusions (10- to 20-mL blood/kg), antibiotic administration, changes to the diet, and oral administration of antacid agents.[26,27] Increasing the luminal pH with antacids aims to provide a more favorable healing environment for ulcers.

Aluminum hydroxide/magnesium hydroxide ($Al(OH)_3$/$Mg(OH)_2$) antacids neutralize acid in the abomasum and require multiple doses (three times) per day. Antacids are an inexpensive option for treatment of cattle with ulcers and have a potential therapeutic advantage. $Al(OH)_3$ directly absorbs pepsin, thus decreasing the proteolytic action of pepsin in the stomach.[28] Also $Al(OH)_3$ and $Mg(OH)_2$ bind bile acids, thus protecting against ulceration caused by bile reflux.[28] Ahmed and colleagues[29] found that healthy calves given oral antacids had a transient increase in abomasal luminal pH. This effect appeared to be dose related and the extent of the acid neutralization was increased when not given with milk replacer.

Histamine type 2 receptor antagonists reduce acid secretion of parietal cells by selective and competitive antagonism of histamine at H-2 receptors on the parietal cells. Cimetidine and ranitidine are synthetic H-2 antagonists that inhibit basal as well as pentagastrin- and cholinergic-stimulated gastric acid secretion. Daily oral administration of cimetidine at 10 mg/kg for 30 days in veal calves was found to aid healing of abomasal ulcers.[27] Oral administration of cimetidine (50 to 100 mg/kg every 8 hours) and ranitidine (10 to 50 mg/kg, every 8 hours) causes a dose-dependent increase in abomasal luminal pH, and ranitidine has greater potency than cimetidine.[25]

Proton-pump inhibitors, such as omeprazole, act by preventing acid secretion. Omeprazole has a prolonged duration of action, which provides for easy daily dosing regimes. In a study by Ahmed and colleagues,[30] once daily oral administration of omeprazole to calves increased the mean 24-hour luminal pH by 1.3 pH units. However, this increase in pH was less pronounced with subsequent daily treatments.

Surgical repair of ulcers can be performed on selected cases. Calves need to be in an operable condition and have isolated ulcers. Surgery needs to be performed early in the disease process. Typically, ulcers are diagnosed during a laparotomy and can be either resected or the serosa can be inverted with a mattress suture. One study reported a survival rate of 74% following surgical repair (with survival being defined as calves living at least 3 months past surgery date or dying because of another disease).[1]

Prevention

Because the cause of abomasal ulcers is not well understood and few animals in a herd show signs of ulcers or die from ulcers, design of prevention strategies is difficult. Focus should be on assessing trace mineral supplementation, particularly copper. This may require assessment of sulfur and molybdenum concentrations in the diet and water. Liver biopsies for copper concentration from a percentage of the animals may be necessary.

Stressors, such as comingling of groups of animals, should be reduced, and appropriate housing, feed, and water should be provided. More research on abomasal ulcers in calves is needed to fill in the gaps in our knowledge so we can move on from vague recommendations based on "theory" to more solid advice that more reliably addresses the disease.

ABOMASAL DILATION AND TYMPANY

Abomasal dilation and tympany is a syndrome in young calves characterized by anorexia, abdominal distension, bloat, and often death in 6 to 48 hours. At necropsy, most of these calves have abomasal tympany, forestomach and abomasal edema, hemorrhage, mucosal necrosis, and, occasionally, mural emphysema. This condition occurs most commonly in dairy calves and seems to occur sporadically with some farms having multiple outbreaks at times. Risk factors can include feeding a large volume of milk in a single daily feeding, cold milk (or milk replacer), not offering water to calves, erratic feeding schedules, and failure of passive transfer.

Recently, the abomasal bloat syndrome was experimentally reproduced by drenching young Holstein calves with a carbohydrate mixture containing milk replacer, corn starch, and glucose mixed in water.[31] The investigators proposed that the pathophysiology of abomasal bloat is primarily excess fermentation of high-energy gastrointestinal contents. Gas-producing bacteria, such as *C perfringens*, *Sarcina ventriculi*, or *Lactobacillus* spp have also been thought to play a role in this syndrome.[31,32] Although the exact pathogenesis of abomasal bloat is not completely understood, the disease is likely to be mutifactorial in origin. Large amounts of fermentable carbohydrate in the abomasum (from milk, milk replacer, or high-energy oral electrolyte solutions) along with the fermentative enzymes (produced by bacteria) would likely lead to gas production and bloat. This process would be exacerbated by anything that slowed abomasal emptying or that caused gastrointestinal ileus. Thus, control of this disease should rely on dietary management more than on therapeutic or prophylactic medications.

Abomasal dilation can be caused by feed, fluid, or gas accumulation following mechanical obstruction of outflow from the abomasum at the level of the pylorus (eg, ulceration, foreign body) or by disturbance of the muscular activity of the abomasum through damage to the ventral nerve trunk of the vagus nerve. An increase in abomasal luminal pressure reduces blood flow to the abomasal mucosa and submucosa through mechanical compression of the vasculature, thus predisposing the gastric mucosa to injury and ulceration from back diffusion of hydrogen ions.[33]

Clinical signs are often mild and may inconsistently include diarrhea, mild abdominal distention with fluid and gas, splashing on abdominal succession, and mild depression (**Fig. 7**). Hyperglycemia (189–516 mg/dL) with an accompanying glucosuria (1000–2000 mg/dL) consistently develops.[31] In severe cases, calves are usually dehydrated,

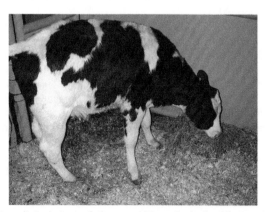

Fig. 7. A calf showing clinical signs of abomasal bloat, including depression and abdominal distension.

show signs of colic, have prominent abdominal distention, experience diarrhea, and become recumbent. Gross lesions include hemorrhage, edema, and necrosis of abomasal and ruminal mucosa. Occasional emphysematous bullae may be present in the stomach wall.[32] Pathogens isolated include alpha streptococci, other *Streptococcus* spp, *E coli*, and *Clostridium*, *Sarcina*, and *Candida* spp.

Treatment generally involves placing the calf in dorsal recumbency and inserting a needle or catheter into the abomasum to relieve the gas.[34] Attempting to deflate the bloat in a standing calf is often unrewarding and may result in leakage of abomasal contents into the abdomen. Antibiotic therapy is also indicated in these calves (most likely parenteral procaine penicillin or oral β-lactam antibiotics to target *Clostridium* bacteria).

SUMMARY

Many factors have been associated with abomasal ulcer development in calves. Ulcers are common in veal calves but rarely result in clinical disease. Perforating ulcers can cause acute sudden death in suckling beef calves on pasture. The etiology is uncertain but is probably associated with prolonged inappetence and sustained low abomasal pH. Ulcers appear to be a multifactorial disease requiring a management approach to minimize the risk in calves. More research is required to find economical prevention strategies for control of abomasal ulcers in calves.

Bacteria appear to have some role in abomasal tympany, which can result in ulceration if the acute bloat does not kill the animal. Control of this disease should rely on dietary management. Specifically, this calls for a consistent feeding schedule and care in the use of very high osmolality milk replacer or electrolyte products that could slow abomasal emptying and facilitate bacterial fermentation in the abomasum.[35]

REFERENCES

1. Katchuik R. Abomasal disease in young beef calves. Surgical findings and management factors. Can Vet J 1992;33:459–61.
2. Wensing T, Breukink HJ, Van Dijk S. The effect of feeding pellets of different types of roughage on the incidence of lesions in the abomasum of veal calves. Vet Res Commun 1986;10:195–202.
3. Welchman D de B, Baust G. A survey of abomasal ulceration in veal calves. Vet Rec 1987;121:586–90.
4. Aukema JJ, Breukink HJ. Abomasal ulcer in adult cattle with fatal hemorrhage. Cornell Vet 1974;64:303–17.
5. Hemmingsen I. Erosiones et ulcera bomasi bovis. Nord Vet Med 1966;18:354–65.
6. Jensen R, Deane HM, Cooper LJ, et al. The rumenitis-liver abscess complex in beef cattle. Am J Vet Res 1954;15:202–16.
7. Jensen R, Pierson RE, Braddy PM, et al. Fatal abomasal ulcers in yearling feedlot cattle. J Am Vet Med Assoc 1976;169:524–6.
8. Smith DF, Munson L, Erb HN. Abomasal ulcer disease in adult dairy cattle. Cornell Vet 1983;73:213–24.
9. Breukink HJ, Wensing T, van Dijk S, et al. The effect of clenbuterol on the incidence of abomasal ulcers in veal calves. Vet Rec 1989;125:109–11.
10. Pearson GR, Welchman D de B, Wells M. Mucosal changes associated with abomasal ulceration in veal calves. Vet Rec 1989;120:557–9.
11. Ooms L, Oyaert W. Electromyographic study of the abomasal antrum and proximal duodenum in cattle. Zentralbl Veterinarmed A 1978;25:464–73.

12. Jelinski MD, Ribble CS, Chirino-Trejo M, et al. The relationship between the presence of *Helicobacter pylori, Clostridium perfringens* type A, *Campylobacter* spp, or fungi and abomasal ulcers in unweaned beef calves. Can Vet J 1995;36: 379–82.

13. Jelinski MD, Ribble CS, Campbell JR, et al. Investigating the relationship between abomasal hairballs and perforating abomasal ulcers in unweaned beef calves. Can Vet J 1996;37:23–6.

14. Lilley CW, Hamar DW, Gerlach M, et al. Linking copper and bacteria with abomasal ulcers in beef calves. Vet Med 1985;80:85–8.

15. Ahmed AF, Constable PD, Misk NA. Effect of feeding frequency and route of administration on abomasal luminal pH in dairy calves fed milk replacer. J Dairy Sci 2002;85:1502–8.

16. Constable PD, Ahmed AF, Misk NA. Effect of suckling cow's milk or milk replacer on abomasal luminal pH in dairy calves. J Vet Intern Med 2005;19:97–102.

17. Walker DE. Suckling and grazing behavior of beef heifers and calves. N.Z.J. Agric Res 1962;5:331–8.

18. Odde KG, Kiracofe GH, Schalles RR. Suckling behavior in range beef calves. J Anim Sci 1985;61(1):307–9.

19. Roeder BL, Chengapa MM, Nagaraja TG, et al. Experimental induction of abdominal tympany, abomasitis, and abomasal ulceration by intraruminal inoculation of *Clostridium perfringens* type A in neonatal calves. Am J Vet Res 1988;49:201–7.

20. Mills KW, Johnson JL, Jensen RL, et al. Laboratory findings associated with abomasal ulcers/tympany in range calves. J Vet Diagn Invest 1990;2:208–12.

21. Jelinski MD, Ribble CS, Campbell JR, et al. Descriptive epidemiology of fatal abomasal ulcers in Canadian beef calves. Prev Vet Med 1996;26:9–15.

22. Assis RA, Lobato FCF, Facury Filho EJ, et al. Isolation of *Clostridium perfringens* type D from a suckling calve with ulcerative abomasitis. Arch Med Vet 2002;2: 287–92.

23. Mesaric M. Role of serum pepsinogen in detecting cows with abomasal ulcer. Vetarinarski Arhiv 2005;75(2):111–8.

24. Mesaric M, Zadnik T, Klinkon M. Comparison of serum pepsinogen activity between enzootic bovine leucosis (EBL) positive beef cattle and cows with abomasitis. Slov Vet Res 2002;39(3/4):227–32.

25. Ahmed AF, Constable PD, Misk NA. Effect of orally administered cimetidine and ranitidine on abomasal luminal pH in clinically normal milk-fed calves. Am J Vet Res 2001;62(10):1531–8.

26. Braun U, Bretscher R, Gerber D. Bleeding abomasal ulcers in dairy cows. Vet Rec 1991;129:279–84.

27. Dirksen GU. Ulceration, dilatation and incarceration of the abomasum in calves: clinical investigations and experiences. Bov Pract 1994;28:127–35.

28. Maton PN, Burton ME. Antacids revisited. A review of their clinical pharmacology and recommended therapeutic use. Drugs 1999;57(6):855–70.

29. Ahmed AF, Constable PD, Misk NA. Effect of an orally administered antacid agent containing aluminum hydroxide and magnesium hydroxide on abomasal luminal pH in clinically normal milk-fed calves. J Am Vet Med Assoc 2002b;220(1):74–9.

30. Ahmed AF, Constable PD, Misk NA. Effect of orally administered omeprazole on abomasal luminal pH in dairy calves fed milk replacer. J Vet Med A 2005;52: 238–43.

31. Panciera RJ, Boileau MJ, Step DL. Tympany, acidosis, and mural emphysema of the stomach in calves: report of cases and experimental induction. J Vet Diagn Invest 2007;19:392–5.

32. Songer JG, Miskimins DW. Clostridial abomasitis in calves: case report and review of the literature. Anaerobe 2005;11:290–4.
33. Constable PD, St-Jean G, Koenig GR, et al. Abomasal luminal pressure in cattle with abomasal volvulus or left displaced abomasum. J Am Vet Med Assoc 1992; 201(10):1564–8.
34. Kümper H. [New therapy for acute abomasal tympany in calves]. Tierarzti Prax 1994;22(1):25–7.
35. Nouri M, Constable PD. Comparison of two oral electrolyte solutions and route of administration on the abomasal emptying rate of Holstein-Friesian calves. J Vet Intern Med 2006;20:620–6.

Neonatal Immunology

Victor S. Cortese, DVM, PhD

KEYWORDS

- Immunology • Neonatal • Calf • Vaccination • Development

The field of neonatal immunology continues to be an area of active research in human and veterinary medicine. New and advanced methods for assessing immune status and function are being used widely to re-evaluate some of the old beliefs about the young animal's immune system. Although much more research is still needed, these new studies are shedding light on a mysterious and critical time in the immunologically frail newborn.

DEVELOPMENT OF THE PRENATAL IMMUNE SYSTEM

The immune system of all species of mammals begins development fairly early in gestation. As the fetus grows, the immune system goes through many changes as cells appear and become specialized. In general, the shorter the gestation period, the less developed the immune system is at birth.[1] The fetus does become immunocompetent while in utero to many diseases, however. In calves, this has been demonstrated with a wide variety of diseases.[2–5] For these types of diseases, precolostral titers from the neonate can be used for diagnostic determination of fetal exposures. The primordial thymus can be seen in fetal lambs and calves between days 27 and 30 of gestation as an epithelial chord.[6,7] As a percentage of body weight, the thymus reaches its maximum size near midgestation and then rapidly decreases after birth. Actual regression of the thymus begins around puberty, and the extent and speed at which it regresses vary by husbandry practices and genetics. By the time of first heat cycle, the thymus' function as an immune gland is almost completely gone.

The cells that initially infiltrate the thymus are of unknown origin, but thymic development and differentiation of thymocytes into specific T cell lines occur during gestation. Some of this development and differentiation can occur in secondary lymphoid organs as well. B cells, by contrast, develop and differentiate in the fetal bone marrow. There is a steady increase in the peripheral lymphocytes throughout gestation.[8] Most of these circulating fetal lymphocytes are T cells. At the same time that lymphocytes are developing in the fetus, development and expansion of other white blood cell populations are occurring.

NEONATAL IMMUNE SYSTEM

The immune system is fully developed, albeit immature, in the neonate at the time of birth. Susceptibility of newborns to pathogens is not attributable to any inherent

Cattle Immunology, Pfizer Animal Health, 746 Veechdale Road, Simpsonville, KY 40067, USA
E-mail address: victor.cortese@pfizer.com

Vet Clin Food Anim 25 (2009) 221–227
doi:10.1016/j.cvfa.2008.10.003
0749-0720/08/$ – see front matter © 2009 Elsevier Inc. All rights reserved.

inability to mount an immune response but is caused by the fact that their immune system is unprimed.[9] Although there are greater numbers of phagocytic cells in the neonate, the function of these cells is decreased (in calves, these deficiencies are found up to 4 months of age).[10] Complement is from 12% to 60% of adult levels at birth. Complement does not reach adult levels in calves until they are 6 months of age. There is a slow maturation of the immune system in mammals. As an animal approaches sexual maturity and begins to cycle, the immune system also matures. In cattle, most of the immune system maturity is seen by 5 to 8 months of age. For example, T cells (CD4+, CD8+ and TCRγδ+ cells) do not reach peak levels until the animal is 8 months of age.[11] This does not mean that a young calf cannot respond to antigens, but the response is weaker, slower, and easier to overcome. For all practical purposes, this immaturity may lead to moderation of disease rather than to complete prevention. Because the placenta is of the epitheliochorial type in food animal species (eg, cattle, pigs, sheep), there is no transplacental transfer of antibodies or white blood cells. Therefore, no discussion on bovine neonatal immunology is complete without a discussion on an important component of the newborn calf's defense mechanism, colostrum.

COLOSTRUM

Colostrum is the most important example of passive immunity. Defined as the "first" secretions from the mammary gland present after birth, colostrum has many known and unknown properties and components. The information on the short- and long-term impacts of colostrum in calves continues to grow. Not only does good passive transfer have an impact on morbidity and mortality in the young calf,[12–14] but it has a positive impact on long-term health and production.[15–17] Constituents of colostrum include concentrated levels of antibodies and many of the immune cells (B cells, CD cells, macrophages, and neutrophils), which are fully functional after absorption by the calf.[18] Additional components of the immune system, such as interferon, are transferred by means of colostrum,[19] along with many important nutrients.[20] The primary colostral antibody in most domestic species is IgG; in ruminants, this is further defined as IgG1. The functions of the various cells found in colostrum are still undergoing much research. The cells are known to enhance defense mechanisms in the newborn animal in the following ways: transfer of cell-mediated immunity, enhanced passive transfer of immunoglobins, local bactericidal and phagocytic activity in the digestive tract, and increased lymphocyte activity.[12,21] Research in swine has shown higher absorption of these white blood cells when the sow is the true dam as compared with grafted piglets. Similar studies have not been done in ruminants. These cells are destroyed by freezing and naturally disappear from the calf between 3 and 5 weeks of age.[12] The long-term impact of these cells on health or production of calves is not well understood at this time.

COLOSTRUM ABSORPTION

When calves are born, the epithelial cells that line the digestive tract allow absorption of colostral proteins by means of pinocytosis. As soon as the digestive tract is stimulated by ingestion of any material, this population of cells begins to change to those that no longer permit absorption. By 6 hours after birth, only approximately 50% of the absorptive capacity remains; by 8 hours, 33%; and by 24 hours, no absorption is typically seen.[12] Colostrum transfer is thus a function of quality and quantity of the colostrum in addition to the timing of colostral administration. In the Holstein breed, the first feeding should be a minimum of 3 qt (3 L) and preferably 4 qt of high-quality clean colostrum. Also, colostrum high in red blood cells may exacerbate any diarrhea caused by gram-negative bacteria.[22] In spite of all the information regarding the importance of colostrum administration to the calf, some degree of failure of passive transfer is common even in beef calves.[13,23] Colostral supplements are available, in addition to products for oral or systemic administration, that contain specific antibodies or general IgG concentrations. There is tremendous variability in the IgG concentration of colostral supplements.[24] Although mixed results pertaining to the efficacy of these products have been observed,[25] they may have significant value in decreasing the mortality or the severity of disease in colostrum-deprived calves.

VACCINATION TO IMPROVE COLOSTRAL QUALITY

It has long been thought that vaccines administered to a cow before calving increase colostral antibodies against those specific antigens. This has been best demonstrated with vaccines that are administered to cows against neonatal diarrhea pathogens. These vaccines are designed to increase the colostral antibody concentration against specific organisms that cause diarrhea in calves, such as *Escherichia coli*, rotavirus, and coronavirus.[26–28] Little research has been done looking at other vaccines and their impact on colostral antibodies, however. Although one study demonstrated that vaccinating cows with a modified-live viral vaccine increased colostral antibodies,[29] a recent study with inactivated viral vaccination of cows did not show the same response.[30] One Israeli study actually demonstrated decreased colostral antibodies when cows were vaccinated before calving.[31] If a vaccine is being designed primarily to improve colostral transfer of antibodies, studies should be requested that demonstrate the vaccine's ability to produce the desired effect.

MATERNAL ANTIBODY INTERFERENCE REVISITED

One of the commonly held beliefs in neonatal immunology is that the presence of maternal antibody blocks the immune responses associated with vaccination. This has been based on vaccinating animals, followed by evaluating subsequent levels of antibody titers. It is clear from many studies that if animals are vaccinated in the presence of high levels of maternal antibody to that antigen, they may not display increased antibody titers after vaccination.[32,33] Nevertheless, recent studies have shown the formation of B-cell memory responses[34–36] and cell-mediated immune responses in the face of maternal antibody[28] when attenuated vaccines were used. Similar responses have been reported in laboratory animals as well.[37–39] It is clear from these studies that maternal antibody interference of vaccines is not as absolute as once thought. The immune status of the animal, particularly against that antigen; the specific antigen; and presentation of that antigen should be considered when trying to design vaccination programs when maternal antibody may be present. In summary, work published to date (and cited previously) has demonstrated that vaccination against diseases that have a primary cell-mediated protective mechanism may be more likely to stimulate an immune response in the face of maternal antibody than those in which humoral immunity is the primary protective mechanism (**Table 1**).

IMPACT OF STRESS

Stress has an impact on the calf's immune system as it does in older animals. There are several factors that can affect the immune system and are unique to the neonatal animal. The calving process has a dramatic impact on the newborn's immune system because of corticosteroid release. Furthermore, the newborn has an increased

Table 1
Diseases with research that has assessed maternal antibody interference in cattle

Primarily Cell-Mediated Protection: Vaccination not Blocked by Maternal Antibody	Primary Antibody Protection: Vaccination Blocked by Maternal Antibody
BRSV	Bovine viral diarrhea
BHV-1	*Mannheimia haemolytica*
Parainfluenza virus	*Pasteurella multocida*
Leptospira borgpetersennii	—
Pseudorabies	—

number of suppressor T cells. These factors, along with others, dramatically decrease systemic immune responses for the first week of life. Recent research has demonstrated that there is actually a decrease in the immune response of neonatal calves. From birth, there is a decrease in immune responses until day 3, when they are at their lowest levels (**Fig. 1**).[40] By day 5, these responses are back to the level of immune responses seen on the day of birth. Systemically administered vaccinations during this time should be avoided because of these decreased responses. Vaccination immediately after birth may even have undesired effects.[41] Furthermore, other stresses should be avoided in the young calf to try and maintain immune system integrity in the immunologically frail newborn. Procedures like castration, dehorning, weaning, and movement need to be considered as stresses that have the potential to decrease immune system function temporarily.

VACCINATION

As discussed previously, the vaccination of the young calf is being revisited. Many different types of vaccines are routinely used in veal, dairy beef, and dairy replacement heifers in addition to branding/turnout vaccinations in beef calves. The effectiveness of these programs is attributable to an interaction among several factors, including antigen (ie, infectious bovine rhinotracheitis [IBR] versus *Pasteurella haemolytica*) and vaccine type (ie, modified-live or inactivated), age of the calf, presence of maternal

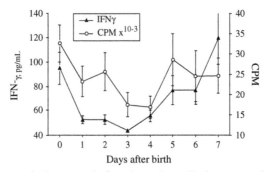

Fig. 1. Graph illustrates the immune dysfunction present in the neonatal calf and shows diminished cytokine (interferon-γ [IFNγ]) production and blastogenic responses in the first few days after birth. CPM, counts per minute. (*Data from* Marcus Kehrli, DVM, PhD, Ames, IA.)

antibody, other stress factors present at the time of vaccination, and timing of disease agent exposure. Vaccines that use the mucosal immune system have been tested and licensed for use in the young calf, including the newborn. These vaccines include modified-live vaccines; intranasal IBR/PI3 vaccines; modified-live vaccines; oral rotavirus/coronavirus vaccines; and new intranasal vaccines containing bovine viral diarrhea virus (BVDV) types 1 and 2, bovine herpesvirus (BHV)-1, PI3 and bovine respiratory syncytial virus (BRSV), or BRSV in combination with PI3. For BRSV in which limited replication occurs with systemic modified-live vaccination, intranasal administration may be the most effective route.[42] Exact timing of early vaccination varies somewhat depending on antigen and presentation. In human immunology, times during which antigen exposure may cause a predominance of IgE production have been shown. Similar immune responses have not been demonstrated in food animals. One study has shown that initial systemic vaccination for the four primary viral diseases (BVDV, infectious bovine rhinotracheitis [IBRV], BRSV, and PI3) has little impact when administered during the 3-week-old to 5-week-old age window in dairy calves, however.[42] The author's own work has seen the same problems with vaccination during this time. This corresponds to the time frame in which maternal T cells are disappearing from the calf.[18,21] Several other studies have looked at vaccinating calves before 3 weeks of age, with good response.[28,43,44] In general, vaccination in the young calf should precede anticipated or historical times of disease by at least 10 days, allowing the immune system to respond before exposure. If a booster dose is required, the booster should be given at least 10 days before the expected disease occurrence. Although in its infancy, the use of vaccination programs in young food animals is gaining popularity and more research is needed to define protection and the timing required by different vaccines in the neonate further.

SUMMARY

The neonatal immune system is a complex and interrelated system containing components from the dam and the newborn. Although the system is capable of responding and inferring varying degrees of protection, it is this combination of passive and active immunity together that provides protection to the neonate.

REFERENCES

1. Halliwell REW, Gorman NT. Neonatal immunology. In: Veterinary clinical immunology. Philadelphia: WB. Saunders Co.; 1989. p. 193–205.
2. Mullaney TP, Newman LE, Whitehair CK. Humoral immune response of the bovine fetus to in utero vaccination with attenuated bovine coronavirus. Am J Vet Res 1988;49:156–9.
3. Pare J, Fecteau JG, Fortin M, et al. Seroepidemiologic study of Neospora caninum in dairy herds. J Am Vet Med Assoc 1998;213:1595–7.
4. Ellsworth MA, Fairbanks KK, Behan S, et al. Fetal protection following exposure to calves persistently infected with bovine viral diarrhea virus type 2 sixteen months after primary vaccination of the dams. Vet Ther 2006;7:295–304.
5. Casaro APE, Kendrick JW, Kennedy PC. Response of the bovine fetus to bovine viral diarrhea-mucosal disease virus. Am J Vet Res 1971;32:1543–62.
6. Jordan HK. Development of sheep thymus in relation to in utero thymectomy experiments. Eur J Immunol 1976;6:693–8.
7. Anderson EI. Pharyngeal derivatives in the calf. Anat Rec 1922;24:25–37.
8. Senogles DR, Muscoplat CC, Paul PS, et al. Ontogeny of circulating B lymphocytes in neonatal calves. Res Vet Sci 1978;25:34–6.

9. Tizard I. Immunity in the fetus and newborn. In: Veterinary immunology, an intro-duction. 4th edition. Philadelphia: WB. Sanders Co.; 1992. p. 248–260.

10. Hawser MA, Knob MD, Wroth JA. Variation of neutrophil function with age in calves. Am J Vet Res 1986;47:152–3.

11. Hein WR. Ontogeny of T cells. In: Goddeeris BML, Morrison WI, editors. Cell mediated immunity in ruminants. Boca Raton (FL): CRC press; 1994. p. 19–36.

12. Rischen CG. Passive immunity in the newborn calf. Iowa State Univ Vet 1981; 12(2):60–5.

13. Boland W, Cortese VS, Steffen D. Interactions between vaccination, failure of passive transfer, and diarrhea in beef calves. Agri Practice 1995;16:25–8.

14. Robison AD, Stott GH, DeNise SK. Effects of passive immunity on growth and survival in the dairy heifer. J Dairy Sci 1988;71:1283–7.

15. Faber SN, Pas Faber NE, et al. Case study: effects of colostrum ingestion on lactational performance. Professional Animal Scientist 2005;21:420–5.

16. Wittum TE, Perino LJ. Passive immune status at postpartum hour 24 and long-term health and performance of calves. Am J Vet Res 1995;56:1149–54.

17. Dewell RD, Hungerford LL, Keen JE, et al. Association of neonatal serum immu-noglobulin G1 concentration with health and performance in beef calves. J Am Vet Med Assoc 2006;228:914–21.

18. Riedel-Caspari G, Schmidt FW. The influence of colostral leukocytes on the immune system of the neonatal calf. I. Effects on lymphocyte responses (p. 102–7). II. Effects on passive and active immunization (p. 190–4). III. Effects on phagocytosis (p. 330–4). IV. Effects on bactericidity, complement and inter-feron. Synopsis (p. 395–8). Dtsch Tierarztl Wochenschr 1991;98:102–398.

19. Jacobsen KL, Arbtan KD. Interferon activity in bovine colostrum and milk. In: Proceedings of the XVII World Buiatrics/XXV American Association of Bovine Practitioners Congress. Minneapolis (MN); 1992. p. 1–2.

20. Schnorr KL, Pearson LD. Intestinal absorption of maternal leukocytes by newborn lambs. J Reprod Immunol 1984;6:329–37.

21. Duhamel GE. Characterization of bovine mammary lymphocytes and their effects on neonatal calf immunity. Ann Arbor (MI): UMI Dissertation Services; 1993.

22. Riedel-Caspari G. The influence of colostral leukocytes on the course of an exper-imental Escherichia coli infection and serum antibodies in neonatal calves. Vet Immunol Immunopathol 1993;35:275–88.

23. United States Department of Agriculture. Transfer of maternal immunity to calves. National Animal Health Monitoring System 2002.

24. Haines DM, Chelack BJ, Naylor JM. Immunoglobulin concentrations in com-mercially available colostrum supplements for calves. Can Vet J 1990;31: 36–7.

25. Godden S. Colostrum management for dairy calves. Vet Clin North Am Food Anim Pract 2008;24:19–39.

26. Saif LJ, Smith KL, Landmeier BJ, et al. Immune response of pregnant cows to bovine rotavirus immunization. Am J Vet Res 1984;45:49–58.

27. Saif LJ, Redmen DR, Smith KL, et al. Passive immunity to bovine rotavirus in newborn calves fed colostrum supplements from immunized or nonimmunized cows. Infect Immun 1983;41:1118–31.

28. Murakami T, Hirano N, Inoue A, et al. Transfer of antibodies against viruses of calf diarrhea from cows to their offspring via colostrum. Japan Journal of Veter-inary Science 1985;47:507–10.

29. Ellis JA, Hassard LE, Cortese VS, et al. Effects of perinatal vaccination on humoral and cellular immune responses in cows and young calves. J Am Vet Med Assoc 1996;208:393–9.
30. Osterstock JB, Callan RJ, Van Metre DC. Evaluation of dry cow vaccination with a killed viral vaccine on post-colostral antibody titers in calves. In: Proceedings of the American Association of Bovine Practitioners. Columbus (OH); 2003. p.163–4.
31. Brenner J, Samina I, Machanai B, et al. Impact of vaccination of pregnant cows on colostral IgG levels and on term of pregnancy. Field observations. Israel Journal of Veterinary Medicine 1997;52:56–9.
32. Brar JS, Johnson DW, Muscoplat CC, et al. Maternal immunity to infectious bovine rhinotracheitis and bovine viral diarrhea: duration and effect on vaccination in young calves. Am J Vet Res 1978;39:241–4.
33. Menanteau-Horta AM, Ames TR, Johnson DW, et al. Effect of maternal antibody upon vaccination with infectious bovine rhinotracheitis and bovine virus diarrhea vaccines. Can J Comp Med 1985;49:10–4.
34. Parker WL, Galyean ML, Winder JA, et al. Effects of vaccination at branding on serum antibody titers to viral agents of bovine respiratory disease (BRD) in newly weaned New Mexico calves. In: Proceedings of the Western Section of the American Society of Animal Science. Spokane (WA); 1983. p. 44.
35. Kimman TG, Westenbrink F, Straver PJ. Priming for local and systematic antibody memory responses to bovine respiratory syncytial virus: effect of amount of virus, viral replication, route of administration and maternal antibodies. Vet Immunol Immunopathol 1989;22:145–60.
36. Pitcher PM. Influence of passively transferred maternal antibody on response of pigs to pseudorabies vaccines. In: Proceedings of the American Association of Swine Practitioners. Ames (IA); 1996. p. 57–62.
37. Ridge JP, Fuchs EJ, Matzinger P. Neonatal tolerance revisited: turning on newborn T cells with dendritic cells. Science 1996;271:1723–6.
38. Sarzotti M, Robbins DS, Hoffman FM. Induction of protective CTL responses in newborn mice by a murine retrovirus. Science 1996;271:1726–8.
39. Forsthuber T, Hualin CY, Lewhmann V. Induction of T_H1 and T_H2 immunity in neonatal mice. Science 1996;271:1728–30.
40. Rajaraman V, Nonnecke BJ, Horst RL. Effects of replacement of native fat in colostrum and milk with coconut oil on fat-soluble vitamins in serum and immune function in calves. J Dairy Sci 1997;80:2380–90.
41. Bryan LA. Fatal, generalized bovine herpesvirus type-1 infection associated with a modified-live infectious bovine rhinotracheitis/parainfluenza-3 vaccine administered to neonatal calves. Can Vet J 1994;35:223–8.
42. Eliis J, Gow S, West K, et al. Response of calves to challenge exposure with virulent bovine respiratory syncytial virus following intranasal administration of vaccines formulated for parenteral administration. J Am Vet Med Assoc 2007; 230:233–43.
43. Cortese VS, West KH, Hassard LE, et al. Clinical and immunologic responses of vaccinated and unvaccinated calves to infection with a virulent type-II isolate of bovine viral diarrhea virus. J Am Vet Med Assoc 1998;213:1312–9.
44. Cortese VS. Clinical and immunologic responses of cattle to vaccinal and natural bovine viral diarrhea virus (BVDV) [PhD thesis]. Western College of Veterinary Medicine, University of Saskatchewan; 1998.

Index

Note: Page numbers of article titles are in **boldface** type.

A

Abomasal dilation and tympany, in calves, 217–218
Abomasal ulceration, of calves, **209–220**
    clinical signs of, 214
    control of, 215–216
    described, 209–210
    diagnostic tests for, 214–215
    effects of, 210–211
    factors related to, 211–214
    prevention of, 216
    treatment of, 215–216
"Absorbants," intestinal, in calf diarrhea management, 13
Acidosis
    ion, strong, assessment of, laboratory tests in, 78–79
    D-lactic, clinical assessment of, in assessment of need for intravenous fluid therapy in
        calf diarrhea management, 79–81
    metabolic
        clinical assessment of, in assessment of need for intravenous fluid therapy in calf
            diarrhea management, 79
        intravenous fluid therapy in calf diarrhea management for, 75–77
Age, as factor in abomasal ulceration of calves, 211
Alkalinizing ability, in diarrhea in calves management, 62–66
Alkalinizing solutions, in calf diarrhea management, 83–84
Analgesia/analgesics, 6–7
Anaphylaxis, in bovine neonates, 130–131
Ancillary treatments, in calf diarrhea management, **1–20**
Anti-inflammatory agents, in calf diarrhea management, 6–7
Antimicrobial agents, in calf diarrhea management, **1–20**
Asphyxia, in newly born calves, metabolic acidosis in, intravenous fluid therapy in calf
    diarrhea management for, 78
Aspiration pneumonia, in bovine neonates, 125–126
Auricular vein catheterization, in calves, 85–90
Azithromycin, for cryptosporidiosis, 8–9

B

Bacteremia, intravenous fluid therapy in calf diarrhea management for, 78
Bacterial pneumonia, in bovine neonates, 126–130
Bovine(s), respiratory disease in, **121–137**. See also *Respiratory disease, in bovine
    neonates.*
Breath(s), first, 179–180

Vet Clin Food Anim 25 (2009) 229–237
doi:10.1016/S0749-0720(09)00009-7
0749-0720/09/$ – see front matter © 2009 Elsevier Inc. All rights reserved.
vetfood.theclinics.com

Our issues help you manage *yours*

Every year brings you new clinical challenges

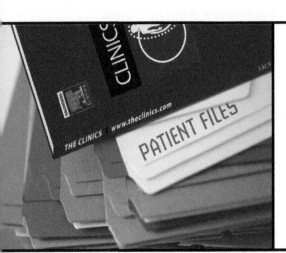

Every **Clinics** issue brings you **today's best thinking** on the challenges you face

Whether you purchase these issues individually, or order an annual subscription (which includes searchable access to past issues online), the **Clinics** offer you an efficient way to update your know how…one issue at a time.

DISCOVER THE CLINICS IN YOUR SPECIALTY!

Veterinary Clinics of North America: Equine Practice.
Publishes three times a year.
ISSN 0749-0739.

Veterinary Clinics of North America: Exotic Animal Practice.
Publishes three times a year.
ISSN 1094-9194.

Veterinary Clinics of North America: Food Animal Practice.
Publishes three times a year.
ISSN 0749-0720.

Veterinary Clinics of North America: Small Animal Practice.
Publishes bimonthly.
ISSN 0195-5616.

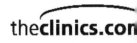

Moving?

Make sure your subscription moves with you!

To notify us of your new address, find your **Clinics Account Number** (located on your mailing label above your name), and contact customer service at:

E-mail: elspcs@elsevier.com

800-654-2452 (subscribers in the U.S. & Canada)
314-453-7041 (subscribers outside of the U.S. & Canada)

Fax number: 314-523-5170

Elsevier Periodicals Customer Service
11830 Westline Industrial Drive
St. Louis, MO 63146

*To ensure uninterrupted delivery of your subscription, please notify us at least 4 weeks in advance of move.

Printed and bound by CPI Group (UK) Ltd, Croydon, CR0 4YY

03/10/2024

01040464-0002